LAW & ETHICS
for the Health Professions

sixth edition

Karen Judson

Carlene Harrison

Hodges University

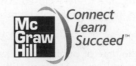

Mc
Graw
Hill

Connect
Learn
Succeed™

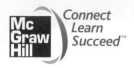

The McGraw·Hill Companies

Connect
Learn
Succeed™

LAW AND ETHICS FOR MEDICAL CAREERS

Published by McGraw-Hill, a business unit of The McGraw-Hill Companies, Inc., 1221 Avenue of the Americas, New York, NY, 10020. Copyright © 2013 by The McGraw-Hill Companies, Inc. All rights reserved. Printed in the United States of America. Previous editions © 1994, 1999, 2003, 2006, and 2010. No part of this publication may be reproduced or distributed in any form or by any means, or stored in a database or retrieval system, without the prior written consent of The McGraw-Hill Companies, Inc., including, but not limited to, in any network or other electronic storage or transmission, or broadcast for distance learning.

Some ancillaries, including electronic and print components, may not be available to customers outside the United States.

This book is printed on acid-free paper.

1 2 3 4 5 6 7 8 9 0 RMN/RMN 1 0 9 8 7 6 5 4 3 2

ISBN 978-0-07-337471-0
MHID 0-07-337471-7

Editorial Director: *Michael Ledbetter*
Vice president/Director of marketing: *Alice Harra*
Publisher: *Kenneth S. Kasee, Jr.*
Sponsoring editor: *Jonathan Joyce*
Managing development editor: *Christine Scheid*
Director, digital products: *Crystal Szewczyk*
Marketing manager: *Mary B. Haran*
Digital development editor: *Katherine Ward*
Director, Editing/Design/Production: *Jess Ann Kosic*
Project manager: *Jean R. Starr*
Buyer: *Nicole Baumgartner*
Senior designer: *Srdjan Savanovic*

Lead photo research coordinator: *Carrie K. Burger*
Manager, digital production: *Janean A. Utley*
Media project manager: *Brent dela Cruz*
Media project manager: *Cathy L. Tepper*
Outside development house: *Jodie Bernard, Laserwords*
Cover design: Cody Wallis
Interior design: Cara Hawthorne
Typeface: 10/12 ITC Garamond
Compositor: *Laserwords Private Limited*
Printer: R.R. Donnelley/Menasha
Cover credit: © Thomas Barwick, Getty Images

Credits: The credits section for this book begins on page 441 and is considered an extension of the copyright page.

Library of Congress Cataloging-in-Publication Data
Judson, Karen, 1941-
  Law & ethics for health professions/Karen Judson, Carlene Harrison. — 6th ed.
    p. ; cm.
  Law and ethics for health professions
  Rev. ed. of: Law & ethics for medical careers/Karen Judson, Carlene Harrison.
5th ed. c2010.
  Includes index.
  ISBN-13: 978-0-07-337471-0 (alk. paper)
  ISBN-10: 0-07-337471-7 (alk. paper)
  I. Harrison, Carlene. II. Judson, Karen, 1941- Law & ethics for medical careers.
III. Title. IV. Title: Law and ethics for health professions.
  [DNLM: 1. Legislation, Medical—United States. 2. Ethics, Medical—United States.
3. Health Personnel—United States. W 32.5 AA1]
  174.2—dc23

                                                    2011032111

Law & Ethics for the Health Professions, sixth edition, is an educational tool, not a law practice book. Since the law is in constant change, no rule or statement of law in this text should be relied upon for any service to any client. The reader should always consult standard legal sources for the current rule or law. If legal counseling or other expert advice is needed, the services of appropriate professionals should be sought. Between the time that Web site information is gathered and published, it is not unusual for some sites to have closed. Also, the transcription of the URLs can result in typographical errors. Text changes will be made in reprints when possible.

The Internet addresses listed in the text were accurate at the time of publication. The inclusion of a Web site does not indicate an endorsement by the authors or McGraw-Hill, and McGraw-Hill does not guarantee the accuracy of the information presented at these sites.

www.mhhe.com

BRIEF CONTENTS

CONTENTS

ABOUT THE AUTHORS

Karen Judson, BS

Karen Judson taught biology laboratories at Black Hills University in Spearfish, South Dakota, high school sciences in Idaho, and grades one and three in Washington State. She is also a former laboratory and X-ray technician and completed two years of nurses' training while completing a degree in biology.

Judson has worked as a science writer since 1983. She has written relationship, family, and psychology articles for a variety of magazines, including a series of high school classroom magazines, making a total of 500 articles published. Judson writes science and relationship books for teenagers (Enslow and Marshall Cavendish publishers). Her book for teens, *Sports & Money: It's a Sell Out,* made the New York City Public Library's list of best books for teens in 1995. Her book for teens, *Genetic Engineering,* was chosen by the National Science Teachers' Association as one of the best science books for children in 2001 and was featured on the NSTA Web site.

Carlene Harrison, EdD, CMA

Carlene Harrison is dean of the School of Allied Health at Hodges University and is also program director for the Masters in Health Administration. She has been a member of the faculty at Hodges University since 1992, but came on board full time in 2000, serving first as chair of the Medical Assisting Program. As dean of the School of Allied Health, she has over all responsibility for five degree programs: Health Administration, Health Studies, Medical Assisting, Health Information Management, and Physical Therapist Assistant. Her doctorate is from Argosy University. Her dissertation research looked at improvement in critical thinking in adult learners.

Before becoming a full-time educator, Dr. Harrison worked for over 20 years in the health care field as an administrator. Employed mostly in the outpatient setting, she has worked in the for-profit, not-for-profit, and public health sectors.

TO THE STUDENT

As you study to become a health care practitioner, you have undoubtedly realized that patients are more than the sum of their medical problems. In fact, they are people with loved ones, professions, worries, hobbies, and daily routines that are probably much like your own. However, because patients' lives and well-being are at stake as they seek and receive health care, in addition to seeing each patient as an individual you must carefully consider the complex legal, moral, and ethical issues that will arise as you practice your profession, and you must learn to resolve such issues in an acceptable manner.

Law & Ethics for the Health Professions, sixth edition, provides an overview of the laws and ethics you should know to help you give competent, compassionate care to patients that is also within acceptable legal and ethical boundaries. The text can also serve as a guide to help you resolve the many legal and ethical questions you may reasonably expect to face as a student and, later, as a health care practitioner.

To derive maximum benefit from *Law & Ethics for the Health Professions,* sixth edition:

- Review the Learning Outcomes and Key Terms at the beginning of each chapter for an overview of the material included in the chapter.

- Complete all Check Your Progress questions as they appear in the chapter and correct any incorrect answers.

- Review the legal cases to see how they apply to topics in the text, and try to determine why the court ruled as it did.

- Study the Ethics Issues at the end of each chapter, and answer the discussion questions.

- Complete the Review questions at the end of the chapter, correct incorrect answers and review the material again.

- Review the Case Studies and use your critical thinking skills to answer the questions.

- Complete the Internet Activities at the end of the chapter to become familiar with online resources and to see what additional information you can find about selected topics.

- Study each chapter until you can answer correctly questions posed by the Learning Outcomes, Check Your Progress, and Review questions.

Chapter Structure

Each chapter begins with a page that previews topics you will study.

Learning Outcomes The learning outcomes describe the basic knowledge you can acquire by studying the chapter. Their importance to you is to indicate what general categories of knowledge you should derive from the chapter.

Learning Outcomes

After studying this chapter, you should be able to:

LO 3.1 Define *licensure, certification, registration,* and *accreditation.*

LO 3.2 Demonstrate an understanding of how physicians are licensed, how physicians are regulated, and the purpose of a medical board.

LO 3.3 Discuss the composition of the health care team and the roles of its members.

LO 3.4 Define the major types of medical practice management systems.

LO 3.5 Define the different types of managed care health plans.

LO 3.6 Discuss the federal legislation that impacts health care reimbursement and prohibits fraud and abuse in health care billing.

LO 3.7 Define *telemedicine, cybermedicine,* and *e-health,* and discuss their roles in today's health care environment.

Key Terms This alphabetic list is of important vocabulary terms found in the chapter. This is a list of key words that you should be familiar with after reading each chapter. The terms are printed in boldface when they first appear in the chapter text and are listed in the margin of the page on which the term is introduced to provide you with a quick definition of each term.

[KEY TERMS]

accreditation

allopathic

associate practice

certification

corporation

cybermedicine

e-health

endorsement

Federal False Claims Act

gatekeeper physician

group practice

Health Care and Education Reconciliation Act (HCERA)

Health Care Quality Improvement Act (HCQIA) of 1986

Healthcare Integrity and Protection Data Bank (HIPDB)

Health Insurance Portability and Accountability Act (HIPAA) of 1996

health maintenance organization (HMO)

indemnity

individual (or independent) practice association (IPA)

licensure

managed care

medical boards

medical practice acts

National Practitioner Data Bank (NPDB)

open access plan

partnership

Patient Protection and Affordable Care Act (PPACA)

physician-hospital organization (PHO)

point-of-service (POS) plan

preferred provider association (PPA)

preferred provider organization (PPO)

primary care physician (PCP)

reciprocity

registration

sole proprietorship

telemedicine

tertiary care settings

Ethics Issues This feature at the end of each chapter is based on interviews conducted with ethics counselors within the professional organizations for health care practitioners, and interviews with bioethics experts. The discussion questions are derived from real-life experiences and ethical dilemmas from a variety of health care practitioners. Read the Ethics Issues, and decide how they are relevant to the health care profession you will practice. Answer the discussion questions to help clarify your personal ethical viewpoint concerning each situation.

[ETHICS ISSUES Working in Health Care]

Ethics ISSUE 1: The "Code of Ethical Business and Professional Behavior" for the Cleveland Clinic Health System states under the heading "I. Conflicts of Interest" that "Each component of the system maintains policies that require disclosure of potential conflicts of interest to ensure that such conflict does not inappropriately influence business or professional decision-making."

Discussion Question

1. Assume you are an orthopedic surgeon working under the previously mentioned ethical guidelines. You own shares in a company called

Chapter Review Each chapter review includes Applying Knowledge questions that review facts presented and points made in the text. Use these questions to test your comprehension of the material; then review appropriate sections of the text as necessary to reinforce the learning outcomes.

[CHAPTER 3 REVIEW]

Applying Knowledge

LO 3.1

Write "L" for licensure, "C" for certification, "R" for registration, and "A" for accreditation in the space provided to indicate which is applicable in the following descriptions.

_____ 1. Involves a mandatory credentialing process established by law, usually at the state level.

_____ 2. Involves simply paying a fee.

_____ 3. Involves a voluntary credentialing process, usually national in scope, most often sponsored by a private-sector group.

_____ 4. Required of all physicians, dentists, and nurses in every state.

_____ 5. Consists simply of an entry in an official record.

_____ 6. A process that implies that health care facilities or HMOs have met certain standards.

Case Studies Each case study is followed by exercises that allow you to practice your critical thinking skills and use knowledge gained from reading the text to decide how to resolve the real-life situations or theoretical scenarios presented.

[CASE STUDIES]

Use your critical thinking skills to answer the questions that follow each case study.

LO 3.1

Physician assistants (PAs) are employed in physician offices throughout the United States. Although the PA provides direct patient care, he or she is under the supervision of a licensed physician. Duties include taking patients' medical histories, performing physical examinations, ordering diagnostic and therapeutic procedures, providing follow-up care, and teaching and counseling patients. In most states, PAs may write prescriptions. The PA may be the only health care practitioner a patient sees during his or her visit to the physician office. Therefore, patients often refer to a PA as "the doctor." Ned, a PA for five years, says the patients he sees often address him as "doctor."

Similarly, Marie, a long-time employee of a physician in private practice, is often called "the doctor's nurse." Although Marie has never had the training necessary to become a certified medical assistant or a registered nurse, she sometimes refers to herself as the "office nurse."

35. What legal and ethical considerations are evident in these situations?

Internet Activities Each activity includes exercises that are designed to increase your knowledge of topics related to the chapter material and to gain expertise in using the Internet as a research tool. Keep a resource notebook to record useful Web sites as they are found. To locate new Web sites, conduct a subject search as needed to help you answer the questions that follow each activity.

[INTERNET ACTIVITIES LO 3.4 & LO 3.7]

Complete the activities and answer the questions that follow.

39. Conduct a Web search for "patient care partnership." This document, published by the American Hospital Association, replaces the previous Patients' Bill of Rights. What six points are listed under "What You Can Expect"?

Text Features

The following special features are found in the student text/workbook for *Law & Ethics for the Health Professions,* sixth edition. These features are designed to stimulate classroom discussion, provide supplementary facts and examples to the text material, introduce you to Internet research, and provide a review of the text material covered.

From the Perspective of . . . This feature illustrates real-life experiences that are related to the text. Each quotes health care practitioners in various locations throughout the United States as they encounter problems or situations relevant to the material discussed in the text. Imagine how you would respond in the same or similar situations, and answer the questions at the end of the feature.

from the perspective of . . .

MELODY, A CERTIFIED NURSING ASSISTANT (CNA), works in a skilled nursing care facility caring for elderly patients. "I like the hands-on care," she says, "and I love just visiting with my patients. They come from all walks of life, and some of them have traveled all over the world."

The part of her job she dislikes the most, Melody adds, "is the demanding patients, who want everything right now. Demanding relatives can also be unreasonable. A daughter will tell me, 'I want you to respond immediately whenever my mother calls for you.' They don't understand, or don't care, that I have several patients to look after."

Once, Melody recalls, several family members were visiting their elderly relative. "I walked in to check my patient, and one of his granddaughters asked me to get her a soda. There was a vending machine in the visitors' lounge, and I debated telling the woman I'm not a waitress, and she could get her own drink. I didn't, though. I got her the drink, but I resented being asked to do it. I'm just a CNA, but I'm not there to wait on patients' relatives."

From Melody's perspective, her job did not include providing refreshments for patients' visitors. What does her remark that she is "just a CNA" reveal about Melody's attitude concerning her work?

From the demanding visitor's perspective, perhaps Melody's job is to serve all needs of anyone in the patient's room. In your opinion, would Melody's registered nurse (RN) supervisor have expected her to fulfill the visitor's request for a soda? Why or why not?

How should Melody respond to patients and their visitors who seem unreasonably demanding?

Check Your Progress This feature is a short quiz that allows you to test your comprehension of the material just read. Answer the questions, correct incorrect answers, and then review appropriate sections to be sure you understand the material.

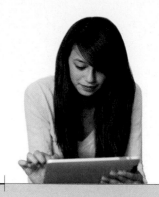

check your **progress**

1. Define *registration*.

_____

_____

2. Define *licensure*.

_____

_____

Court Case Each case summarizes a lawsuit that illustrates points made in the text. In each case, consider the relevance of the case to your health care specialty area and note the outcome. Determine why the court made its particular ruling. The legal citations at the end of each court case indicate where to find the complete text of a case. "Landmark" cases are those that established ongoing precedent.

COURT CASE

Physician Disciplined by Board of Medical Examiners

A licensed pharmacist and a state pharmacy board investigator called a state's Board of Medical Examiners to express concern about a physician's prescription practices. The board investigated and found the physician had deviated from accepted standard of care by

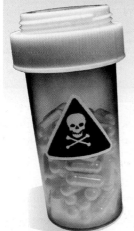

▸ Inadequately evaluating patients before prescribing antidepressants and failing to document reasons for prescriptions or following up on patients' use of the prescribed medications.

▸ Prescribing antibiotics for prolonged periods as treatment for urinary tract infections without determining that the infections had recurred or documenting the recurrence of the infections. The physician had also prescribed several antibiotics to a patient at once, allowing the patient to choose which antibiotic was the most effective.

▸ Prescribing narcotic and anxiolytic medications (drugs that relieve anxiety) to patients with nonterminal chronic pain without adequately pursuing and documenting use of available alternatives to narcotics and controlled medications.

Based on the above findings, the Board of Medical Examiners placed the physician on probation for two years and ordered him to secure 60 hours of continuing education in

Source: Miller v. Board of Medical Examiners, 609 N.W.2d 478, 2000 Iowa Sup.

What's New

1. The From the Perspective of . . . feature at the beginning of each chapter replaces Voice of Experience. This feature encourages students to see situations from the perspective of the various participants and determine how they would react if faced with similar situations.

2. Chapter 2, "Making Ethical Decisions," is new content and discusses prominent theories about ethics development and how one arrives at ethical decisions. This chapter provides students with several different decision-making models to help process information and move toward action.

3. All statistics are updated, as well as content relevant to laws passed since the fifth edition, court cases, and lists in the appendixes.

4. New case studies are added. We made an effort to include a variety of allied health professions in case studies and other examples throughout the text, even more so than in previous editions of the book.

Teaching and Learning Supplements

Introducing *Connect*

McGraw-Hill's new *Connect* is a revolutionary online assignment and assessment solution, providing instructors and students with tools and resources to maximize their success.

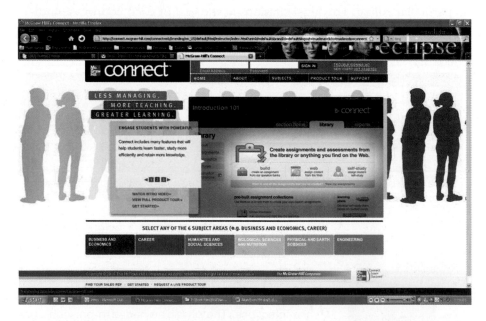

Simple Assignment Management With *Connect,* creating assignments is easier than ever, so you can spend more time teaching and less time managing. The assignment management function enables you to:

- Create and deliver assignments easily with selectable interactives, vocabulary exercises, end-of-chapter questions and test bank items.

- Streamline lesson planning, student progress reporting, and assignment grading to make classroom management more efficient than ever.

- Go paperless with the eBook and online submission and grading of student assignments.

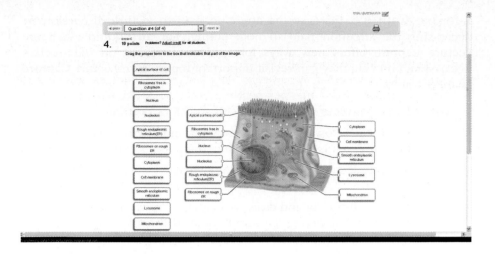

Smart Grading When it comes to studying, time is precious. *Connect* helps students learn more efficiently by providing feedback and practice material when they need it, where they need it. When it comes to teaching, your time also is precious. The grading function enables you to:

- Have assignments scored automatically, giving students immediate feedback on their work and side-by-side comparisons with correct answers.

- Access and review each response; manually change grades or leave comments for students to review.

- Reinforce classroom concepts with practice tests and instant quizzes.

Instructor Library The *Connect* Instructor Library is your repository for additional resources to improve student engagement in and out of class. You can select and use any asset that enhances your lecture. The *Connect* Instructor Library includes:

- *Instructor's Manual*
- *Test bank*
- *PowerPoint presentation*
- *Videos–ethical vignettes*
- *eBook*
  - Fully integrated, allowing for anytime, anywhere access to the textbook.
  - Dynamic links between the exercises or questions you assign to your students and the location in the eBook where that exercise or question is covered.
  - A powerful search function to pinpoint and connect key concepts in a snap.

Student Progress Tracking *Connect* keeps instructors informed about how each student, section, and class is performing, allowing for more productive use of lecture and office hours. The progress-tracking function enables you to:

- View scored work immediately, and track individual or group performance with assignment and grade reports.

- Access an instant view of student or class performance relative to learning objectives.

Lecture Capture Increase the attention paid to lecture discussion by decreasing the attention paid to note taking. For an additional charge Lecture Capture offers new ways for students to focus on the in-class discussion, knowing they can revisit important topics later. Lecture Capture enables you to:

- Record and distribute your lecture with a click of button.
- Record and index PowerPoint presentations and anything shown on your computer so it is easily searchable, frame by frame.
- Offer access to lectures anytime and anywhere by computer, iPod, or mobile device.
- Increase intent listening and class participation by easing students' concerns about note-taking. Lecture Capture will make it more likely you will see students' faces, not the tops of their heads.

Online Learning Center www.mhhe.com/judson6e The Online Learning Center offers an extensive array of teaching tools for the instructor, including the Test Bank and PowerPoint presentations for each chapter, and the Instructor's Manual. The **Instructor's Manual** provides instructors with guidance in how to interpret court case citations, helpful Web site links, correlation charts, course syllabi, teaching strategies, answers to Check Your Progress, answers to Ethics Issue discussion questions, and answers to Applying Your Knowledge, Case Studies, and Internet Activities questions.

ACKNOWLEDGMENTS

Author Acknowledgments

Karen Judson

Thank you to the editorial team and production staff at McGraw-Hill, and all the reviewers and sources who contributed their time and expertise to making the sixth edition of Law & Ethics for the Health Professions *the best ever. Thank you, too, Carlene, for your hard work on this sixth edition.*

Carlene Harrison

A big thank you to Karen Judson for getting me started on this marvelous adventure called writing. To our reviewers, your contributions really make a difference. The editorial and production staff at McGraw-Hill did a great job. And last, to my husband Bill, your support and love keeps me going.

Reviewer Acknowledgments
Reviewers for the Sixth Edition

Diane Alagna, RN, RMA Medical Assisting Program Director   *Branford Hall Career Institute*

Jeanne C. Ambrosio, BSN   *Goodwin College*

Norma Bird, MEd, CMA (AAMA)   *Idaho State University*

Rebecca Bonefas, MA   *Kaplan University*

Joey L. Brown, MA/MOA   *Great Lakes Institute of Technology*

Martina Forte Brown, CCMA, CPT, CET   *Brookstone College*

Lynn Callister, RN, PhD, FAAN   *Brigham Young University*

Cindy Caviness, CRT, CMA (AAMA) AHI, Director/Senior Instructor, Medical Assisting–AAS   *Montgomery Community College*

Linda Ciarleglio, BS   *Stone Academy*

Rebecca Complin, BS, RDH, RDMS, RVT   *American Career College*

Deborah Eid   *Carrington College*

Christine Enz, CCS-P   *Bryant & Stratton College*

Cynthia Ferguson, AAS   *Texas State Technical College*

Rebecca Anne French   *Allen County Community College*

Jill Frost   *Tennessee Technology Center- Murfreesboro*

Deborah Galanski-Maciak, MS, RHIT   *Davenport University Online*

Debbie Gilbert   *Dalton State College*

James Goss, MHA, MICP   *Loma Linda University*

Grant Iannelli, BS, DC   *Kaplan University School of Health Sciences*

Wendyanne Jex, BA, MPA-HS   *Kaplan University School of Health Sciences*

Carrie Kaye, BA, MA   *The Salter School*

Katin Keirstead   *Seacoast Career Schools*

Mary Koloski, CBCS, CHI   *Florida Career College*

Michelle Lovings, BA   *Missouri College*

Loreen W. MacNichol, BS   *Kaplan University, Maine*

Loreen MacNichol, CMRS, RMC, CCS-P   *Andover College*

Robert Micallef, MA   *Madonna University*

Lane Miller, MBA/HCM   *Medical Careers Institute*

Kathleen Olewinski, MS RHIA, NHA, FACHE   *Bryant & Stratton College*

Sherry Pearsall, RN, MSN, CAS   *Bryant & Stratton College*

Kim Rock   *Branford Hall Career Institute*

Elizabeth Salazar, AS, BS   *Centura College*

Tammy L. Shick,   *Great Lakes Institute of Technology*

Tammy Summerson, BSN   *Westwood College*

Marlene Suvada, MHPE, RRT   *National-Louis University*

Mary M. Zulaybar, BS, CBCS   *ASA Institute, Division of Health Disciplines*

Reviewers of Previous Editions

Carol Adams-Turner   *Lamar State College–Orange*

Thomas Ankeney, BA, RCP, RRT, CPFT, AE-C, NCPT   *Maric College*

Shkelzen Badivuku   *Gibbs College*

Julette Barta, CphT, BSIT   *SJVC*

Rebecca Britt   *Northwestern State University*

Lou Brown   *Wayne Community College*

Rita Bulington, RN, AS   *Ivy Tech Community College*

Christine M. Cole, CCA   *Williston State College*

Barbara Desch   *San Joaquin Valley College, Inc.*

Terri Fleming   *Ivy Tech Community College*

Tammy B. Foles   *Antonelli College*

William D. Goren, JD, LLM   *Northwestern Business College*

Beulah A. Hofmann, RN, MSN   *Ivy Tech Community College*

Carol Lee Jarrell   *Brown Mackie College*

Karmon Kingsley, CMA, CHI   *Cleveland State Community College*

Christine Malone, MHA   *Everett Community College*

Lynne M. Muñoz, Med   *Everett Community College*

Matthew R. Panzio, MD   *Gibbs College*

Cindy Pavel   *Ivy Tech Community College*

Pamela B. Primrose, MLFSC, ABD, MT, ASCP   *Ivy Tech Community College*

Pat Stettler, CMT, FAAMT   *Everett Community College*

Constance Winter   *Bossier Parish Community College*

Previous Reviewers

Cindy A. Abel, BS, CMA, PBT (ASCP)   *Ivy Tech State College*

Barbara C. Berger, BSN, RN, CMA, MS   *Northwestern Connecticut Community College*

Amelia Broussard, PhD, RN, MPH, Associate Professor   *Clayton College & State University*

Christine M. Cole   *Williston State College*

Dawn Felice Dannenbrink, MHA   *High-Tech Institute*

Dena A. Evans, BSN, MPH, RN, CMA   *Richmond Community College*

Kim Ford, CMA   *Catawba Valley Community College*

Gardiner M. Haight, BS Comm, JD   *Bryant and Stratton College*

Janet K. Henderson, CMA, AAT   *North Georgia Technical College*

Beulah A. Hofmann   *Ivy Tech State College*

Joyce S. Johnson, Department Head, Office Systems Technology   *Alamance Community College*

Lynda M. Konecny   *New York City College of Technology*

Norma Mercado, MAHS, RHIA   *Austin Community College*

Helen L. Myers   *Hagerstown Community College*

Michael W. Posey, PhD   *Franklin University*

Joan Renner, BSN, RNBC, Adjunct Faculty   *Cecil Community College*

Sharon M. Roberts, MBA, MS, PTA   *Newbury College*

Diane P. Roche, CMA, BSHCA, MSA   *South Piedmont Community College*

James Steen, MBA, SS, RHIA   *San Jacinto College North*

Rita Stoffel, BS, MT, MBA   *Red Rocks Community College*

Nina Thierer, CMA, BS, CPC   *Ivy Tech State College–Fort Wayne*

Geraldine M. Todaro, MSTE, CMA, CLPlb   *Stark State College of Technology*

Tova R. Wiegand-Green   *Ivy Tech State College*

part one

The Foundations of Law and Ethics

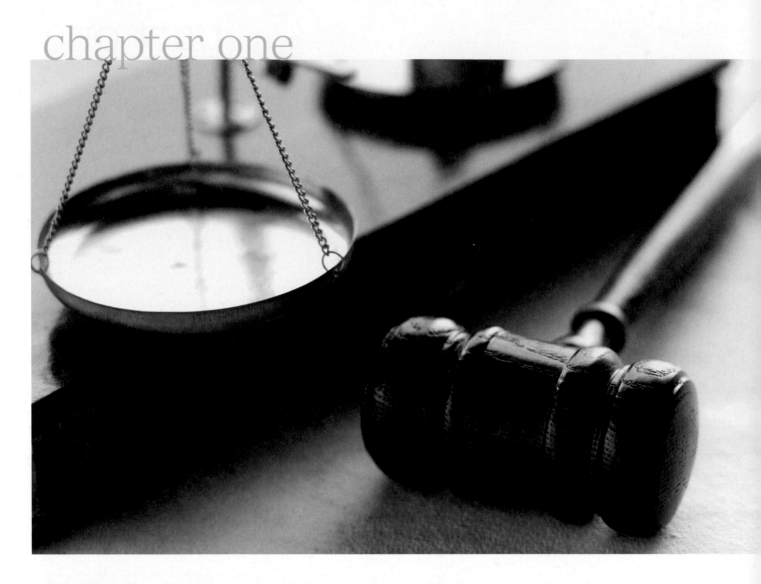

INTRODUCTION TO LAW AND ETHICS

Learning Outcomes

After studying this chapter, you should be able to:

LO 1.1 Explain why knowledge of law and ethics is important to health care practitioners.

LO 1.2 Distinguish among law, ethics, bioethics, etiquette, and protocol.

LO 1.3 Define *moral values* and explain how they relate to law, ethics, and etiquette.

LO 1.4 Discuss the characteristics and skills most likely to lead to a successful career in one of the health care professions.

Cases in This Chapter

BARBARA, AN EXPERIENCED CERTIFIED MEDICAL ASSISTANT (CMA) in a medical office with a walk-in clinic, instructs new employees in the reception area of the office to follow the medical office procedures whenever possible and prudent, but, above all, to use common sense in dealing with patients.

Barbara told Elaine, a new receptionist in the medical office, to politely ask walk-in patients why they needed to see a doctor. Elaine had been on the job for two weeks when an elderly man who was hard of hearing approached her, and she dutifully asked him the purpose for his visit. He was obviously too embarrassed to reply, but Elaine persisted, finally raising her voice. When the man shouted "I can't pee," all heads in the busy waiting room turned toward Elaine and the patient. A red-faced Elaine turned to arrange for the man to see a physician, but he quickly left the building. Barbara criticized Elaine's patient-handling technique, but the crux of the matter was that the patient left without seeing a doctor for his medical problem.

"Patients' needs always trump office routine," Barbara emphasizes. "If we somehow hurt or hinder a patient while doggedly sticking to a set routine, we may have risked legal liability, but more important, we haven't done our job."

From Barbara's perspective as the person responsible for training medical office personnel, Elaine failed to use common sense in communicating with a patient, and as a result, the man did not receive the medical treatment he needed.

From Elaine's perspective, she followed Barbara's instructions to the letter, and she failed to understand why Barbara had criticized her. She hadn't meant to embarrass the man, so was it her fault that he left without making an appointment?

From the patient's perspective as an elderly gentleman who seldom discussed personal matters, the young woman who was his first contact in the medical office embarrassed him, and he left rather than face further humiliation.

How would using "common sense" have helped Elaine communicate with the elderly gentleman? Do you see a way to remedy this situation, once the patient left the clinic?

As you progress through *Law & Ethics for Medical Careers*, try to interpret the court cases, laws, case studies, and other examples or situations cited from the perspectives of everyone involved.

Why Study Law and Ethics?

There are two important reasons for you to study law and ethics:

- To help you function at the highest possible professional level, providing competent, compassionate health care to patients.
- To help you avoid legal entanglements that can threaten your ability to earn a living as a successful **health care practitioner.**

We live in a **litigious** society, where patients, relatives, and others are inclined to sue health care practitioners, health care facilities, manufacturers of medical

LO 1.1

Explain why knowledge of law and ethics is important to health care practitioners.

health care practitioners
Those who are trained to administer medical or health care to patients.

equipment and products, and others when medical outcomes are not acceptable. This means that every person responsible for health care delivery is at risk of being involved in a health care–related lawsuit. It is important, therefore, for you to know the basics of law and ethics as they apply to health care, so you can recognize and avoid those situations that might not serve your patients well, or that might put you at risk of legal liability.

In addition to keeping you at your professional best and helping you avoid litigation, knowledge of law and ethics can also help you gain perspective in the following three areas:

1. *The rights, responsibilities, and concerns of health care consumers.* Health care practitioners not only need to be concerned about how law and ethics impact their respective professions, but they must also understand how legal and ethical issues affect the patients they treat. With the increased complexity of medicine has come the desire of consumers to know more about their options and rights and more about the responsibilities of health care providers. Today's health care consumers are likely to consider themselves partners with health care practitioners in the healing process and to question fees and treatment modes. They may ask such questions as, Do I need to see a specialist? If so, which specialist can best treat my condition? Will I be given complete information about my condition? How much will medical treatment cost? Will a physician treat me if I have no health insurance?

   In addition, as medical technology has advanced, patients have come to expect favorable outcomes from medical treatment, and when expectations are not met, lawsuits may result.

2. *The legal and ethical issues facing society, patients, and health care practitioners as the world changes.* Nearly every day the media report news events concerning individuals who face legal and ethical dilemmas over biological/medical issues. For example, a grief-stricken husband must give consent for an abortion in order to save the life of his critically ill and unconscious wife. Parents must argue in court their decision to terminate life-support measures for a daughter whose injured brain no longer functions. Patients with HIV/AIDS fight to retain their right to confidentiality.

   While the situations that make news headlines often involve larger social issues, legal and ethical questions are resolved daily, on a smaller scale, each time a patient visits his or her physician, dentist, physical therapist, or other health care practitioner. Questions that must often be resolved include these: Who can legally give consent if the patient cannot? Can patients be assured of confidentiality, especially since telecommunication has become a way of life? Can a physician or other health care practitioner refuse to treat a patient? Who may legally examine a patient's medical records?

   Rapid advances in medical technology have also influenced laws and ethics for health care practitioners. For example, recent court cases have debated these issues: Does the husband or the wife have ownership rights to a divorced couple's frozen embryos? Will a surrogate mother have legal visitation rights to the child she carried to term? Should modern technology be used to keep those patients alive who are diagnosed as brain-dead and have no hope of recovery? How should parenthood disputes be resolved for children resulting from reproductive technology?

3. *The impact of rising costs on the laws and ethics of health care delivery.* Rising costs, both of health care insurance and of medical treatment in general, lead to questions concerning access to health care services and allocation of medical treatment. For instance, should the

uninsured or underinsured receive government help to pay for health insurance? And should everyone, regardless of age or lifestyle, have the same access to scarce medical commodities such as organs for transplantation or very expensive drugs?

Court Cases Illustrate Risk of Litigation

As you will see in the court cases used throughout this text, sometimes when a lawsuit is brought, the trial court or a higher court must first decide if the **plaintiff** has a legal reason to sue, or if the **defendant** is **liable.** When a court has ruled that there is a standing (reason) to sue and that a defendant can be held liable, the case may proceed to resolution. Often, once liability and a standing to sue have been established, the two sides agree on an out-of-court settlement. Depending on state law, an out-of-court settlement may not be published. For this reason, the final disposition of a case is not always available from published sources. The published cases that have decided liability, however, are still case law, and such cases have been used in this text to illustrate specific points.

In addition, sometimes it takes time after the initial trial for a case to be settled. For example, perhaps a patient dies after surgery in 1998, and

plaintiff The person bringing charges in a lawsuit.

defendant The person or party against whom criminal or civil charges are brought in a lawsuit.

liable Legally responsible or obligated.

COURT CASE

Patient Sues Hospital

In August 1997, a patient admitted to a Louisiana medical center for the treatment of bronchitis and back pain called the nurses' station to ask for someone to fix the television set and the window blinds. In response, two maintenance workers came to the patient's room and removed the television set. The workers examined the blinds, but informed the patient they could not fix them. The workers then left, promising to replace the television set, but not commenting on the window blinds.

The patient continued to ask for someone to adjust the window blinds to keep out the sun. She said that when she was in pain, light was unpleasant to her. No one came to fix the blinds.

The patient eventually tried to close the blinds herself. Dressed in street clothes and sandals, she climbed on a recliner chair with lockable wheels located in her room, and reached high above her head in an attempt to turn the slats of the blinds. The patient fell off the chair and sustained an injury to her left shoulder, upper back, and cervical spine.

The patient then sued the medical center for the injuries she had suffered. The trial court granted summary judgment for the defendant. An appeals court reversed the trial court's decision, holding that a legal relationship between the parties existed, due to the fact that Lichti was a patient at Schumpert Medical Center, thus establishing a duty for the hospital to exercise the necessary patient care and to protect Lichti from dangers within the hospital's control.

The appeals court determined: "It is not unforeseeable that a patient experiencing discomfort due to bright light entering the room, and who has obtained no relief through repeated requests for aid, might decide to take matters into her own hands and attempt to close the broken blinds. Furthermore, because the top of the blinds is located above the easy reach of the average person, it is not unforeseeable that the patient would attempt to use a chair to reach the top of the blinds."

Source: Lichti v. Schumpert Medical Center, No. 32,620-CA, Court of Appeal of Louisiana, Second Circuit, January 26, 2000.

In your opinion, were the hospital employees summoned to help the patient in any way responsible for her injuries? Explain your answer.

Remember Barbara in this chapter's opening scenario? Would such training in patient communication have helped the dispatcher in the next case, "County Liable in Ambulance Delay"?

precedent Decisions made by judges in the various courts that become rule of law and apply to future cases, even though they were not enacted by a legislature; also known as case law.

summary judgment A decision made by a court in a lawsuit in response to a motion that pleads there is no basis for a trial.

the family files a wrongful death suit soon after. The case may go through several appeals and finally be settled in 2001.

It is also important to remember that while the final result of a case is important to the parties involved, from a legal standpoint the most important aspect of a court case is not the result, but whether the case represents good law and will be persuasive as other cases are decided.

Although the most recent cases published have been sought for illustration in this text, sometimes a dated case (1995, 1985, 1970, etc.) is used because it established important **precedent.**

Court cases appear throughout each chapter of the text to illustrate how the legal system has decided complaints brought by or against health care service providers and product manufacturers. Some of these cases involve **summary judgment.** Summary judgment is the legal term for a decision made by a court in a lawsuit in response to a motion that pleads there is no basis for a trial because there is no genuine issue of material

COURT CASE

County Liable in Ambulance Delay

In 1991 an Indiana man suffered a heart attack while mowing the lawn. He took two nitroglycerin tablets while his wife called an ambulance. The emergency operator took the wife's call at 2:10 PM and said an ambulance would be dispatched. Seven minutes later the ambulance had not arrived, so the wife called a nearby fire station, where the local branch of the emergency medical squad was holding a meeting. An ambulance was sent immediately when this call was received, and it arrived at the patient's house in one minute.

The patient later learned that the emergency operator who had first been called had never dispatched an ambulance to his home. The chief deputy sheriff of the county explained that the officer taking emergency calls was inexperienced as a dispatcher. The officer had been the only one assigned to monitor the emergency line on that day because the sheriff's department was having its annual picnic.

The patient sued the county for negligence in operating the 911 emergency service. He claimed he had suffered permanent heart damage because of the operator's failure to promptly dispatch an ambulance.

The county moved for summary judgment based on the fact that it had no relationship with the man that created a duty of care to him. The trial court granted the motion, but an appellate court reversed the judgment. It held that the call to the emergency operator, in which the man's wife spoke of her husband's heart attack and the immediate need for an ambulance, was sufficient to establish knowledge that inaction could be harmful.

When the operator said an ambulance would be dispatched, he established that the county explicitly agreed to assist the patient. Accordingly, the court held, the county had assumed a private duty to the man and could be held liable for failure to dispatch an ambulance.

Source: Koher v. Dial, Ind.Ct.App. (1995).

From the perspective of the man suffering a heart attack, should he have expected an ambulance to arrive promptly, as promised? Why or why not?

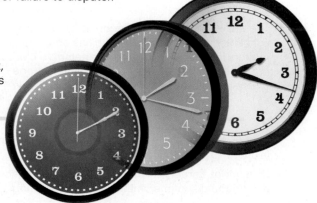

fact. In other words, a motion for summary judgment states that one party is entitled to win as a matter of law. Summary judgment is available only in a civil action. (Chapter 4 distinguishes between criminal and civil actions.)

The following court cases illustrate that a wide variety of legal questions can arise for those engaged directly in providing health care services, whether in a hospital, in a medical office, or in an emergency situation. Health care equipment and product dealers and manufacturers can be held indirectly responsible for defective medical devices and products through charges of the following types:

- Breach of warranty.

- Statements made by the manufacturer about the device or product that are found to be untrue.

- Strict liability, for cases in which defective products threaten the personal safety of consumers.

- **Fraud** or intentional deceit. (Fraud is discussed in further detail in Chapter 4.)

fraud Dishonest or deceitful practices in depriving, or attempting to deprive, another of his or her rights.

The extent of liability for manufacturers of medical devices and products may be changing, however, since a 2008 U.S. Supreme Court decision held that makers of medical devices such as implantable defibrillators or

COURT CASE

Supreme Court Shields Medical Devices from Lawsuits

An angioplasty was performed on a patient, Charles Riegel, in New York. During the procedure, the catheter used to dilate the patient's coronary artery failed, causing serious complications. The patient sued the catheter's manufacturer, Medtronic, Inc., under New York state law, charging negligence in design, manufacture, and labeling of the device, which had received FDA approval in 1994. Medtronic argued that Riegel could not bring state law negligence claims because the company was preempted from liability under Section 360k(a) of the Medical Device Amendments (MDA) of the U.S. Food, Drug, and Cosmetic Act. (State requirements are preempted under the MDA only to the extent that they are "different from, or in addition to" the requirements imposed by federal law. Thus, 360k(a) does not prevent a state from providing a damages remedy for claims premised on a violation of FDA regulations; the state duties in such a case "parallel," rather than add to, federal requirements (*Lohr*, 518 U.S., at 495, 116 S.Ct. 2240).

The *Riegel* case reached the U.S. Supreme Court, where the question to be decided was this: Does Section 360k(a) of the Medical Device Amendments to the Food, Drug, and Cosmetic Act preempt state law claims seeking damages for injuries caused by medical devices that received premarket approval from the Food and Drug Administration?

In February 2008, the U.S. Supreme Court held in this case that makers of medical devices are immune from liability for personal injuries as long as the FDA approved the device before it was marketed and it meets the FDA's specifications.

Sources: Appeals Court Case: *Riegel v. Medtronic, Inc.,* 451 F.3d 104 (2006);
Supreme Court Case: *Riegel v. Medtronic, Inc.,* 552 U.S. 312, 128 S.Ct. 999, 2008.

In your opinion, why was this case so decided?

Do you concur with the Supreme Court's decision in this case? Why or why not?

breast implants are immune from liability for personal injuries as long as the Food and Drug Administration (FDA) approved the device before it was marketed and it meets the FDA's specifications. (See the previous *Medtronic Inc.* case.)

Drugs and medical devices are regulated under separate federal laws, and an important issue in deciding drug injury cases is whether or not the drug manufacturer made false or misleading statements to win FDA approval. For example, the case *Warner-Lambert Co. v. Kent*, filed in 2006, involved a group of Michigan residents who claimed injury after taking Warner-Lambert's Rezulin diabetes drug. The case was brought under a Michigan tort reform law that said a drug company could be liable for product injury if it had misrepresented the product to win FDA approval. In this case, the question before the court was, Does a federal law prohibiting fraudulent communications to government agencies preempt a state law permitting plaintiffs to sue for faulty products that would not have reached the market absent the fraud?

A federal appeals court eventually heard the case and ruled that the Michigan "fraud on the FDA" law was preempted by a federal law that allowed the FDA itself to punish misrepresentations. This decision was appealed to the U.S. Supreme Court, and in a March 2008 decision, the Roberts Supreme Court affirmed the appeals court, thus leaving the previous state of the law unchanged and unclarified.

In this case, the people who sued the drug manufacturer were not allowed to collect damages. But when courts find that drugs are misrepresented so that developers can win FDA approval, drug manufacturers could be held legally responsible and forced to pay damages.

Examples of how drug manufacturers could be held legally responsible before any Supreme Court decision protecting them from liability were the many lawsuits filed against Merck & Company, a pharmaceutical firm that manufactured the drug Vioxx, once widely recommended for pain relief for arthritis sufferers. The drug was suspected of causing heart attacks and strokes in some patients, and from 1999, the year Vioxx went on the market, to 2007, Merck faced lawsuits from 47,000 plaintiffs, including patients, health providers, unions, and insurers. Many of the lawsuits alleged that Merck knew of the drug's potentially harmful side effects when the company placed the drug on the market.

In November 2007, Merck agreed to settle most of the lawsuits relating to Vioxx for a total of $4.85 billion. The settlement was open to plaintiffs who filed cases before November 8, 2007, who could provide medical proof of their heart attack or stroke, and who could prove they had used at least 30 Vioxx pills within 14 days prior to their illness. In March 2010, Merck and the Securities and Exchange Commission (SEC) announced that all payouts through the settlement process would be paid out by the end of June 2010.

Merck anticipated that some plaintiffs would opt out of the settlement, continuing to fight the company on a case-by-case basis. The company projected that remaining claims could cost the firm between $2 and $3 billion, and those claims are still being litigated.

Federal preemption—a doctrine that can bar injured consumers from suing in state court when the products that hurt them had met federal standards—has become an important concern in product liability law. One such case, *Wyeth v. Levine*, decided by the U.S. Supreme Court in 2009, will become precedent for future cases involving drug manufacturers and consumers.

COURT CASE

Patient Sues over Drug Labeling Issue

In 2000, Diana Levine, a Vermont woman in her fifties, sought medical help for migraine headaches. As part of the treatment, the antinausea drug Phenergan, made by Wyeth, was injected in her arm. An artery was accidentally damaged during the injection, gangrene set in, and Levine's right arm was amputated. The amputation was devastating for Levine, a professional musician who had released 16 albums, and she filed a personal injury action against Wyeth in Vermont state court.

Levine asserted that Wyeth should have included a warning label describing the possible arterial injuries that could occur from negligent injection of the drug. Wyeth argued that because the warning label had been deemed acceptable by the FDA, a federal agency, any Vermont state regulations making the label insufficient were preempted by the federal approval. The Superior Court of Vermont found in favor of Levine and denied Wyeth's motion for a new trial. Levine was awarded $7 million in damages for the amputation of her arm. The Supreme Court of Vermont affirmed this ruling on appeal, holding that the FDA requirements merely provide a floor, not a ceiling, for state regulation. Therefore, states are free to create more stringent labeling requirements than federal law provides.

The U.S. Supreme Court eventually heard the case and issued a decision in March 2009. Wyeth had argued that because the warning label had been accepted by the FDA, any Vermont state regulations making the label insufficient were preempted by the federal approval. The U.S. Supreme Court affirmed the Vermont Supreme Court, holding that federal law did not preempt Levine's state law claim that Wyeth's labeling of Phenergan failed to warn of the dangers of intravenous administration.

Source: Wyeth v. Levine, 555 U.S 555, 129 S.Ct. 1187 (2009).

used in a inapromted matter!

Comparing Aspects of Law and Ethics

To understand the complexities of law and ethics, it is helpful to define and compare a few basic terms. Table 1-1 summarizes the terms described in the following sections.

Law

A **law** is defined as a rule of conduct or action prescribed or formally recognized as binding or enforced by a controlling authority. Governments enact laws to keep society running smoothly and to control behavior that could threaten public safety. Laws are considered the minimum standard necessary to keep society functioning.

Enforcement of laws is made possible by penalties for disobedience, which are decided by a court of law or are mandatory as written into the law. Penalties vary with the severity of the crime. Lawbreakers may be fined, imprisoned, or both. Sometimes lawbreakers are sentenced to probation. Other penalties appropriate to the crime may be handed down by the sentencing authority, as when offenders must perform a specified number of hours of volunteer community service or are ordered to repair public facilities they have damaged.

LO 1.2 and LO 1.3

Distinguish among law, ethics, bioethics, etiquette, and protocol.

Define *moral values* and explain how they relate to law, ethics, and etiquette.

law Rule of conduct or action prescribed or formally recognized as binding or enforced by a controlling authority.

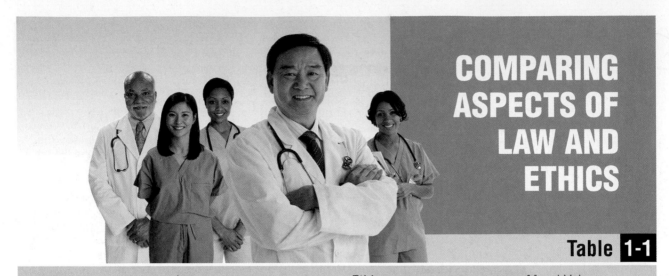

COMPARING ASPECTS OF LAW AND ETHICS

Table 1-1

	Law	Ethics	Moral Values
Definition	Set of governing rules	Principles, standards, guide to conduct	Beliefs formed through the influence of family, culture, and society
Main purpose	To protect the public	To elevate the standard of competence	To serve as a guide for personal ethical conduct
Standards	Minimal — promotes smooth functioning of society	Builds values and ideals	Serves as a basis for forming a personal code of ethics
Penalties of violation	Civil or criminal liability. Upon conviction: fine, imprisonment, revocation of license, or other penalty as determined by courts	Suspension or eviction from medical society membership, as decided by peers	Difficulty in getting along with others

	Bioethics	Etiquette	Protocol
Definition	Discipline relating to ethics concerning biological research, especially as applied to medicine	Courtesy and manners	Rules of etiquette applicable to one's place of employment
Main purpose	To allow scientific progress in a manner that benefits society in all possible ways	To enable one to get along with others	To enable one to get along with others engaged in the same profession
Standards	Leads the highest standards possible in applying research to medical care	Leads to pleasant interaction	Promotes smooth functioning of workplace routines
Penalties of violation	Can include all those listed under "Law," "Ethics," and "Etiquette"; as current standards are applied and as new laws and ethical standards evolve to govern medical research and development, penalties may change	Ostracism from chosen groups	Disapproval of one's professional colleagues; possible loss of business

Many laws affect health care practitioners, including criminal and civil statutes as well as state medical practice acts. Medical practice acts apply specifically to the practice of medicine in a certain state. Licensed health care professionals convicted of violating criminal, civil, or medical practice laws may lose their licenses to practice. (Medical practice acts are discussed further in Chapter 3. Laws and the court system are discussed in more detail in Chapter 4.)

Ethics

An illegal act by a health care practitioner is always unethical, but an unethical act is not necessarily illegal. **Ethics** are concerned with standards of behavior and the concept of right and wrong, over and above that which is legal in a given situation. **Moral values**—formed through the influence of the family, culture, and society—serve as the basis for ethical conduct.

The United States is a culturally diverse country, with many residents who have grown up within vastly different ethnic environments. For example, a Chinese student in the United States brings to his or her studies a unique set of religious and social experiences and moral concepts that will differ from that of a German, Japanese, Korean, French, Italian, or even Canadian classmate. Therefore, moral values and ethical standards can differ for health care practitioners, as well as patients, in the same setting.

In the American cultural environment, however, acting morally toward another usually requires that you put yourself in that individual's place. For example, when you are a patient in a physician office, how do you like to be treated? As a health care provider, can you give care to a person whose conduct or professed beliefs differ radically from your own? In an emergency, can you provide for the patient's welfare without reservation?

ethics Standards of behavior, developed as a result of one's concept of right and wrong.

moral values One's personal concept of right and wrong, formed through the influence of the family, culture, and society.

code of ethics A list of principles intended to govern behavior—here, the behavior of those entrusted with providing care to the sick.

Codes of Ethics and Ethics Guidelines

While most individuals can rely on a well-developed personal value system, organizations for the health occupations also have formalized **codes of ethics** to govern behavior of members and to increase the level of competence and standards of care within the group. Included among these are the American Nurses Association Code for Nurses, American Medical Association Code of Medical Ethics, American Health Information Management Association Code of Ethics, American Society of Radiologic Technologists Code of Ethics, and the Code of Ethics of the American Association of Medical Assistants. Codes of

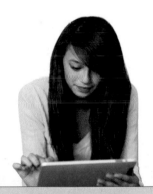

check your **progress**

1. Name two important reasons for studying law and ethics.

2. Which state laws apply specifically to the practice of medicine?

3. What purpose do laws serve?

4. How is the enforcement of laws made possible?

5. What factors influence the formation of one's personal set of ethics and values?

6. Define the term *moral values*.

7. Explain how one's moral values affect one's sense of ethics.

ethics guidelines Publications that detail a wide variety of ethical situations that professionals (in this case, health care practitioners) might face in their work and offer principles for dealing with the situations in an ethical manner.

Hippocratic oath A pledge for physicians, developed by the Greek physician Hippocrates circa 400 B.C.E.

ethics generally consist of a list of general principles, and are often available to laypersons as well as members of health care practitioner organizations.

Many professional organizations for health care practitioners also publish more detailed **ethics guidelines,** usually in book form, for members. Generally, ethics guideline publications detail a wide variety of ethical situations that health care practitioners might face in their work and offer principles for dealing with the situations in an ethical manner. They are routinely available to members of health care organizations, and are typically available to others for a fee.

One of the earliest medical codes of ethics, the code of Hammurabi, was written by the Babylonians around 2250 B.C.E. This document discussed the conduct expected of physicians at that time, including fees that could be charged.

Sometime around 400 B.C.E., Hippocrates, the Greek physician known as the *father of medicine*, created the **Hippocratic oath,** a pledge for physicians that remains influential today (see Figure 1-1).

> **Figure 1-1**

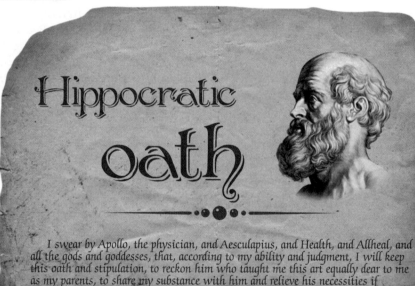

Hippocratic oath

I swear by Apollo, the physician, and Aesculapius, and Health, and Allheal, and all the gods and goddesses, that, according to my ability and judgment, I will keep this oath and stipulation, to reckon him who taught me this art equally dear to me as my parents, to share my substance with him and relieve his necessities if required; to regard his offspring as on the same footing with my own brothers, and to teach them this art if they should wish to learn it, without fee or stipulation; and that by precept, lecture, and every other mode of instruction, I will impart a knowledge of the art to my own sons and to those of my teachers, and to disciples bound by a stipulation and oath, according to the law of medicine, but to none other.

I will follow that method of treatment which, according to my ability and judgment, I consider for the benefit of my patients, and abstain from whatever is deleterious and mischievous. I will give no deadly medicine to anyone if asked, nor suggest any such counsel; furthermore, I will not give to a woman an instrument to produce abortion.

With purity and holiness I will pass my life and practice my art. I will not cut a person who is suffering with a stone, but will leave this to be done by practitioners of the work. Into whatever houses I enter I will go into them for the benefit of the sick and will abstain from every voluntary act of mischief and corruption; and further from the seduction of females or males, bond or free.

Whatever, in connection with my professional practice, or not in connection with it, I may see or hear in the lives of men which ought not to be spoken abroad, I will not divulge, as reckoning that all such should be kept secret.

While I continue to keep this oath unviolated, may it be granted to me to enjoy life and the practice of the art, respected by all men at all times, but should I trespass and violate this oath, may the reverse be my lot.

Percival's Medical Ethics, written by the English physician and philosopher Thomas Percival in 1803, superseded earlier codes to become the definitive guide for a physician's professional conduct. Earlier codes did not address concerns about experimental medicine, but according to Percival's code, physicians could try experimental treatments when all else failed, if such treatments served the public good.

When the American Medical Association met for the first time in Philadelphia in 1847, the group devised a code of ethics for members based on Percival's code. The resulting ***American Medical Association Principles,*** currently called the *American Medical Association Principles of Medical Ethics,* has been revised and updated periodically to keep pace with changing times (see Figure 1-2). The *American Medical Association Principles of Medical Ethics* briefly summarizes the position of the American Medical Association (AMA) on ethical treatment of patients, while the more extensive *Code of Medical Ethics: Current Opinions with Annotations* provides more detailed coverage.

American Medical Association Principles A code of ethics for members of the American Medical Association, written in 1847. (American Medical Association Web site: **www.ama-assn.org/ama/pub/physicianresources/medical-ethics/code-medical-ethics/principles-medical-ethics.page**.)

> **Figure 1-2**

Preamble

The medical profession has long subscribed to a body of ethical statements developed primarily for the benefit of the patient. As a member of this profession, a physician must recognize responsibility to patients first and foremost, as well as to society, to other health professionals, and to self. The following Principles adopted by the American Medical Association are not laws, but standards of conduct which define the essentials of honorable behavior for the physician.

A physician shall be dedicated to providing competent medical care, with compassion and respect for human dignity and right.

A physician shall uphold the standards of professionalism, be honest in all professional interactions, and strive to report physicians deficient in character or competence, or who engage in fraud or deception, to appropriate entities.

A physician shall respect the law and also recognize a responsibility to seek changes in those requirements which are contrary to the best interests of the patient.

A physician shall respect the rights of patients, colleagues, and other health professionals and shall safeguard patient confidences and privacy within the constraints of the law.

A physician shall continue to study, apply, and advance scientific knowledge, maintain commitment to medical education, make relevant information available to patients, colleagues, and the public, obtain consultation, and use the talents of other health professionals when indicated.

A physician shall, in the provision of appropriate patient care, except in emergencies, be free to choose whom to serve, with whom to associate, and the environment in which to provide care.

A physician shall recognize a responsibility to participate in activities contributing to the improvement of the community and the betterment of public health.

A physician shall, while caring for a patient, regard responsibility to the patient as paramount.

A physician shall support access to medical care for all people.

AMERICAN MEDICAL ASSOCIATION PRINCIPLES OF MEDICAL ETHICS

Source: American Medical Association, *Code of Medical Ethics, Current Opinions with Annotations,* current issue.

When members of professional associations such as the AMA and the AAMA are accused of unethical conduct, they are subject to peer council review and may be censured by the organization (see Figure 1-3). Although a professional group cannot revoke a member's license to practice, unethical members may be expelled from the group, suspended for a period of time, or ostracized by other members. Unethical behavior by a medical practitioner can result in loss of income and eventually the loss of a practice if, as a result of that behavior, patients choose another practitioner.

bioethics A discipline dealing with the ethical implications of biological research methods and results, especially in medicine.

Bioethics

Bioethics is a discipline dealing with the ethical implications of biological research methods and results, especially in medicine. As biological research

> **Figure 1-3**

The Code of Ethics of AAMA shall set forth principles of ethical and moral conduct as they relate to the medical profession and the particular practice of medical assisting.

Members of AAMA dedicated to the conscientious pursuit of their profession and thus desiring to merit the high regard of the entire medical profession and the respect of the general public which they serve, do pledge themselves to strive always to:

A. render service with full respect for the dignity of humanity;

B. respect confidential information obtained through employment unless legally authorized or required by responsible performance of duty to divulge such information;

C. uphold the honor and high principles of the profession and accept its disciplines;

D. seek to continually improve the knowledge and skills of medical assistants for the benefit of patients and professional colleagues;

E. participate in additional service activities aimed toward improving the health and well-being of the community.

I. I believe in the principles and purposes of the profession of medical assisting.

II. I endeavor to be more effective.

III. I aspire to render greater service.

IV. I protect the confidence entrusted to me.

V. I am dedicated to the care and well-being of all people.

VI. I am loyal to my employer.

VII. I am true to the ethics of my profession.

VIII. I am strengthened by compassion, courage, and faith.

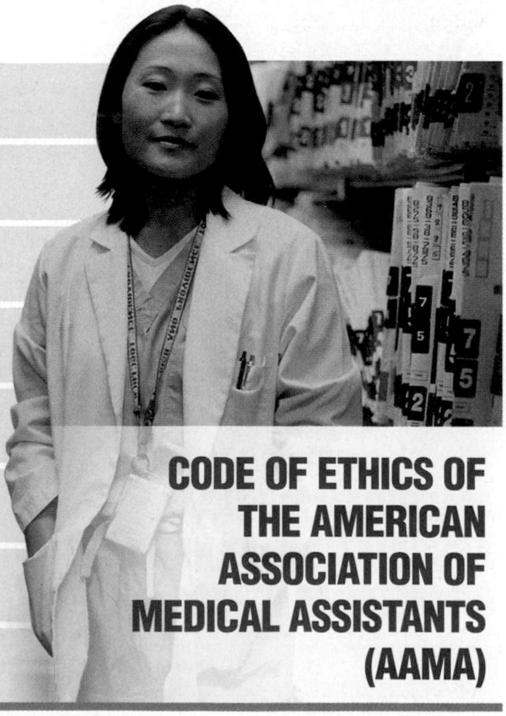

CODE OF ETHICS OF THE AMERICAN ASSOCIATION OF MEDICAL ASSISTANTS (AAMA)

Source: http://www.aama-ntl.org/aboutcode_creed.aspx

has led to unprecedented progress in medicine, medical practitioners have had to grapple with issues such as these:

- What ethics should guide biomedical research? Do individuals own all rights to their body cells, or should scientists own cells they have altered? Is human experimentation essential, or even permissible, to advance biomedical research?

- What ethics should guide organ transplants? Although organs suitable for transplant are in short supply, is the search for organs dehumanizing? Should certain categories of people have lower priority than others for organ transplants?

- What ethics should guide fetal tissue research? Some say such research, especially stem cell research, is moral because it offers hope to disease victims, while others argue that it is immoral.

- Do reproductive technologies offer hope to the childless, or are they unethical? Are the multiple births that sometimes result from taking fertility drugs an acceptable aspect of reproductive technology, or are those multiple births too risky for women and their fetuses and even immoral in an allegedly overpopulated world?

- Should animals ever be used in research?

- How ethical is genetic research? Should the government regulate it? Will genetic testing benefit those at risk for genetic disease, or will it lead to discrimination? Should cloning of human organs for transplantation be permitted? Should cloning of human beings ever be permitted?

Society is attempting to address these questions, but because the issues are complicated, many questions may never be completely resolved.

The Role of Ethics Committees

Health care practitioners may be able to resolve the majority of the ethical issues they face in the workplace from their own intuitive sense of moral values and ethics. Some ethical dilemmas, however, are not so much a question of right or wrong but more a question like, "Which of these alternatives will do the most good and the least harm?" In these more ambiguous situations, health care practitioners may want to ask the advice of a medical ethicist or members of an institutional ethics committee.

Medical ethicists or **bioethicists** are specialists who consult with physicians, researchers, and others to help them make difficult decisions, such as whether to resuscitate brain-damaged premature infants or what ethics should govern privacy in genetic testing. Hospital or medical center **ethics committees** usually consist of physicians, nurses, social workers, clergy, a patient's family, members of the community, and other individuals involved with the patient's medical care. A medical ethicist may also sit on the ethics committee if such a specialist is available. When difficult decisions must be made, any one of the individuals involved in a patient's medical care can ask for a consultation with the ethics committee. Larger hospitals have standing ethics committees, while smaller facilities may form ethics committees as needed.

When a case is referred to the ethics committee, the members meet and review the case. The committee does not make binding decisions, but helps the physician, nurse, patient, patient's family, and others clarify the issue and understand the medical facts of the case and the alternatives available to resolve the situation. Ethics committees may also help with conflict resolution among parties involved with a case. They do not, however, function as institutional review boards or morals police looking for health care workers who have committed unethical acts.

See Chapter 2 for a more detailed discussion of the processes involved in making ethical decisions.

> **medical ethicist or bioethicist** Specialists who consult with physicians, researchers, and others to help them make difficult ethical decisions regarding patient care.

> **ethics committee** Committee made up of individuals who are involved in a patient's care, including health care practitioners, family members, clergy, and others, with the purpose of reviewing ethical issues in difficult cases.

Etiquette

etiquette Standards of behavior considered to be good manners among members of a profession as they function as individuals in society.

While professional codes of ethics focus on the protection of the patient and his or her right to appropriate, competent, and humane treatment, **etiquette** refers to standards of behavior that are considered good manners. Every culture has its own ideas of common courtesy. Behavior considered good manners in one culture may be bad manners in another. For example, in some Middle Eastern countries it is extremely discourteous for one male acquaintance to ask another, "How is your wife?" In Western culture, such a question is well received. Similarly, within nearly every profession, there are recognized practices considered to be good manners for members.

Most health care facilities have their own policies concerning professional etiquette that staff members are expected to follow. Policy manuals written especially for the facility can serve as permanent records and as guidelines for employees in these matters.

protocol A code prescribing correct behavior in a specific situation, such as a situation arising in a medical office.

By the same token, health care practitioners are expected to know **protocol,** standard rules of etiquette applicable specifically to their place of employment. For example, when another physician telephones, does the receptionist put the call through without delay? What is the protocol in the diagnostic testing office when the technicians get behind because of a late patient or a repair to an X-ray machine?

Within the health care environment, all health care practitioners are, of course, expected to treat patients with the same respect and courtesy afforded others in the course of day-to-day living. Politeness and appropriate dress are mandatory.

LO 1.4

Discuss the characteristics and skills most likely to lead to a successful career in one of the health care professions.

Qualities of Successful Health Care Practitioners

Successful health care practitioners have a knowledge of techniques and principles that includes an understanding of legal and ethical issues. They must also acquire a working knowledge of and tolerance for human nature and individual characteristics, since daily contact with a wide variety of individuals with a host of problems and concerns is a significant part of the work. Courtesy, compassion, and common sense are often cited as the "three Cs" most vital to the professional success of health care practitioners.

Courtesy

courtesy The practice of good manners.

The simplest definition of **courtesy** is the practice of good manners. Most of us know how to practice good manners, but sometimes circumstances make us forget. Maybe we're having a rotten day—we overslept and dressed in a hurry but were still late to work; the car didn't start so we had to walk, making us even more late; we were rebuked at work for coming in late . . . and on and on. Perhaps we're burned out, stressed out, or simply too busy to think. Regardless of a health care practitioner's personal situation, however, patients have the right to expect courtesy and respect, including self-introduction. ("Hi, I'm Maggie and I'll be taking care of you," is one nursing assistant's way of introducing herself to new patients in the nursing home where she works.)

Think back to experiences you have had with health care practitioners. Did the receptionist in a medical office greet you pleasantly, or did he or she make you feel as though you were an unwelcome intruder? (Remember Elaine in the chapter's opening scenario?) Did the laboratory technician or phlebotomist who drew your blood for testing put you at ease or make you more anxious than you already were? If you were hospitalized, did health care practitioners carefully explain procedures and treatments before performing them, or were you left wondering what was happening to you?

Chances are that you know from your own experiences how important common courtesy can be to a patient.

Compassion

Compassion is empathy—the identification with and understanding of another's situation, feelings, and motives (Figure 1-4). In other words, compassion is temporarily putting oneself in another's shoes. It should not be confused with sympathy, which is feeling sorry for another person's plight—typically a less deeply felt emotion than compassion. While "I know how you feel" is not usually the best phrase to utter to a patient (it too often earns the retort, "No, you don't"), compassion means that you are sincerely attempting to know how the patient feels.

> **compassion** The identification with and understanding of another's situation, feelings, and motives.

Common Sense

Common sense is simply sound practical judgment. It is somewhat difficult to define, because it can have different meanings for different people, but it generally means that you can see which solution or action makes good sense in a given situation. For example, if you were a nursing assistant and a gasping, panicked patient told you he was having trouble breathing, common sense would tell you to immediately seek help. You wouldn't simply enter the patient's complaint in his medical chart and wait for a physician or a nurse to see the notation. Likewise, if a patient spilled something on the floor, common sense would tell you to wipe it up (even if you were not a member of the housekeeping staff) before someone stepped in it and possibly slipped and fell. While it's not always immediately obvious that someone has common sense, it usually doesn't take long to recognize its absence in an individual.

> **common sense** Sound practical judgment.

Additional capabilities that are helpful to those who choose to work in the health care field include those that are listed in the following sections "People Skills" and "Technical Skills."

People Skills

People skills are those traits and capabilities that allow you to get along well with others and to relate well to patients or clients in a health care setting. They include such attributes as the following:

- A relaxed attitude when meeting new people.
- An understanding of and empathy for others.
- Good communication skills, including writing, speaking, and listening.
- Patience in dealing with others and the ability to work as a member of a health care team (see Figure 1-5).
- Tact.
- The ability to impart information clearly and accurately.
- The ability to keep information confidential.
- The ability to leave private concerns at home.
- Trustworthiness and a sense of responsibility.

Technical Skills

Technical skills include those abilities you have acquired in your course of study, including but not limited to the following:

- Computer literacy.
- Proficiency in English, science, and mathematics.

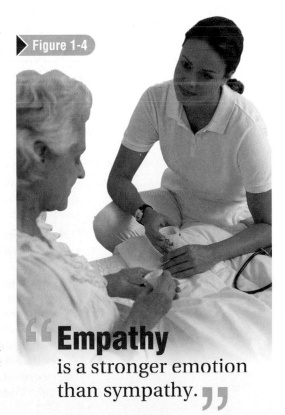

▶ Figure 1-4

"**Empathy** is a stronger emotion than sympathy."

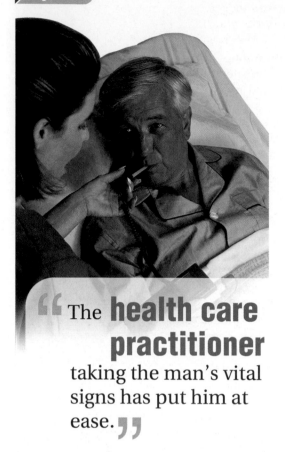

Figure 1-5

" The **health care practitioner** taking the man's vital signs has put him at ease. "

critical thinking   The ability to think analytically, using fewer emotions and more rationality.

- A willingness to learn new skills and techniques.
- An aptitude for working with the hands.
- Ability to document well.
- Ability to think critically.

Critical Thinking Skills

When faced with a problem, most of us worry a lot before we finally begin working through the problem effectively, which means using fewer emotions and more rational thinking skills. As a health care practitioner, you will be expected to approach a problem at work in a manner that lets you act as ethically, legally, and helpfully as possible. Sometimes solutions to problems must also be found as quickly as possible, but solutions must always be within the scope of your training, licensure, and capabilities. This problem-solving process is called **critical thinking.** Here is a five-step aid for approaching a problem using critical thinking:

1. **Identify and clarify the problem.** It's impossible to solve a problem unless you know the exact nature of the problem. For example, imagine that patients in a medical office have frequently complained that the wait to see physicians is too long, and several have protested loudly and angrily that their time "is valuable too." Rhea is the waiting room receptionist and the person who faces angry patients first, so she would like to solve this problem as quickly as possible. Rhea has recognized that a problem exists, of course, but her apologies to patients have been temporary fixes, and the situation continues.

2. **Gather information.** In the previous situation, Rhea begins to gather information. She first checks to see exactly why patients have been kept waiting, and considers the following questions: Are all the physicians simply oversleeping and beginning the day behind schedule? (Not likely, but an easy solution if this were the case would be to buy the physicians new alarm clocks.) Are the physicians often delayed in surgery or because of hospital rounds? Is the clinic understaffed? How long, on average, has each patient who has complained been left waiting beyond his or her appointment time?

3. **Evaluate the evidence.** Rhea evaluates the answers she has gathered to the earlier questions and determines that too many patients are, indeed, waiting too long beyond appointment times to see their physicians. The next step in the critical thinking process is to consider all possible ways to solve the problem.

4. **Consider alternatives and implications.** Rhea has determined that the evidence supports the fact that a problem exists and begins to formulate alternatives by asking herself these questions: Could the waiting room be better supplied with current reading material or perhaps television sets and a children's corner, so that patients both with and without children are less likely to complain about waiting? Is the waiting room cheery and comfortable, so waiting does not seem interminable? What solution would best serve the goals of physicians, other medical office personnel, and patients? Rhea must consider costs of, objections to, and all others' opinions of each alternative she considers.

5. **Choose and implement the best alternative.** Rhea selects an alternative and implements it. As a medical office receptionist, she cannot act alone, but she has brought the problem to the attention of those who can help, and her suggestions have been heard. As a result of Rhea's research, acceptable solutions to patients' complaints that they are forced to wait too long to see physicians might include the following:

- Patients are asked to remind receptionists when they have been waiting over 15 minutes so receptionists can check to see what is causing the delay.

- Additional personnel are hired to see patients.

- The waiting room is stocked with current news publications, television sets, and/or a child play center for patient comfort while waiting.

Critical thinking is not easy, but, like any skill, it improves with practice.

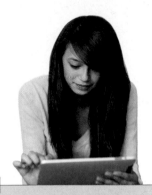

check your **progress**

8. Tell how each of the following characteristics relates to law and ethics in the health care professions:

   The ability to be a good communicator and listener.
   The ability to keep information confidential.
   The ability to impart information clearly and accurately.
   The ability to think critically.

9. List and discuss each of the steps helpful to developing critical thinking skills.

10. Explain how you, as a health care practitioner, would use the critical thinking steps listed above to reach a solution to the following problem: A patient from a different culture believes he has been cursed with a "liver demon" and will die unless the organ is surgically removed.

_____

_____

_____

_____

_____

_____

_____

_____

Determining If a Decision Is Ethical

While considering the legality of a certain act, health care practitioners must also consider ethical implications. According to many ethics experts, the following questions can help you determine if an act you have decided on via critical thinking skills is ethical:

- If you perform this act, have you followed relevant laws, and kept within your employing company's policy?

- Will this act promote a win–win situation for as many of the involved individuals as possible?

- How would you feel if this act were to be publicized in the newspapers or other media?
- Would you want your family members to know?
- If you perform this act, can you look at yourself in a mirror?

The health care practitioner who demonstrates these qualities and skills, coupled with a working knowledge of law and ethics, is most likely to find success and job satisfaction in his or her chosen profession.

[CHAPTER SUMMARY]

LO 1.1 Why study law and ethics?

- Health care practitioners who function at the highest possible levels have a working knowledge of law and ethics.
- Knowing the law relevant to your profession can help you avoid legal entanglements that threaten your ability to earn a living. Court cases illustrate how health care practitioners, health care facilities, and drug and medical device manufacturers can be held accountable in a court of law.
- A knowledge of law and ethics will also help familiarize you with the following areas:
  - The rights, responsibilities, and concerns of health care consumers.
  - The legal and ethical issues facing society, patients, and health care practitioners as the world changes.
  - The impact of rising costs on the laws and ethics of health care delivery.

LO 1.2 and LO 1.3 What are the basic aspects of law and ethics, and how do they compare?

- Laws are considered the minimum standard necessary to keep society functioning. Many laws govern the health care professions, including criminal and civil statutes and medical practice acts.
- Ethics are principles and standards that govern behavior. Most health care professions have a code of ethics members are expected to follow.
- Bioethics is the discipline dealing with the ethical implications of biological research methods and results, especially in medicine.
- Moral values define one's personal concept of right and wrong.
- Etiquette refers to manners and courtesy.
- Protocol is a code prescribing correct behavior in a specific situation, such as in a medical office.

LO 1.4 What characteristics and skills will most likely help a health care practitioner achieve success?

- People skills, such as listening to others and communicating well, are an asset to health care practitioners.
- Technical skills, including a basic knowledge of computers, and a foundation in science and math are necessary to achieve an education in the health care sciences.

- Critical thinking skills are required for you to correctly assess a situation and provide the proper response. Solving problems through critical thinking involves:

  1. Identifying and clarifying the problem.
  2. Gathering information.
  3. Evaluating the evidence.
  4. Considering alternatives and implications.
  5. Choosing and implementing the best alternative.

  What questions can help you decide if a decision is ethical?

  1. If you perform this act, have you followed relevant laws and kept within your employing company's policy?
  2. Will this act promote a win–win situation for as many of the involved individuals as possible?
  3. How would you feel if this act were to be publicized in the newspapers or other media?
  4. Would you want your family members to know?
  5. If you perform this act, can you look at yourself in a mirror?

LO 1.4 Exercise: Assessing Your Strengths and Weaknesses

Think carefully about each of the following statements, then put a check mark next to the statement that most accurately describes you. This is not a test, and there are no correct or incorrect answers; it is intended solely to help you evaluate those areas where you excel or need improvement.

❏ I like meeting new people and willingly place myself in situations where I can interact with someone new.

❏ I often make excuses in order to decline social invitations that would require me to meet and interact with new people.

❏ I can visit with anyone, and I enjoy listening to the opinions and experiences of others.

❏ I often have trouble initiating a conversation, and if forced to listen too long, my mind wanders or I find myself concentrating on my response, rather than on the conversation.

❏ If someone complains to me and I am in a position to help, I willingly explore solutions with the person who complains.

❏ I go out of my way to avoid people who chronically complain.

❏ I can tactfully tell a person the truth when necessary, without hurting feelings or fostering anger.

❏ I believe it's best to always tell others the truth, even if it risks making them angry or hurting their feelings.

❏ I know correct grammar, and always use it when writing reports or conversing with others.

❏ I can get my meaning across without always using good grammar.

❏ On the job I can listen to another person's complaints or criticism without becoming angry.

❏ Complaining about or criticizing my work always makes me angry.

❏ I can always keep private information about others to myself.

- ❏ One of my most endearing qualities is my inability to keep a secret.
- ❏ In stressful situations I keep my composure and think about the best way to proceed.
- ❏ I avoid stressful situations, because I tend to panic and would rather rely on someone else to tell me what to do.
- ❏ I am familiar with computers and enjoy learning new applications.
- ❏ I don't like using computers.
- ❏ I like science and math, and get good grades in those subjects.
- ❏ Science and math turn me off, and I avoid those courses whenever possible.
- ❏ Using my own words, both orally and in writing, I can explain technical or complicated material in a way others can easily understand.
- ❏ I don't like explaining complicated material to others, either orally or in writing.

ETHICS ISSUES Introduction to End-of-Chapter Ethics Discussions

Learning Outcomes for the Ethics Issues Feature at the End of Each Chapter

After studying the material in each chapter's Ethics Issues feature, you should be able to:

1. Discuss current ethical issues of concern to health care practitioners.
2. Compare ethical guidelines to the law as discussed in each chapter of the text.
3. Practice critical thinking skills as you consider medical, legal, and ethical issues for each situation presented.
4. Relate the ethical issues presented in the text to the health care profession you intend to practice.

Health care practitioners are bound by state and federal laws, but they are also bound by certain ethical standards—both personal standards and those set forth by professional codes of ethics and ethical guidelines, and by bioethicists. Many professional organizations for health care practitioners employ an ethics consultant who is available to speak with organization members who need help with an ethical dilemma. "We serve as a third party who can stand outside a situation and facilitate communication," says Dr. Carmen Paradis, an ethics consultant with the Cleveland Clinic's Department of Bioethics. At the Cleveland Clinic, ethics consultations are available to health care practitioners, patients, family members, and others involved with patient decisions.

Medical facility ethics committees can also serve as consultants. In larger health care facilities such committees usually deal with institutional matters, but in smaller communities where ethics consultants may not be available, members of an ethics committee may also function as ethics consultants.

Keep in mind as you read the Ethics Issues feature for each chapter that ethical guidelines are not law, but deal solely with ethical conduct for health care practitioners. Most guidelines published for professional health care practitioner organizations emphasize this difference. For example, as stated in *Guidelines for Ethical Conduct for the Physician Assistant Profession,* "Generally, the law delineates the minimum standard of acceptable behavior in our society. Acceptable ethical behavior is usually less clearly defined than law and often places greater demands on an individual. . . .

"Ethical guidelines for health care practitioners are not meant to be used in courts of law as legal standards to which practitioners will be held. Ethical guidelines are, rather, meant to guide health care practitioners and to encourage them to think about their individual actions in certain situations."

The ethical guidelines for various health care professions have several points in common, but first and foremost is that health care practitioners are obligated to provide the best care possible for every patient, and to protect the safety and welfare of every patient.

State and federal law may differ somewhat from an ethical principle. For example, a state's law may not require physicians to routinely inquire about physical, sexual, and psychological abuse as part of a patient's medical history, but the physician may feel an ethical duty to his or her patients to do so.

Furthermore, the fact that a health care practitioner who has been charged with illegal conduct is acquitted or exonerated does not necessarily mean that the health care practitioner acted ethically.

The term *ethical* as used here refers to matters involving the following:

1. Moral principles or practices.
2. Matters of social policy involving issues of morality in the practice of medicine.

The term *unethical* refers to professional conduct that fails to conform to these moral standards or policies.

The ethical issues raised are from the real-life experiences of a variety of health care practitioners and are recounted throughout the text to raise awareness of the ethical dilemmas many practitioners face daily, and to stimulate discussion.

[ETHICS ISSUES Introduction to Law and Ethics]

Ethics ISSUE 1: A physician assistant in a medical practice with several physicians contacts his professional association, the American Academy of Physician Assistants (AAPA), to report that one of his employing physicians often recommends chiropractic treatment for patients with persistent back pain issues that have resisted medical solutions. The PA knows it is legal to refer a patient for chiropractic treatments, but he adamantly opposes the practice, considering it "bogus medicine." The physician declines to discuss the matter.

Discussion Questions

1. In your opinion, how might the situation be resolved?

_____

_____

2. Is it ethical for the PA to continue working for the physician when their opinions differ so widely on this issue?

_____

_____

Ethics ISSUE 2: A registered nurse calls her professional organization's ethics consultant to ask for resources she can present to her employing medical clinic to support her intention to quit working with a physician she feels is providing sloppy and possibly dangerous care.

Discussion Questions

1. What is the most important principle for the nurse to consider here?

_____

_____

2. In your opinion, are there legal issues inherent in this situation, as well as ethical issues? Explain your answer.

_____

_____

Ethics Issue 3: A physician assistant (PA) has been helping treat a patient awaiting a heart transplant. The patient is depressed, and says he no longer wants to live. The PA is doubtful that the patient will cooperate in the demanding regimen required for posttransplantation patients.

Discussion Question

1. Is it ethical for the PA to say nothing to the patient's attending physician, or should he chart the patient's remarks and discuss the matter with the patient's physician?

_____

_____

Ethics Issue 4: Family members of a certified medical assistant (CMA) employed by a medical clinic in a small community often ask the CMA for medical advice. Two of her family members have asked her to bring antibiotic samples home for them.

Discussion Question

1. In your opinion, would it be ethical for the CMA to give medical advice to her own family members? To bring drug samples home for them? Explain your answers.

_____

_____

Ethics Issue 5: A radiology technician practicing in a small community is interested in dating a person he has seen as a patient.

_____

_____

Discussion Question

1. In your opinion, would it be ethical for the radiology technician to date one of his patients? Would it be ethical for him to date a coworker? Explain your answers.

_____

_____

Go to **www.mhhe.com/judson6e** to practice your case review skills. Then read on for more information.

American Medical Association Principles

bioethicists

bioethics

code of ethics

common sense

compassion

courtesy

critical thinking

defendant

ethics

ethics committees

ethics guidelines

etiquette

fraud

health care practitioners

Hippocratic oath

law

liable

litigious

medical ethicists

moral values

plaintiff

precedent

protocol

summary judgment

CHAPTER 1 REVIEW

Applying Knowledge

LO 1.1

Answer the following questions in the spaces provided.

1. List three areas where health care practitioners can gain insight through studying law and ethics.

_____

_____

_____

_____

2. Define *summary judgment*.

_____

_____

_____

_____

LO 1.2

Answer the following questions in the spaces provided.

3. Define *bioethics*.

_____

_____

4. Define *law*.

_____

_____

5. Define *ethics*.

_____

_____

6. How is unethical behavior punished?

_____

_____

7. Define _etiquette._

_____

_____

8. How are violations of etiquette handled?

_____

_____

9. What is the purpose of a professional code of ethics?

_____

_____

10. Name five bioethical issues of concern in today's society.

_____

_____

11. What duties might a medical ethicist perform?

_____

_____

12. Decisions made by judges in the various courts and used as a guide for future decisions are called what?

_____

_____

_____

_____

Circle the correct answer for each of the following questions.

13. Written codes of ethics for health care practitioners
  a. Evolved primarily to serve as moral guidelines for those who provided care to the sick
  b. Are legally binding
  c. Did not exist in ancient times
  d. None of the above

14. What Greek physician is known as the father of medicine?
  a. Hippocrates
  b. Percival
  c. Hammurabi
  d. Socrates

15. Name the pledge for physicians that remains influential today.
  a. Code of Hammurabi
  b. Babylonian Ethics Code
  c. Hippocratic oath
  d. None of the above

16. What ethics code superseded earlier codes to become the definitive guide for a physician's professional conduct?
  a. Code of Hammurabi
  b. Percival's Medical Ethics

c. Hippocratic oath

d. Babylonian Ethics Code

17. Unethical behavior is always
    a. Illegal
    b. Punishable by legal means
    c. Unacceptable
    d. None of the above

18. Unlawful acts are always
    a. Unacceptable
    b. Unethical
    c. Punishable by legal means
    d. All of the above

19. Violation of a professional organization's formalized code of ethics
    a. Always leads to prosecution in a court of law
    b. Is ignored if one's membership dues in the organization are paid
    c. Can lead to expulsion from the organization
    d. None of the above

20. Law is
    a. The minimum standard necessary to keep society functioning smoothly
    b. Ignored if transgressions are ethical, rather than legal
    c. Seldom enforced by controlling authorities
    d. None of the above

21. Conviction of a crime
    a. Cannot result in loss of license unless ethical violations also exist
    b. Is always punishable by imprisonment
    c. Always results in expulsion from a professional organization
    d. Can result in loss of license

22. Sellers and manufacturers can be held legally responsible for defective medical devices and products through what charges?
    a. Fraud
    b. Breach of warranty
    c. Misrepresentation of the product through untrue statements made by the manufacturer or seller
    d. All of the above

23. The basis for ethical conduct includes
    a. One's morals
    b. One's culture
    c. One's family
    d. All of the above

LO 1.2 and LO 1.3

24. What is bioethics concerned with?
    a. Health care law
    b. Etiquette in medical facilities
    c. The ethical implications of biological research methods and results
    d. None of the above

LO 1.4

25. Critical thinking skills include
    a. Assessing the ethics of a situation
    b. First clearly defining a problem
    c. Determining the legal implications of a situation
    d. None of the above

CASE STUDIES

LO 1.2 and LO 1.3

Use your critical thinking skills to answer the questions that follow each case study. Indicate whether each situation is a question of law, ethics, protocol, or etiquette.

You are employed as an assistant in an ophthalmologist's office. Your neighbor asks you to find out for him how much another patient was charged for an eye examination at the eye clinic that employs you. Your neighbor also asks you how much the patient was charged for his prescription eyeglasses (the eye clinic also sells lenses and frames).

26. Can you answer either of your neighbor's questions? Explain your answer.

_____

_____

A physician employs you as a medical assistant. Another physician comes into the medical office where you work and asks to speak with your physician/employer.

27. Should you seat the physician in the waiting room, or show her to your employer's private office? Why?

_____

_____

You are employed as a licensed practical nurse (LPN) in a small town. (In California and Texas, the term for this profession is "licensed vocational nurse"—abbreviated as LVN.) A woman visits the clinic where you work, complaining of a rash on her body. She says she recently came in contact with a child who had the same symptoms, and she asks, "What did this child see the doctor for, and what was the diagnosis?" She explains that she needs to know, so that she can be immunized if necessary. You explain that you cannot give out this information, but another LPN overhears, pulls the child's chart, and gives the woman the information she requested.

28. Did both LPNs in this scenario act ethically and responsibly? Explain your answer.

_____

_____

LO 1.4

A physician admitted an elderly patient to the hospital, where she was treated for an irregular heartbeat and chest pain. The patient was competent to make her own decisions about a course of treatment, but her opinionated and outspoken daughter repeatedly second-guessed the physician's recommendations with medical information she had obtained from the Internet.

29. In your opinion, what responsibilities, if any, does a physician or other health care practitioner have toward difficult family members or other third parties who interfere with a patient's medical care?

_____

_____

30. What might the physician in this situation have said to her patient's daughter to help resolve the situation?

_____

_____

[INTERNET ACTIVITIES LO 1.1 and LO 1.2]

Complete the activities and answer the questions that follow.

31. Use a search engine to conduct a search for Web sites on the Internet concerned with bioethics. Name two of those sites you think are reliable sources of information. Explain your choices. How does each site define the term *bioethics?*

_____

_____

32. Locate the Web site for the organization that represents the health care profession you intend to practice. Does the site provide guidance on ethics? If so, how? Does the site link to other sites concerning ethics? If so, list three ethics links; then explore these links.

_____

_____

33. Visit the Web site sponsored by the National Institutes of Health called Bioethics Resources (**http://bioethics.od.nih.gov/casestudies.html**). Click on the "Case Studies" link, and pick a case study and review it. Do you agree or disagree with the conclusions reached about the issue? Explain your answer.

_____

_____

RESOURCES

Differences among law, ethics, and etiquette:

Answers.com Web site: **http://wiki.answers.com/Q/How_do_medical_ ethics_differ_from_medical_etiquette.**

Yeh, Elizabeth, Ethel Taylor, and June Eastmond. *Nursing Assistant Fundamentals: A Patient-Centered Approach.* New York: McGraw-Hill, 1998.

Critical thinking:

Sanchez, M. A. "Using Critical-Thinking Principles as a Guide to College-Level Instruction." *Teaching of Psychology* 22, no 1. (1995), pp. 72–74.

Telephone interview November 5, 2007, with Dr. Carmen Paradis, Dept. of Bioethics, Cleveland Clinic.

University of Dayton School of Law Web site: **http://academic.udayton. edu/legaled/CTSkills/CTskills01.htm.**

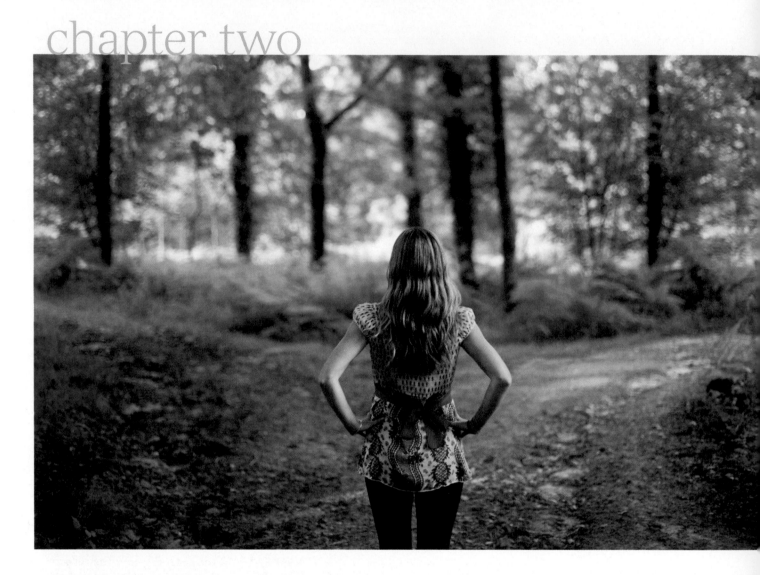

MAKING ETHICAL DECISIONS

Learning Outcomes

After studying this chapter, you should be able to:

LO 2.1 Describe and compare need and value development theories.

LO 2.2 Identify the major principles of contemporary consequence-oriented, duty-oriented, and virtue ethics reasoning.

LO 2.3 Define the basic principles of health care ethics.

TOM AND BILL ARE RADIOLOGY TECHNICIANS at a 300-bed hospital in a large metropolitan area. Tom has been employed by the hospital for 10 years, and Bill is a recent graduate from radiology technician school and has been on the job for four months. Their supervisor, Anna, has been with the hospital for 20 years, moving up the ranks from radiology technician to manager of the department. Because they are short staffed, Anna has been helping the staff complete the required X-rays throughout the day.

One afternoon, Bill notices that Anna is late coming back from lunch. He doesn't give it a second thought because Anna is the boss and often has lunch meetings. However, while working with her that afternoon, Bill realizes that he smells alcohol on Anna's breath. He decides not to say anything. Several days later, Bill once again smells alcohol when around Anna.

Bill decides to talk with Tom about the problem. Tom confirms that he has noticed the problem also. Tom advises Bill not to say anything and offers three pieces of advice. First, Anna's behavior is not Bill's problem. Second, Anna is a supervisor, and it is difficult to understand the pressure she is under. For his final piece of advice, Tom reminds Bill that the last person hired is often the first person fired.

From Bill's perspective, he has seen a clear violation of hospital policy on the part of his supervisor.

From Tom's perspective, he has already decided he doesn't want to get involved in what could be a messy situation. The department is already short staffed, and if Anna were fired, that would mean he would have to work even harder until a new manager was found.

From Anna's perspective, she may not realize that she has a problem with alcohol. Even if she does realize that she has a problem, she may believe that the problem is not serious or she would never be fired because she has been with the hospital for so long.

What should Bill do? Even if patient safety were not an issue, is it his responsibility to report what he has observed? Should not Anna's supervisor also have noticed?

As health care practitioners, we have the responsibility to report problems. But what if by reporting the problem, another person could lose his or her job? How do you decide what to do?

Ethical decision making requires you to tap into your values, morals, and sense of fair play, so that you can be comfortable with the decisions you implement, and so that your decisions do not harm others. Study the following theories for further understanding of your own decision-making process.

Value Development Theories

In Chapter 1, the differences between law, ethics, and etiquette were briefly discussed. Ethics was defined as standards of behavior, developed as a result of one's concept of right and wrong. One's personal concept of right and wrong, called moral values, is formed through the influence of the family, culture, and society. Because each individual experiences different family, cultural, and societal influences, like Tom and Bill in the opening scenario, individuals may see the same situation, yet determine different methods to handle the problem.

LO 2.1

Describe and compare need and value development theories.

Psychologists, philosophers, and social scientists all study human behavior. Many subscribe to the idea that human behavior is a reflection of our attention to our needs or to our values. A classic work by Abraham Maslow, *Motivation and Personality,* first published in 1954, identified a hierarchy of needs that motivates our actions (see Figure 2-1). According to Maslow's theory, there are five stages of need that influence our behavior. We must satisfy each need in order, and the resulting progression is called a hierarchy. Maslow defined needs 1 to 3 as *deficiency,* or D-needs. Needs 4 and 5 are growth needs, also known as *being,* or B-needs.

1. The need for *basic life*—food and shelter.
2. The need for a *safe and secure environment.*
3. The need to *belong and to be loved.*
4. The need for *esteem,* where status, responsibility, and recognition are important.
5. The need for *self-actualization*, for personal growth and fulfillment.

Originally, Maslow believed that the needs followed a strict order, but in his later years he allowed for the possibility that some people may not require meeting all the D-needs before moving on to the B-needs.

Figure 2-1 Maslow's Hierarchy of Needs Pyramid

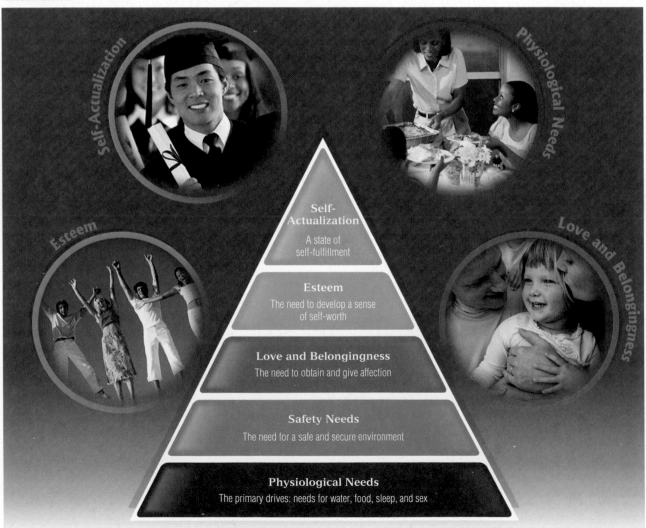

Self-Actualization

Physiological Needs

Esteem

Love and Belongingness

Self-Actualization
A state of
self-fulfillment

Esteem
The need to develop a sense
of self-worth

Love and Belongingness
The need to obtain and give affection

Safety Needs
The need for a safe and secure environment

Physiological Needs
The primary drives: needs for water, food, sleep, and sex

Maslow's theory may help us understand what motivates people, but it does not always help us determine how we developed the values that guide us in ethical decision making.

Many psychologists believe that individuals move from **needs-based motivation** to a personal value system that develops from childhood. When we are born, we have no values. The value system we develop as we grow and mature is dependent on the cultural framework in which we live. If one grows up in an Asian culture, for example, honoring ancestors and tradition may emerge as prominent values; growing up in a Western culture, such as in the United States, may encourage one to place more value on materialism.

A variety of theories exist about how we develop values. Most focus on our stages of development from childhood to adulthood. One of the most famous researchers in this area is Jean Piaget (see Figure 2-2). By observing children at play, Piaget described four levels of moral development.

Lawrence Kohlberg modified and expanded Piaget's work, laying the groundwork for modern studies on moral development. Consistent with Piaget, he proposed that children form ways of thinking through their experiences that include understandings of moral concepts such as justice,

needs-based motivation
The theory that human behavior is based on specific human needs that must often be met in a specific order. Abraham Maslow is the best-known psychologist for this theory.

> **Figure 2-2** Stages of Development from Childhood to Adulthood

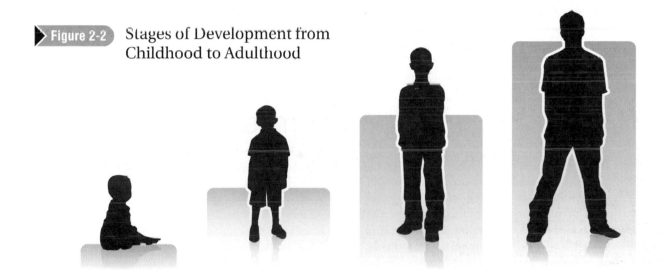

1. The first stage occurs from birth to age 2 and is called the *sensorimotor* stage, during which the child is totally self-centered. Children at this stage of development explore the world with their five senses, and cannot yet see from another's point of view.

2. As infants grow, they develop an awareness of things and people even if not in their direct sight, leading to the second stage, called the *preoperational* or egocentric stage, which extends from ages 2 to 7. During this time period, the child views the world from his or her own perspective. For example, when playing a game, the child is not particularly concerned with rules of play; the focus is on fun, not rules.

3. The third stage of Piaget's theory is called the *concrete operational* stage, extending from ages 7 to 12. In this stage, children tend to see things as either right or wrong, and to see adults as powerful and controlling.

4. Finally, during the *formal operational* stage, children develop abstract thought and begin to understand that there may be different degrees of wrongdoing. For example, children in earlier stages of development, when asked why telling a lie is wrong, may simply reply "because it's bad" whereas children in the formal operational stage can explain "because a lie isn't true." During this stage and through adulthood, intentions, such as lying (I intend to deceive you) and stealing (I intend to take that object) are central to decisions made.

rights, equality, and human welfare. Kohlberg differed from Piaget in that he followed the development of moral judgment beyond the ages studied by Piaget, and he determined that the process of attaining moral maturity took longer and was more gradual than Piaget had proposed.

Kohlberg suggested that moral reasoning can best be understood as sequenced in six stages, grouped into three major levels:

1. Kohlberg's first major level is called *pre-conventional morality*. In the early stages of this level, children from ages 2 to 7 are egocentric, as in Piaget's first stage, and they accept the authority of others. Nearing the end of this stage, children begin to recognize their own interests, which they see in terms of rewards and punishments. They generally avoid breaking rules and committing physical acts backed by punishment, and may avoid obedience for the sake of obedience.

2. The second level in Kohlberg's theory is called *conventional morality,* and is characterized by moral reciprocity—Hit me and I'll hit you back. Do something nice for me and I'll do something nice for you. Children are now in school (ages 7 to 12) and in the first stages of this level are capable of conforming to expectations of family or of a group of people to win approval. The last stage of this level focuses on rules, social order, and respect for authority. Children in this stage of development believe it is their duty to do things right. According to Kohlberg, many of us stay in this stage our entire lives.

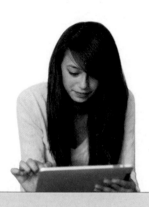

check your **progress**

A pharmacist/researcher has invented a drug that is very effective against a certain type of cancer. He determines that he will sell the drug for $3,000 a treatment. The drug is effective only if it is taken once every week. Harry's young wife is dying from this specific type of cancer. Harry sells everything he can and borrows money from anyone who will lend it to him, but cannot come up with enough money to pay for the drug. He approaches the pharmacist asking if the pharmacist will agree to payments or a lower fee. The pharmacist refuses, stating that he had worked very hard for many years to develop the drug and was entitled to profit from it. Harry decides to break into the pharmacy and steal the drug. (This dilemma was outlined in Kohlberg's writings and used as an example of how different levels of moral reasoning could be identified.)

1–6. Using Kohlberg's levels of pre-conventional, conventional, and post-conventional moral reasoning, complete the following table by filling in the moral reasoning.

Level	In Favor of Stealing the Drug	Against Stealing the Drug
Pre-conventional—reward and punishment		
Conventional—please others and maintain a good society		
Post-conventional—moral principles broader than any society		

3. *Post-conventional morality* (ages 12 and above) is the last level of Kohlberg's moral development theory. There are two stages to this level:

   a. The first stage of post-conventional morality focuses on the social contract and individual rights. A social contract is accepted when people freely enter into work for the benefit of all and for a pleasant society. During this stage individuals explore how to balance individual rights and a fair society for all.

   b. The second stage of post-conventional morality is called universal principles. In this stage, the individual makes a personal commitment to such universal principles as social justice, equal rights, and respect for the dignity of all people and realizes that conventional norms and conventions are necessary to uphold society. If there is a conflict between these values and the social contract, the individual follows his or her basic principles. For example, some people want strict control of U.S. borders so that immigrants cannot cross into America illegally, and they want all illegal immigrants deported. Other individuals want people who cross into America illegally to have a fair route to citizenship.

Kohlberg's theory has recently been criticized, since much of his data were gathered from observing young males. As a result, he has revised his research methodology to account for possible gender bias.

Value Choices Theories

LO 2.2

Identify the major principles of contemporary consequence-oriented, duty-oriented, and virtue ethics reasoning.

Maslow, Piaget, and Kohlberg devised theories to help explain how we develop our values, but their theories do not tell us why moral individuals often come to different conclusions based on reasoning. Tom and Bill, the radiology technicians presented in the chapter's opening scenario, illustrate how two moral individuals can reach different solutions for a problem they both face.

As health care practitioners we know how to perform the tasks required in doing our jobs. That is, we know the right way to take a patient's history, give an injection, take an X-ray, draw blood, or bill the insurance company for the services provided. We know what is right or wrong in performing each medical procedure. That part of the job is straightforward.

Our values, however—our concepts of right or wrong, good or evil as related to our behavior—can be subjective. Universal ethics—problems such as abortion, stem cell research, and euthanasia—are discussed in later chapters, but it is the everyday problems like Bill and Tom faced that are frustrating. They frustrate us because individuals often come to different conclusions, and thus actions, based on their personal beliefs. When faced with a difficult problem, some of us will draw conclusions based on formal religious beliefs or philosophies, while others will place more emphasis on weighing the outcomes of actions, and still others will rely heavily on past experience.

Because no professional code of ethics can address every situation found in health care, we may often find ourselves facing a problem that has no perfect and specific right or wrong solution. Moral people may agree to differ; therefore, it is important to determine a common framework for examining our value decisions.

At least three frameworks or theories exist in the literature that determine how value choices are made: teleological or consequence-oriented theory, deontological or duty-oriented theory, and virtue ethics.

Teleological or Consequence-Oriented Theory

teleological or consequence-oriented theory Decision-making theory that judges the rightness or wrongness based on the outcomes or predicted outcomes.

Teleological or consequence-oriented theory judges the rightness of a decision based on the outcome or predicted outcome of the decision. **Utilitarianism** is the most well known of these theories. In *act-utilitarianism*, a person makes value decisions based on results that will produce the greatest balance of good over evil, everyone considered. In *rule-utilitarianism*, a person makes value decisions based on a rule, that if generally followed would produce the greatest balance of good over evil, everyone considered (Mappes and Degrazia, 2006). In Tom and Bill's problem at the beginning of the chapter, Tom is perhaps using act-utilitarianism to decide that nothing should be done as there has been no harm done and by reporting Anna, harm may occur. Bill, on the other hand, may be using rule-utilitarianism because he knows there is a rule against drinking alcohol during work hours and drunken employees are potential safety hazards.

utilitarianism A consequence-oriented theory that states that decisions should be made by determining what results will produce the best outcome for the most people.

Whether one uses act- or rule-utilitarianism, the process is the same. Once the person has described the problem and determined possible solutions, the solution will be based on which solution is best for all concerned. Often when describing utilitarianism, writers indicate that the solution that provides happiness or a net increase in pleasure over pain for those involved should be selected.

principle of utility Used in utilitarianism; requires that the rule used in making a decision must bring about positive results when generalized to a wide variety of situations.

Supporters of the utilitarian theory have created a **principle of utility.** The principle of utility requires that the rule used to make the decision be a rule that brings about positive results when generalized to a wide variety of situations. There are, however, no absolute truths in utilitarianism.

Deontological or Duty-Oriented Theory

deontological or duty-oriented theory Decision-making theory that states that the rightness or wrongness of the act depends on its intrinsic nature and not the outcome of the act.

Deontological or duty-oriented theory focuses on the essential rightness or wrongness of an act, not the consequences of the act. Immanuel Kant (1724–1804) is considered the father of duty-oriented theory. He defined the **categorical imperative** as the guiding principle for all decision making. This principle means that there are no exceptions (categorical) from the rule (imperative). The right action is one based on a determined principle, regardless of outcome. The rule may come from religious or other beliefs, but it is a rule not to be ignored under any circumstances. A priest who maintains the absolute confidentiality of confession even if he knows harm has come to or will come to another human being is an example of using duty-oriented decision making.

categorical imperative A rule that is considered universal law binding on everyone and requiring action.

Kant argued that people may never be used as a means to an end. The Golden Rule ("do unto others as you would have them do unto you") is often cited in support of duty-oriented theory. Duty-oriented theories provide a foundation for rules of morality and for the idea of individual rights. However, critics of Kant find some of his ideas difficult to use in real life. For example, Kant argues that it is not permissible to lie or break a promise in an effort to save a third party from harm. These absolutes may create problems. For example, if a person promises to write a letter of recommendation for someone, but has to stretch the truth in order to write a favorable recommendation, does not writing the letter make the person immoral? A terminally ill patient asks a nurse questions about physician-assisted death and asks that the nurse not say anything to the family about his questions. When the family asks if the patient has asked about euthanasia, should the nurse tell the truth, even if the patient has asked that his questions be kept confidential?

Virtue Ethics

Rather than focusing on decision making or reasoning to arrive at a right action, virtue ethics focuses on the traits, characteristics, and virtues that a moral person should have. Virtue ethicists believe that someone who has appropriate moral virtues such as practical wisdom (common sense), a sense of justice, and courage will make the right decision. Ethicists who support this idea began with Aristole (384 B.C.E.), but Alasdair MacIntrye (1929–present) is the most well known ethicist to write about virtue ethics. MacIntyre argued that our practice of medicine has traditions and standards of practice that apply to every health care practitioner—whether one is a technician, medical assistant, physician, nurse, coder, or other professional. He stated that if we examine our actions in our roles as health care practitioners, we will see that we often follow the dictates of an idealized role. We ask ourselves, What would a perfect medical assistant (or physician or nurse) do in this situation? In virtue ethics, the loyalty to the role we play helps us make our decision. We look to what has been done in the past, assuming that it represents the right answer.

Like the other theories, virtue ethics has its critics. First, the past may not provide the right answer. As an example, the role of nurses or medical assistants even 10 years ago is different than their roles today. Previously, virtues for nurses included always following the physician's orders and never questioning authority. Today, such virtues for nurses have been replaced with playing patient advocacy and education roles. Additionally, there are new situations coming up every day in health care that have never been at issue before, such as the possibility of cloning human organs for transplant, and new medical imaging techniques that utilize the principles of particle physics, so there is no established tradition. Last, practitioners may find themselves with conflicting roles. For example, in the case at the beginning of the chapter, Bill wants to be a team player, but he also may need to report Anna for violation of hospital policy.

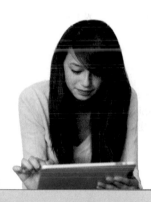

check your **progress**

The following questions involve making a decision. Answer each question with a *yes* or a *no*. Identify whether you arrived at your answer by consequence-oriented, duty-oriented, or virtue ethics.

7. Would it be acceptable to "stretch the truth" on insurance papers so that patients could get the care needed, but could not afford under their current insurance policy?

8. Is it acceptable to date a patient? Does it make a difference if, for example, you are a medical assistant dating a physician?

9. A patient asks about a physician in the community. You think that particular physician is rude and doesn't care about his patients. Should you tell the patient who is asking about the physician what you think?

10. Would a surgical assistant with strong pro-life views be wrong in refusing to take part in a therapeutic abortion for a patient?

11. The radiology technician you work with has just done a chest X-ray on the wrong person. The patient was not hurt. Do you have to report the error to your manager?

12. A pharmacist believes that a prescription for a patient will do little to improve the patient's medical condition and may actually be contraindicated for the patient's problem. Does the pharmacist have a responsibility to talk with the physician?

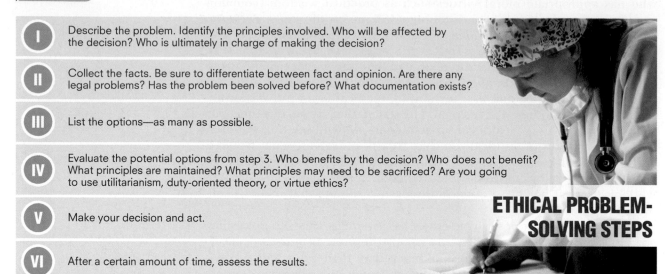

Figure 2-3

I — Describe the problem. Identify the principles involved. Who will be affected by the decision? Who is ultimately in charge of making the decision?

II — Collect the facts. Be sure to differentiate between fact and opinion. Are there any legal problems? Has the problem been solved before? What documentation exists?

III — List the options—as many as possible.

IV — Evaluate the potential options from step 3. Who benefits by the decision? Who does not benefit? What principles are maintained? What principles may need to be sacrificed? Are you going to use utilitarianism, duty-oriented theory, or virtue ethics?

V — Make your decision and act.

VI — After a certain amount of time, assess the results.

ETHICAL PROBLEM-SOLVING STEPS

Making ethical decisions is not easy regardless of what model you choose to use. But whatever ethical framework is used, there are several steps that are common to them all. Figure 2-3 lists six steps to consider.

LO 2.3
Define the basic principles of health care ethics.

The Seven Principles of Health Care Ethics

Several codes of ethics were quoted in Chapter 1. Each code, such as the AAMA Code or the AMA Code, addresses a specific profession, but there are common elements in all health care professional ethics codes. The seven universal principles of health care ethics include the following:

1. Autonomy or Self-Determination

autonomy The capacity to be one's own person and make one's own decisions without being manipulated by external forces.

The word ***autonomy*** comes from the Greek words *auto* (self) and *nomos* (governance). It is generally understood as the capacity to be one's own person, to make decisions based on one's own reasons and motives, not manipulated or dictated to by external forces. Autonomous decisions are characterized by:

- Competency—a person must be competent to make his or her own decision.
- Ability to act on the decision.
- Respect for the autonomy of others.

Chapter 7 discusses informed consent, which derives from the principle of autonomy, as applied to health care. Paternalism, substituting the medical provider's opinion of what is "best" for the patient for the patient's own determination of his or her best interests, often threatens the concept of autonomy in health care. Because patients may disagree with medical providers about what is best, and may not know or understand viable alternatives, informed consent is vital to preserving a health care consumer's autonomy.

Right-to-die cases, as discussed in Chapter 12, deal with a person's autonomy in making critical decisions.

The court case "Physician Charged in Assisted Suicide" is a landmark legal case that dealt with a patient's autonomy, as well as the issues of informed consent and the right to die.

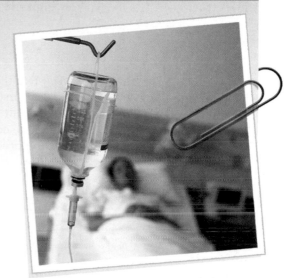
2. Beneficence

Although most dictionaries define **beneficence** as acts of charity and mercy, beneficence means more for the health care provider. Regardless of specialty, health care practitioners perform acts to help people stay healthy or recover from an illness. In fact, their first duty is to promote health for the patient above all other considerations. Modern medicine, however, has given rise to questions about the futility of care when discussing beneficence. For example, is it more beneficial for a patient in his nineties, who is hospitalized after suffering a series of debilitating strokes, to be maintained on a ventilator and drugs during his last days, or to be allowed to die in comfort?

beneficence Acts performed by a health care practitioner to help people stay healthy or recover from illness.

3. Nonmaleficence

Nonmaleficence, as paraphrased from the Hippocratic oath, means the duty to "do no harm." Technology has made this a difficult principle to follow, since many modern-day drugs and treatments have the potential to heal, but also have serious side effects. A common example given when discussing nonmaleficence is the administration of morphine to reduce pain. Morphine is a powerful pain-killer, but it also suppresses respiration. When administering morphine, the provider's intent, of course, is to reduce pain, not to stop the patient's breathing. Accordingly, under the principle of double effect, secondary effects, such as reduced respiration or any other harmful outcome, must never be the intended result of medical treatment. The benefit to the patient must always outweigh the harm.

4. Confidentiality

confidentiality Keeping medical information strictly private.

The Health Information Portability and Accountability Act (HIPAA), discussed in detail in Chapter 8, mandates privacy and **confidentiality** of medical records, but health care practitioners who take care to maintain confidentiality at all times are equally as effective as laws. Health care practitioners mindful of protecting privacy and confidentiality, for example, do not conduct conversations about patients in the hospital hallway, in the medical office break room, or with an acquaintance on the street or in any other public place. They also take care to protect computerized medical information, as detailed in Chapter 7, and when patients ask that information be kept from concerned relatives, such requests are honored.

Health care practitioners are in the most likely position to violate confidentiality rules, but others who have access to protected health care information, as defined under HIPAA, may also violate confidentiality, as in the case "Attorney Guilty of Unauthorized Disclosure."

5. Justice

justice Providing to an individual what is his or her due.

Justice, defined as what is due an individual, seems simple when applied to the U.S. health care system, but it is often complicated. Many would argue, for example, that everyone is entitled to health care, regardless of ability to pay for the care. Others argue that the distribution of scarce resources and the expense of providing them do not allow us to provide all care for all patients. Still others argue that people must take responsibility for their actions before assuming they can have justice. For example, should a lifelong smoker who refuses to quit and develops emphysema and continues to smoke be entitled to all available health care regardless of cost? Should a motorcycle owner who refuses to wear a helmet while riding his or her motorcycle, or an automobile driver who refuses to wear a seatbelt, be entitled to all available health care in the event of an accident, regardless of cost?

Compensatory justice, a concept that applies to medical malpractice lawsuits, refers to an individual's right to seek monetary compensation in the form of damages for a wrong done, and is discussed in more detail in Chapters 5 and 6, respectively. The act of seeking compensatory justice—of suing for damages for medical malpractice—has become an important part of health care today.

Ethics and laws often interconnect, as illustrated in the following Figure 2-4. A third element interconnecting with ethics and the law in health care is risk management—taking steps to minimize danger, hazard,

Attorney Guilty of Unauthorized Disclosure of Medical Information

In January 2003, a man began meeting with a psychiatrist. He confided to his doctor that he was having homicidal thoughts about his wife. The physician determined that his patient had bipolar disorder, and treated him for this condition for the next seven months.

A month into the man's psychiatric treatment, his wife filed for divorce. The man filed a counterclaim, in which he sought legal custody of the couple's minor child. While both the divorce case and the man's psychiatric treatment were ongoing, the man allegedly assaulted his wife at their home, and criminal charges were brought against him. Shortly thereafter, his wife sought and received a civil domestic-violence protection order. The order gave her temporary custody of the couple's child and suspended the man's contact and visitation rights until a full hearing could be held.

In preparation for the hearing, the wife's attorney issued subpoenas to the psychiatrist seeking the production in court of the man's medical records. The attorney mistakenly believed that the man had waived his privilege to his medical records by filing the counterclaim for custody in the divorce action. On the date of the hearing, the wife's attorney met with the prosecutor in the criminal case against the man, and she gave the prosecutor a copy of the man's medical records that she had received from his psychiatrist.

Before the hearing, the man and his wife reached a separation agreement, and the man's medical records were therefore never admitted into evidence in the divorce/protection-order case. Likewise, the man's medical records were not admitted in the criminal matter, and the man was ultimately acquitted.

The man brought an action against his wife's attorney, his ex-wife, his psychiatrist, and his psychiatrist's employer, alleging improper disclosure of his medical records without his authorization. Charges against the defendants were dropped, but a court of appeals eventually held that the ex-wife's attorney "over-stepped her bounds as [the ex-wife's] attorney when she disseminated information regarding the man's psychiatric condition to the prosecution."

The court held that by giving the psychological records she obtained in the divorce case to the prosecutor in the criminal case against Hageman, attorney Belovich violated Hageman's rights to keep that information confidential. Allowing attorneys with such information obtained through discovery to treat the information as public would violate the policy of maintaining the confidentiality of individual medical records. The court therefore recognized that waiver of medical confidentiality for litigation purposes is limited to the specific case for which the records are sought, and that an attorney who violates this limited waiver by disclosing the records to a third party unconnected to the litigation may be held liable for these actions

Source: Hageman v. Southwest General Health Center, 119 Ohio St. 3rd, 185, 893 N.E.2d 153 (2008).

In your opinion, was the psychiatrist in this case also guilty of a breach of confidentiality? Why or why not?

Do you believe the attorney in the above case was also guilty of a breach of ethics in disclosing the health records? Explain your answer.

and liability. Risk management is an important concept in the prevention of medical lawsuits, and is discussed further in Chapter 6.

6. Role Fidelity

All health care practitioners have a specific scope of practice, for which they are licensed, certified, or registered, and from which the law says they

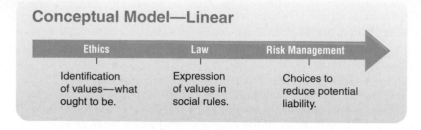

Conceptual Model—Linear

Ethics	Law	Risk Management
Identification of values—what ought to be.	Expression of values in social rules.	Choices to reduce potential liability.

Conceptual Model—Distinctions

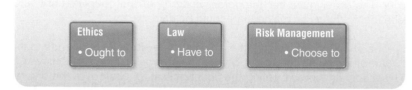

Ethics	Law	Risk Management
• Ought to	• Have to	• Choose to

Conceptual Model—Interconnectedness

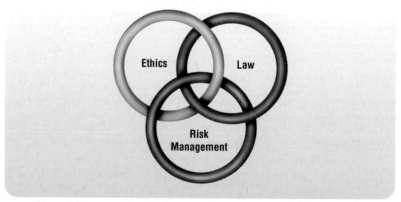

Source: "Law and Medical Ethics," Lisa Vincler, Assistant Attorney General, Washington State, April 11, 2008. **http://depts.washington.edu/bioethx/topics/law. html#ques2**

role fidelity Being faithful to the scope of the services for which you are licensed, certified, or registered.

may not deviate, as discussed in Chapters 3 and 5. In addition to the laws that affect scope of practice, it is a basic ethical principle that a practitioner must be true to (have **fidelity**) to his or her role. For example, a medical assistant should not diagnose a patient's condition, and a nursing assistant should not administer an intravenous drug to a patient, since such acts are not within scope of practice for either profession.

7. Veracity

veracity Truth telling.

Veracity or truth telling has always had an ambiguous place in the health care practitioner's world. Because medical providers want to do what is best for the patient, they may not always tell the whole truth. For example, consider the use of placebos—biologically inert substances that will do no harm, but are sometimes given to patients under the guise of therapeutic treatment. Many studies have proven that if patients believe they are taking a drug that will help them, even if they are taking a placebo, their conditions may improve. In other cases, medical providers take a paternalistic view about truth telling, determining that what the patients don't know won't hurt them.

Health care ethics are drawn from the same pool of basic ethical principles that might be listed for any profession, but the nature of health care provides a unique focus. Primarily because a person's health is paramount to his or her living a successful and satisfying life, health care practitioners are routinely challenged to make sound decisions—concerning not only the appropriate medical care for each patient's condition but also the patient's future health and well-being, and sometimes the health and well-being of the patient's family. In our changing world, the use of technology, scarce resources, and the ever-increasing cost of health care all require that health care practitioners constantly strive to provide the best possible care for patients.

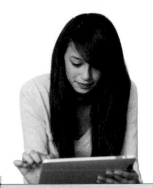

check your **progress**

For each of the following actions, name a principle of health care ethics that was followed or violated, adding whether the principle was followed or violated.

13. A nurse tells a patient faced with the dilemma of deciding for and against debilitating surgery what he thinks is "best" for her.

14. A patient's medical malpractice lawsuit against a physician is dismissed in court because her HMO employer lost the patient's medical records.

15. A physician who knows one of his patients always wants to hear the truth tells him treatment for his cancer has not cured him of the disease, and he has less than a year to live.

16. An 85-year-old woman suffering from congestive heart failure is semiconscious and has been placed on a ventilator. Upon admission to the hospital, she filed a living will with the hospital, detailing her end-of-life requests, and signed a do-not-resuscitate (DNR) order. She is not expected to live beyond a matter of days, but her two daughters arrive from out of state and insist on overriding her DNR request. "Do everything to keep her alive," both daughters insist. The attending physician does not agree with the daughters, but cannot dissuade them and is obligated to comply.

17. A nurse's physician/employer asks her to dress the burn on a patient's hand after debriding the wound. The nurse knows correct procedure for dressing the burn, but she finds gloves uncomfortable and fails to wear them. The patient's burn later becomes infected.

18. A medical assistant believes her mother has a thyroid condition, so she steals samples of the appropriate medication from the clinic where she works and takes them home for her mother.

19. A medical coder who works for a group of physicians knows, through her access to patients' medical records, that Melanie, a single friend, is pregnant. When another friend asks her why Melanie is seeing a doctor, she refuses to admit even that Melanie is a patient of one of her physician/employers.

CHAPTER SUMMARY

LO 2.1 What classic need development theory is discussed in this chapter?

- Abraham Maslow, in *Motivation and Personality* first published in 1954, identified a hierarchy of needs that motivates our actions:

  Deficiency or D-needs:

  1. Need for basic life—food and shelter.
  2. Need for a safe and secure environment
  3. Need to belong and to be loved.

  Being or B-needs:

  4. Need for esteem, where status, responsibility, and recognition are important.
  5. Need for self-actualization, for personal growth and fulfillment.

LO 2.1 What two value development theories are discussed in this chapter?

- Jean Piaget's moral development stages:
  - Sensorimotor stage, during which the child is totally self-centered—birth to age 2.
  - Preoperational or egocentric stage, during which children view the world from their own perspective—ages 2 to 7.
  - Concrete operational stage, when children see things as right or wrong and adults as all powerful—ages 7 to 12.
  - Formal operational state, during which children practice more abstract thinking and learn there may be different degrees of wrongdoing—age 12, often extending into adulthood.

- Lawrence Kohlberg's moral development stages:
  - Pre-conventional morality—children ages 2 to 7 accept others' authority; at end of stage, recognize their own interests.
  - Conventional morality—children ages 7 to 12 conform to others' expectations to win approval; at end of stage, focus on rules and respect for authority.
  - Post-conventional morality (ages 12 and above).
    a. Social contract and individual rights are balanced.
    b. Universal principles—personal commitment to larger issues of society.

LO 2.2 What is consequence-oriented ethics reasoning?

- Best known is utilitarianism—judge the rightness of a decision based on the outcome or predicted outcome.
  - Act-utilitarianism—person makes value decisions based on results that will produce the greatest balance of good over evil.

- Rule-utilitarianism—person makes value decisions based on a rule that should produce greatest balance of good over evil.

LO 2.2 What is the principle of utility?

- Requires that the rule used to make a decision bring about positive results when generalized to a wide variety of situations.

LO 2.2 What is duty-oriented ethics reasoning?

- Focuses on the essential rightness or wrongness of an act, not the consequences of the act.
- The right action is one based on a determined principle, regardless of outcome.

LO 2.2 What is virtue ethics reasoning?

- People who have appropriate moral **virtues** will make the right decisions

> **virtue ethics**   Refers to the theory that people who have moral virtues will make the right decisions.

LO 2.2 What ethical problem-solving steps are discussed in this chapter?

- Describe the problem and identify the principles involved.
- Collect the facts, differentiating between fact and opinion.
- List as many options as possible.
- Evaluate the potential options.
- Make your decision and act.
- After a certain amount of time, assess the results.

LO 2.3 What are the basic principles of health care ethics?

- Autonomy or self-determination
- Beneficence
- **Nonmaleficence**
- Confidentiality
- Justice
- Role fidelity
- Veracity

> **nonmaleficence**   The duty to do no harm.

ETHICS ISSUES Making Ethical Decisions

Ethics ISSUE 1: Joyce Weathers is a 62-year-old patient with emphysema. Mrs. Weathers is a grandmother who has smoked a pack of cigarettes a day for over 40 years. She enjoys smoking and does not want to quit. Her physician has become somewhat insistent that Mrs. Weathers quit. She tries, but each time she becomes nasty and irritable around her family. She lives with her daughter and two young grandchildren. The family members want her to quit, but it becomes very unpleasant at home when Mrs. Weathers tries to quit.

Discussion Questions

1. Using act-utilitarianism as a model, create a pain-avoided, pleasure-gained list to determine if Mrs. Weathers should continue smoking.

_____

_____

2. If your decision is that she should quit smoking, how can Mrs. Weathers's family help her?

_____

_____

Ethics ISSUE 2: An eight-year-old girl is suffering from a rare form of cancer and is in need of a bone marrow transplant. Despite searches for the past year, no donor match has been located. The parents decide to have another child, hoping that the younger child will be a blood marrow match for their eight-year-old. The baby will be born in the next three months.

Discussion Question

1. Compare consequence-oriented decision making and duty-oriented decision making in this case. In your opinion, which method of decision making will lead to the best decision for everyone concerned, or are the methods equal in that both will lead to the optimum decision?

_____

_____

Ethics ISSUE 3: Martha is the administrative assistant to Valerie, the practice manager in a five-physician practice. Salaries of staff are confidential. Since payroll is handled by an outside company, only the practice manager has knowledge of who makes what salary. Valerie has gone to lunch and left her door open. Several people have been in and out of Valerie's office dropping off reports or other information. Martha goes in the office to place a report on Valerie's desk and notices that a budget worksheet, listing all staff salaries, is in clear view. It would be easy to take a quick look, especially since Martha believes she is paid less than other employees with fewer responsibilities. Martha backs out of the office and locks Valerie's door without looking at the sheet. She thinks to herself, If I should not know what everyone else is being paid, then no one else should either.

Curtis is one of the employees who had left information on Valerie's desk before Martha closed the door. He also sees the budget sheet, but does not stop to look at it. It did not occur to him to look at it, although it would have been great to know that he was being paid more than other employees. He puts his file down on Valerie's desk and thinks to himself, I will warn Valerie that she needs to be more careful about what she leaves on her desk for anyone to see.

Discussion Question

1. According to virtue ethics, who is more ethical—Martha, the one tempted to look but doesn't, or Curtis, who isn't even tempted to look? Defend your answer.

_____

_____

Go to **www.mhhe.com/judson6e** to practice your case review skills. Then read on for more information.

KEY TERMS

autonomy

beneficence

categorical imperative

confidentiality

deontological or duty-
oriented theory

justice

needs-based
motivation

nonmaleficence

principle of utility

role fidelity

teleological or
consequence-
oriented theory

utilitarianism

veracity

virtue ethics

CHAPTER 2 REVIEW

Applying Knowledge

Circle the correct answer for each of the following questions.

LO 2.1

1. What is another term for your personal concept of right and wrong?
   a. Utilitarianism
   b. Beneficence
   c. Moral values
   d. Role fidelity

2. Why did Tom and Bill in this chapter's opening scenario come to different decisions?
   a. Because of their age differences
   b. Because of differences in their societal, cultural, and family influences
   c. Because of their different relationships with their supervisor
   d. None of the above

3. How is Abraham Maslow's theory of needs-based motivation best defined?
   a. It is a five-step progression that sees pleasure as the primary motivation for all human behavior.
   b. It is a progression called beneficence.
   c. It is a theory that says human behavior is based on specific human needs that must often be met in a specific order.
   d. It is a system of moral values.

4. Which of the following is *not* true of Jean Piaget's theory of value development?
   a. Children in the sensorimotor stage of development see things as right or wrong.
   b. During the sensorimotor stage of development, children explore the world with their five senses.
   c. Children in the concrete operational stage of development see things as right or wrong.
   d. Children begin to see different degrees of wrong doing during the post-conventional stage.

5. How does Lawrence Kohlberg's theory of moral reasoning differ from Piaget's theory?
   a. Kohlberg theorized that moral development occurs more gradually and takes longer than Piaget proposed.
   b. Kohlberg studied adults instead of children.
   c. Kohlberg studied both boys and girls whereas Piaget did not.
   d. Kohlberg does not break down moral development into stages whereas Piaget did.

6. Which of the following is *not* true of Piaget's stages of value development?
   a. During the sensorimotor stage of development, children use their five senses to explore the world.
   b. The preoperational stage of development is characterized by abstract reasoning.
   c. During the concrete operational stage of development, children see certain behaviors as right or wrong.
   d. None of the above are true of Piaget's theory.

7. Which of the following is true of Lawrence Kohlberg's theory of the development of moral reasoning?
   a. During the pre-conventional morality stage, children reject the authority of others.
   b. A social contract is formed during the post-conventional morality stage.
   c. Children become rebellious during the conventional morality stage.
   d. None of the above are true of Kohlberg's theory of moral reasoning.

LO 2.2

8. Teleological or consequence-oriented theories judge the rightness of a decision based on
   a. The feelings of the person making the decision
   b. The opinions of others who see the results of the decision
   c. How many people agree that the decision was right
   d. The outcome or predicted outcome of the decision

9. Which of the following best defines utilitarianism?
   a. It is the same as pre-conventional morality.
   b. It is a consequence-oriented theory that states that decisions should be made by determining what results will produce the best outcome for the most people.
   c. It is a duty-oriented theory that says everyone has a duty to behave correctly.
   d. It is a consequence-oriented theory that states that each individual should make decisions based on which outcome is best for him or her.

10. Which of the following best defines duty-oriented moral reasoning?
    a. Each individual's duty is to himself or herself first.
    b. Everyone should reject the authority of others and rely solely on self.
    c. It is a decision-making theory that states that the rightness or wrongness of the act depends on its intrinsic nature and not the outcome of the act.
    d. It is a form of post-conventional morality.

11. Immanuel Kant's categorical imperative states that
    a. Every rule has exceptions
    b. Only the outcome is important in decision making
    c. Feelings are not important in decision making
    d. The right action is one based on a determined principle, regardless of outcome

12. Virtue ethics focuses on
    a. The traits, characteristics, and virtues that a moral person should have
    b. The method one uses to make a moral decision
    c. Only the outcome of one's decisions
    d. The rule one uses in making a moral decision

13. Alasdair MacIntrye argues that
    a. All health care practitioners practice duty-oriented ethics reasoning
    b. Virtue ethics is the only theory that makes sense
    c. Individuals who have certain desirable qualities will make the right decisions
    d. None of the above

Answer the following questions in the spaces provided.

LO 2.3

14.–20. List and define the seven basic principles of health care ethics.

_____

_____

CASE STUDIES

Use your critical thinking skills to answer the questions that follow each case study.

LO 2.3

Susan is a nursing student, arguing with her friend Linda, also a nursing student, over the benefits of getting a flu shot.

"I'm not getting a flu shot this year," Linda declares. "I paid $14 for one last year, and I still got sick. I had a horrible sinus infection that kept me out of school for days."

"I remember, but that wasn't the flu," Susan argues. "Since we see so many people in the clinic—especially older people with weakened immune systems—don't you think we, of all people, should be immunized against the flu?"

The argument continues at length, with Linda finally raising her voice and stomping off.

21. In your opinion, is the question of whether or not the nursing students should get a flu vaccine an ethical question? Explain your answer.

_____

_____

22. If you decide that this is an ethical question, which theory of moral reasoning best applies?

_____

_____

Ethan is an orderly in a skilled nursing care facility. He is charged with supervising patients in the dining room on a day when two of his coworkers have called in sick, leaving the facility shorthanded. On this day several patients seem more irritable than usual, and Ethan is kept busy preventing outbursts and calming them. He also worries about patients prone to choking episodes, and finds himself feeling harried and stressed.

Wallace, an 80-year-old confined to a wheelchair, demands that Ethan help him back to his room. "It's a madhouse in here today," he shouts. Ethan knows he cannot leave his post, and panics when Wallace heads for the door.

Ethan runs ahead of Wallace, shuts the double doors to the dining room, and locks them.

23. Has Ethan acted ethically? Explain your answer.

_____

_____

24. What would you do in a similar situation? Use steps one through five for ethical decision making to reach a solution. Describe how each step was used.

_____

_____

25. Do you believe your solution is more ethical than Ethan's? Why or why not?

_____

_____

Complete the activities and answer the questions that follow.

26. Locate the Web site for the organization representing the profession you plan to practice. Check the organization's code of ethics. Does the code conform to the seven principles of health care ethics? Explain your answer.

_____

_____

27. Visit the Web site for the National Center for Ethics in Health Care at **www.ethics.va.gov/resources/ethicsresources.asp.** Under the list of resource links, click on "Professionalism in Patient Care." What topics are listed under this link? How might these resources prove useful to you?

_____

_____

28. Visit Santa Clara University's Web site: **www.scu.edu/ethics/practicing/ decision/framework.html.** List three things that, according to the site, ethics are _not_. Do you agree? Explain your answer. (If this URL is no longer available, do a Web search for "framework for thinking ethically." What was the number one result for this search, and how might you make use of the source?)

_____

_____

[**RESOURCES**]

Edge, R., and J. Groves. _Ethics of Health Care: A Guide for Clinical Practice._ 3rd ed. New York: Thomson Delmar Learning, 2006.

Kohlberg, L. _The psychology of Moral Development: Essays on Moral Development._ Vol. 2. San Francisco: Harper and Row, 1984.

Kohlberg, L., and R. A. Ryncarz. "Beyond Justice Reasoning: Moral Development and Consideration of a Seventh Stage." In _Higher Stages of Human Development: Perspectives on Adult Growth,_ ed. C. N. Alexander and E. J. Langer. New York: Oxford University Press, 1990.

MacIntyre, Alasdair. *After Virtue*. Notre Dame: University of Indiana Press, 1984.

"Making Ethical Decisions," Arizona Character Education Foundation Web site: **www.azcharacteredfoundation.org/ethical.html.**

Mappes, T., and D. Degrazia. *Biomedical Ethics*. 6th ed. Boston: McGraw-Hill, 2006.

Power, F. C., A. Higgins, and L. Kohlberg. *Lawrence Kohlberg's Approach to Moral Education*. New York: Columbia University Press, 1989.

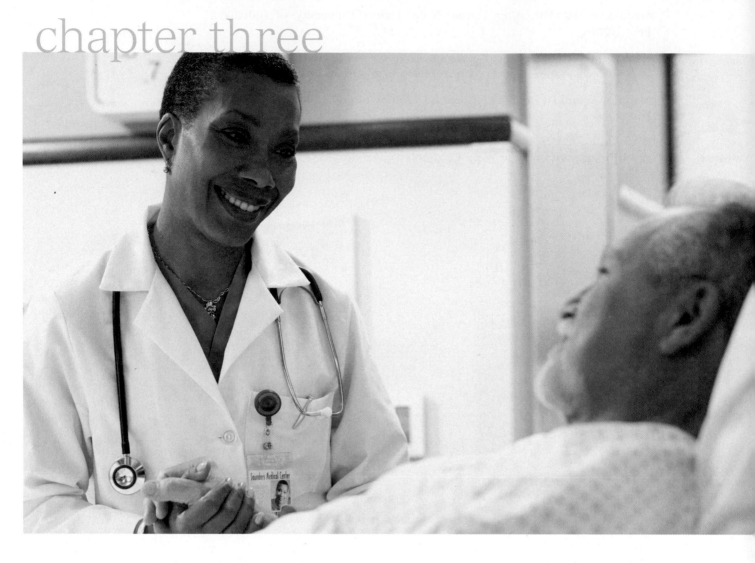

WORKING IN HEALTH CARE

Learning Outcomes

After studying this chapter, you should be able to:

LO 3.1 Define *licensure, certification, registration,* and *accreditation.*

LO 3.2 Demonstrate an understanding of how physicians are licensed, how physicians are regulated, and the purpose of a medical board.

LO 3.3 Discuss the composition of the health care team and the roles of its members.

LO 3.4 Define the major types of medical practice management systems.

LO 3.5 Define the different types of managed care health plans.

LO 3.6 Discuss the federal legislation that impacts health care reimbursement and prohibits fraud and abuse in health care billing.

LO 3.7 Define *telemedicine, cybermedicine,* and *e-health,* and discuss their roles in today's health care environment.

MELODY, A CERTIFIED NURSING ASSISTANT (CNA), works in a skilled nursing care facility caring for elderly patients. "I like the hands-on care," she says, "and I love just visiting with my patients. They come from all walks of life, and some of them have traveled all over the world."

The part of her job she dislikes the most, Melody adds, "is the demanding patients, who want everything right now. Demanding relatives can also be unreasonable. A daughter will tell me, 'I want you to respond immediately whenever my mother calls for you.' They don't understand, or don't care, that I have several patients to look after."

Once, Melody recalls, several family members were visiting their elderly relative. "I walked in to check my patient, and one of his granddaughters asked me to get her a soda. There was a vending machine in the visitors' lounge, and I debated telling the woman I'm not a waitress, and she could get her own drink. I didn't, though. I got her the drink, but I resented being asked to do it. I'm just a CNA, but I'm not there to wait on patients' relatives."

From Melody's perspective, her job did not include providing refreshments for patients' visitors. What does her remark that she is "just a CNA" reveal about Melody's attitude concerning her work?

From the demanding visitor's perspective, perhaps Melody's job is to serve all needs of anyone in the patient's room. In your opinion, would Melody's registered nurse (RN) supervisor have expected her to fulfill the visitor's request for a soda? Why or why not?

How should Melody respond to patients and their visitors who seem unreasonably demanding?

Licensure, Certification, Registration, and Accreditation

LO 3.1
Define *licensure, certification, registration,* and *accreditation.*

With increased medical specialization have come more exacting professional requirements for health care practitioners. Members of the health care team today are usually licensed, registered, or certified to perform specific duties, depending on job classification and state requirements. Furthermore, programs for educating health care practitioners are often accredited. Accreditation is a process education programs may complete that ensures certain standards have been met. Managed care plans may also earn accreditation or certification for excellence.

Licensure is a mandatory credentialing process established by law, usually at the state level. Licenses to practice are required in every state for all physicians and nurses and for many other health care practitioners as well. Individuals who do not have the required license are prohibited by law from practicing certain health care professions.

Certification is a voluntary credentialing process, usually national in scope, and is most often sponsored by a nongovernmental, private-sector group. Certification by a professional organization, usually through an examination, signifies that an applicant has attained a certain level of knowledge and skill. Since the process is voluntary, lack of certification does not prevent an employee from practicing the profession for which he

licensure A mandatory credentialing process established by law, usually at the state level, that grants the right to practice certain skills and endeavors.

certification A voluntary credentialing process whereby applicants who meet specific requirements may receive a certificate.

or she is otherwise qualified. (In the opening scenario, Melody has chosen to fulfill requirements to become a *certified* nursing assistant. In her state she could begin working as a nursing assistant without certification, but at a lower hourly wage.)

registration A credentialing procedure whereby one's name is listed on a register as having paid a fee and/or met certain criteria within a profession.

Registration is an entry in an official registry or record, listing the names of persons in a certain occupation who have satisfied specific requirements. The list is usually made available to health care providers. One way to become registered is simply to add one's name to the list in the registry. Under this method of registration, unregistered persons are not prevented from working in a field for which they are otherwise qualified.

A second way to become registered in a health occupation is to attain a certain level of education and/or pay a registration fee. Under this second method, when there are specific requirements for registration, unregistered individuals may be prevented from working in a field for which they are otherwise qualified.

Under no circumstances may persons claim to be licensed, certified, or registered if they are not.

accreditation Official authorization or approval for conforming to a specified standard.

Accreditation is the process by which health care practitioner education programs, health care facilities, and managed care plans are officially authorized. Two examples of accrediting agencies for health care practitioner education programs are the Commission on Accreditation of Allied Health Education Programs (CAAHEP), discussed in more detail later in the chapter, and the Accrediting Bureau of Health Education Schools (ABHES). Accreditation is usually voluntary, but accredited programs for various disciplines must maintain certain standards to earn and keep accreditation. Most accredited programs for health care education also include an internship or externship (practical work experience) that lasts for a specified period of time.

The Joint Commission (TJC; formerly the Joint Commission on Accreditation of Healthcare Organizations [JCAHO]) accredits health care organizations that meet certain standards. As of 2010, the Joint Commission evaluated and accredited over 17,000 health care organizations and programs in the United States, including the following:

- General, psychiatric, children's, and rehabilitation hospitals.
- Critical access hospitals.
- Health care networks, including health maintenance organizations (HMOs), preferred provider organizations (PPOs), integrated delivery networks, and managed behavioral health care organizations.
- Home care organizations, including those that provide home health services, personal care and support services, home infusion and other pharmacy services, durable medical equipment services, and hospice services.
- Nursing homes and other long-term care facilities, including subacute care programs, dementia special care programs, and long-term care pharmacies.
- Assisted living facilities.
- Behavioral health care organizations.
- Ambulatory care providers, such as outpatient surgery facilities, rehabilitation centers, infusion centers, and group practices, as well as office-based surgery.
- Clinical laboratories, including independent or freestanding laboratories, blood transfusion and donor centers, and public health laboratories.

To earn and maintain TJC accreditation, an organization must undergo an on-site survey by a TJC survey team at least every three years. Laboratories must be surveyed every two years.

A recognized accrediting agency for managed care plans is the National Committee for Quality Assurance (NCQA), an independent, nonprofit organization that evaluates and reports on the quality of the nation's managed care organizations. NCQA evaluates managed care programs in three ways:

1. Through on-site reviews of key clinical and administrative processes.

2. Through the Healthcare Effectiveness Data and Information Set (HEDIS)—data used to measure performance in areas such as immunization and mammography screening rates.

3. Through use of member satisfaction surveys.

Participation in NCQA accreditation and certification programs is voluntary. The organization reported in 2011 that it now evaluates all types of health plans, and "today, more than 100 million Americans, or 70.5% of all health plan members are covered by an NCQA-Accredited health plan."

reciprocity The process by which a professional license obtained in one state may be accepted as valid in other states by prior agreement without reexamination.

Reciprocity

For those professions that require a state license, such as physician, registered nurse, or licensed practical or vocational nurse, **reciprocity** may be granted. This means that a state licensing authority will accept a person's valid license from another state as proof of competency without requiring reexamination.

If a state license is required and reciprocity is not granted when moving to another state, then the health care practitioner must apply to the state licensing authority to take required examinations to obtain a valid license to practice in the new state.

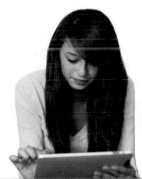

check your **progress**

1. Define *registration*.

_____

_____

2. Define *licensure*.

_____

_____

3. Define *certification*.

_____

_____

4. Define *accreditation*.

_____

_____

5. Define *reciprocity*.

_____

_____

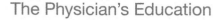

LO 3.2

Demonstrate an understanding of how physicians are licensed, how physicians are regulated, and the purpose of a medical board.

Physicians' Education and Licensing and Medical Practice Acts and Medical Boards

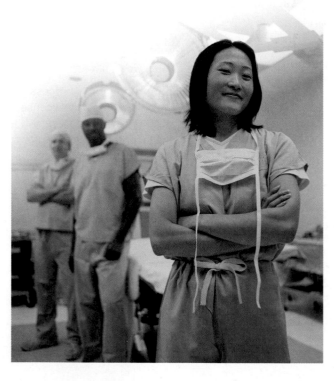

The Physician's Education

Doctor of Medicine (MD) Degree Before a person can be licensed to practice medicine, he or she must complete a rigorous course of study. Programs leading to the doctor of medicine (MD) degree consist of

- Graduation with a bachelor's degree from a four-year, premedicine course, usually with a concentration in the sciences.

- Graduation from a four-year medical school—in the United States, a school accredited by the Liaison Committee on Medical Education. Upon graduation from medical school, students are awarded the doctor of medicine (MD) degree.

After earning the MD degree, the prospective physician must then pass the United States Medical Licensing Examination (USMLE), commonly called "medical boards." Student physicians take Part 1 of the exam after the first year of medical school. They take Part 2 of the exam during the fourth year of medical school, and Part 3 during the first or second year of postgraduate medical training.

The next step in a physician's education is completion of a residency: a period of practical postgraduate training in a hospital. The first year of residency is called an internship.

After completion of the internship and passing the medical boards, the National Board of Medical Examiners (NBME) certifies the physician as an NBME Diplomate.

To specialize, physicians must complete an additional two to six years of residency in the chosen specialty. When the residency is completed, specialists can then apply to the American Board of Medical Specialties (ABMS) to take an exam in their specialty. After passing this exam, physicians are board-certified in their area of specialization. For example, a specialist in oncology becomes a board-certified oncologist, and so on.

Doctor of Osteopathy (DO) Degree All 50 states also license physicians who have obtained a doctor of osteopathy (DO) degree from an accredited medical school, have successfully completed a licensing examination governed by the National Board of Osteopathic Medical Examiners, and have successfully completed the required internship and residency.

MDs and DOs spend 12 years or more training to become physicians. Both medical and osteopathic physicians prescribe drugs and practice surgery. The difference between the two is in their approach to medical treatment. Osteopathic doctors are trained to emphasize the musculoskeletal system of the body and the correction of joint and tissue problems. Medical doctors are trained in **allopathic** medicine which means, literally, "different suffering" and emphasizes intervention in the form of drugs and/or surgery to alleviate symptoms.

Osteopathic and medical doctors can practice as generalists or primary care physicians—a designation that includes primary care specialties in

allopathic Means "different suffering" and refers to the medical philosophy that dictates training physicians to intervene in the disease process, through the use of drugs and surgery.

family medicine/general practice, general internal medicine, and general pediatrics—or they can specialize in a specific type of medicine, such as obstetrics/gynecology, oncology, geriatrics, surgery, orthopedics, or a host of other specialties. Medical and osteopathic physicians may also further specialize in subspecialties, such as abnormalities of the hand within orthopedics, or diseases of the gastrointestinal system within internal medicine.

Recent U.S. government statistics show that in the United States, medical students are three times more likely to specialize than to remain generalists or primary care physicians. This has led to a ratio in the United States of 37.4 percent primary care physicians to 62.6 percent specialists. According to the American Medical Student Association (AMSA), reasons for the preference among medical students to specialize include these:

- Higher financial compensation for specialists (studies have found that a surgeon can earn up to seven times more than a primary care physician, per time spent with the patient).

- Decreased prestige for generalists.

- Medical training most often provided in **tertiary care settings**—those providing highly specialized services.

- Decreased exposure to generalist role models.

- Lack of attractiveness of general practices in, for example, rural and underserved areas because of relative isolation from technology and peer support.

A person educated in a foreign medical school who wants to practice in the United States must serve a residency and must take the Clinical Skills Assessment Exam (CSAE) before being licensed. The CSAE evaluates a candidate's ability to use the English language, to take medical histories, and to interact with patients and treat a case.

The Physician's License and Responsibilities

After physicians have finished their education and obtained licenses to practice medicine, their continued licensure falls under the jurisdiction of state medical boards (see Figure 3-1). Each state's medical board has the authority to grant or to revoke a physician's license. The federal government has no medical licensing authority except for the permit issued by the Drug Enforcement Administration (DEA) for any physician who dispenses, prescribes, or administers controlled substances, including narcotics and non-narcotics (see Chapter 9).

When these conditions are satisfied and a license is granted, the physician who moves out of the licensing state may obtain a license in his or her new state of residence by

- *Reciprocity*—the process by which a valid license from out of state is accepted as the basis for issuing a license in a second state if prior agreement to grant reciprocity has been reached between those states.

- *Endorsement*—the process by which a license may be awarded based on individual credentials judged to meet licensing requirements in the new state of residence.

In some situations, physicians do not need a valid license to practice medicine in a specific state. These situations include the following:

- When responding to emergencies.

- While establishing state residency requirements in order to obtain a license.

tertiary care settings
Those care settings providing highly specialized services.

endorsement The process by which a license may be awarded based on individual credentials judged to meet licensing requirements in a new state.

Figure 3-1

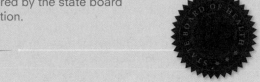

CRITERIA FOR STATE LICENSING OF PHYSICIANS

*The following criteria must be met before
a physician can be granted a state license to practice medicine. He or she*

- Must have reached the age of majority, generally 21.
- Must be of good moral character.
- Must have completed required preliminary education, including graduation from an approved medical school.
- Must have completed an approved residency program.
- Must be a U.S. citizen or have filed a declaration of intent to become a citizen. (Some states have dropped this requirement.)
- Must be a state resident.
- Must have passed all examinations administered by the state board of medical examiners or the board of registration.

- When employed by the U.S. armed forces, Public Health Service, Veterans Administration, or other federal facility.
- When engaged solely in research and not treating patients.

Physicians may be licensed in more than one state. Periodic license renewal is necessary; this usually requires simply paying a fee. However, many states require proof of continuing education units for license renewal; the average is 50 hours annually.

License Revocation or Suspension A physician's license can be revoked (canceled) or suspended (temporarily recalled) for conviction of a felony, unprofessional conduct, or personal or professional incapacity.

A felony is a crime that is punishable by death or a year or more in prison. Conviction of a felony is grounds for revocation or suspension of the license to practice medicine. Felonies include such crimes as murder, rape, larceny, manslaughter, robbery, arson, burglary, violations of narcotic laws, and tax evasion.

Unprofessional conduct is also cause for revoking or suspending a physician's license. Some states substitute the term *gross immorality* for *unprofessional conduct,* but offenses in either category are considered serious breaches of ethics and may also be illegal. Conduct deemed unprofessional includes falsifying records, using unprofessional methods to treat a disease, betrayal of patient confidentiality, fee splitting, and sexual misconduct.

Personal or professional incapacity may be due to senility, injury, illness, chronic alcoholism, drug abuse, or other conditions that impair a physician's ability to practice.

In all 50 states, **medical practice acts** have been established by statute to govern the practice of medicine. Primary mandates of medical practice acts are to

1. Define what is meant by "practice of medicine" in each state.

2. Explain requirements and methods for licensure.

3. Provide for the establishment of medical licensing boards.

4. Establish grounds for suspension or revocation of license.

5. Give conditions for license renewal.

Medical practice acts were first passed in colonial times, but were repealed in the 1800s, when citizens decided that the U.S. Constitution gave anyone the right to practice medicine. Quackery became rampant, and for the protection of the public, medical practice acts were reenacted.

Although laws are in place to protect consumers against medical quackery, even today unscrupulous people attempt to circumvent the law by hawking devices, potions, and treatments they say are "guaranteed" to cure any ailment or infirmity. Each state periodically revises its medical practice acts to keep them current with the times. Medical practice acts can be found in the code of each state, which consists of laws for that state. A copy of the state code is available in most public libraries, in some university libraries, and, in some cases, on the Internet.

Each state's medical practice acts also mandate the establishment of **medical boards,** whose purpose is to protect the health, safety, and welfare of health care consumers through proper licensing and regulation of physicians and, in some jurisdictions, other health care practitioners. Board membership is composed of physicians and others who are, in most cases, appointed by the state's governor. Some boards act independently, exercising all licensing and disciplinary powers, while others are part of larger agencies such as departments of health. Funding for state medical boards comes from licensing and registration fees. Most boards include an executive officer, attorneys, and investigators. Some legal services may be provided by the state's office of the attorney general.

Through licensing, each state medical board ensures that all health care practitioners who work in areas for which licensing is required have adequate and appropriate education and training and that they follow high standards of professional conduct while caring for patients. Applicants for license must generally

- Provide proof of education and training.

- Provide details about work history.

- Pass an examination designed to assess their knowledge and their ability to apply that knowledge and other concepts and principles important to ensure safe and effective patient care.

- Reveal information about past medical history (including alcohol and drug abuse), arrests, and convictions.

Each state's medical practice acts also define unprofessional conduct for medical professionals. Laws vary from state to state, but examples of unprofessional conduct include

- Physical abuse of a patient.

- Inadequate record keeping.

- Failure to recognize or act on common symptoms.

- The prescription of drugs in excessive amounts or without legitimate reason.

medical practice acts
State laws written for the express purpose of governing the practice of medicine.

medical boards Bodies established by the authority of each state's medical practice acts for the purpose of protecting the health, safety, and welfare of health care consumers through proper licensing and regulation of physicians and other health care practitioners.

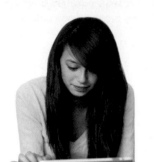

- Impaired ability to practice due to addiction or physical or mental illness.
- Failure to meet continuing education requirements.
- The performance of duties beyond the scope of a license.
- Dishonesty.
- Conviction of a felony.
- The delegation of the practice of medicine to an unlicensed individual.

Minor disagreements and poor customer service do not fall under the heading of misconduct.

check your **progress**

6. Define *medical practice acts*.

_____

7. Where can you find the medical practice acts for your state?

_____

8. What is the primary responsibility of state medical boards?

_____

COURT CASE

Physician Disciplined by Board of Medical Examiners

A licensed pharmacist and a state pharmacy board investigator called a state's Board of Medical Examiners to express concern about a physician's prescription practices. The board investigated and found the physician had deviated from accepted standard of care by

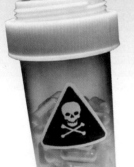

- ‣ Inadequately evaluating patients before prescribing antidepressants and failing to document reasons for prescriptions or following up on patients' use of the prescribed medications.

- ‣ Prescribing antibiotics for prolonged periods as treatment for urinary tract infections without determining that the infections had recurred or documenting the recurrence of the infections. The physician had also prescribed several antibiotics to a patient at once, allowing the patient to choose which antibiotic was the most effective.

- ‣ Prescribing narcotic and anxiolytic medications (drugs that relieve anxiety) to patients with nonterminal chronic pain without adequately pursuing and documenting use of available alternatives to narcotics and controlled medications.

Based on the above findings, the Board of Medical Examiners placed the physician on probation for two years and ordered him to secure 60 hours of continuing education in the treatment of urinary tract infections, medical treatment of the elderly, management of chronic pain patients, and record keeping. He was also ordered to make prescription records available at all times for board inspection and was directed to stop making telephone refills for prescriptions of controlled medications.

Source: Miller v. Board of Medical Examiners, 609 N.W.2d 478, 2000 Iowa Sup.

In 1995 an Ohio appellate court ruled that the state medical board had the authority to revoke a physician's license permanently.

The physician was convicted on two felony counts of theft. Afterward, the state medical board held a hearing and revoked the physician's license. The physician appealed, and a court affirmed.

On further appeal, the case was remanded to the board for further consideration. The board again voted to revoke the physician's license and this time specifically noted that the revocation was permanent. The physician again appealed. The trial court reversed, ruling that the board did not have the statutory authority to revoke the physician's license permanently.

The appellate court overturned the trial court's decision. It held that the board's authority to revoke a license to practice medicine included the authority to revoke such a license permanently.

Source: Roy v. Ohio State Medical Board, 101 Ohio App. 3d 352, 655 N.E.2d 771 Ohio App.Dist. 10, 1995.

State Board of Medical Examiners

Be it known that

Roy, M.D.

License to Practice Medicine Revoked

In Testimony Thereof this license No.0124586 is granted and the seal of the Board of Examiners, the signatures of the President and Secretary-Treasurer thereof are here unto affixed at Denver, Ohio, this 26th day of june A.D. 1995.

Attest:

Secretary-Treasurer

President

The court case "Board Upheld in Permanently Revoking" established legal precedent for a state medical board's authority to *permanently* revoke a physician's license to practice medicine. It continues to be cited as precedent in cases where a state medical board *permanently* revokes a physician's license and the physician appeals the board's decision.

The Health Care Team

Today a growing number of specialized medical practitioners work with physicians as part of the health care team. Nonphysician members of the health care team, called allied health care practitioners, have certain professional characteristics in common. They

- Share responsibility for delivery of health services.
- Generally have received a certificate, associate's degree, bachelor's degree, master's degree, doctoral degree, or postbaccalaureate training in a science related to health care and have met all state requirements concerning licensure, certification, and registration.

Table 3-1 lists various licensed, certified, and registered health care practitioners who work with physicians, dentists, and/or other professionals in providing services to patients in medical offices, dental offices, hospitals, clinics, hospices, extended-care facilities, community programs, schools, and other health care settings. A brief description of each profession is given. When both technicians and technologists are included in the description of a profession, technologists perform duties at a higher level of expertise than technicians. They have either taken a more extensive course of study

LO 3.3

Discuss the composition of the health care team and the roles of its members.

ALLIED HEALTH EDUCATION PROGRAMS

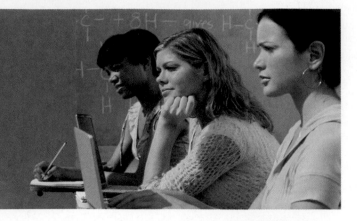

Table 3-1

*Anesthesiologist Assistant. The anesthesiologist assistant assists the anesthesiologist in developing and implementing an anesthesia care plan. Duties can include preoperative and postoperative tasks, as well as operating room assistance.

Athletic Trainer. The athletic trainer works with attending and/or consulting physicians as an integral part of the health care team associated with physical training and sports.

Audiologist. Audiologists are educated in the science of hearing and are qualified to test patients' hearing and to prescribe some types of therapy for hearing problems. Positions require a minimum of a master's degree, plus national certification and state licensing. In 2007, education requirements were moving toward a minimum of a doctorate in audiology (AuD).

*Cardiovascular Technologist. The cardiovascular technologist works under the supervision of physicians to perform diagnostic and therapeutic examinations in the cardiology (heart) and vascular (circulation) areas.

*Cytotechnologist. Cytology is the study of the structure and function of cells. Cytotechnologists work with pathologists to microscopically examine body cells to detect changes that may help diagnose cancer and other diseases.

Dental Hygienist. Dental hygienists perform clinical and educational duties related to hygiene of the mouth and teeth, usually for dentists within a dental office. They may work for one dentist or dental clinic or for several dentists at varying locations.

*Diagnostic Medical Sonographer. The diagnostic medical sonographer administers ultrasound examinations under the supervision of a physician responsible for the use and interpretation of ultrasound procedures.

Dietician and Nutritionist. These specialists work closely with physicians and other medical practitioners to educate and assist patients with special dietary and nutritional needs.

ECG Technician. Electric activity of the heart is measured and recorded by electrocardiographic equipment operated by ECG (electrocardiogram) technicians under the supervision of physicians.

EEG Technician and Technologist. Electroencephalography is the recording and study of the electrical activity of the brain. EEG (electroencephalogram) technicians and technologists work under the supervision of physicians to operate EEG equipment used to perform patient diagnostic tests.

*Electroneurodiagnostic Technologist. Electroneurodiagnostic technology involves the study and recording of the electrical activity of the brain and nervous system. Electroneurodiagnostic technologists work in collaboration with EEG technicians and technologists.

*Emergency Medical Technician (Paramedic). Emergency medical technicians (EMTs), or paramedics, most often work from an ambulance or in a hospital emergency room, providing life-support care to critically ill and injured patients.

Professions marked with an asterisk are currently included in the list of CAAHEP-accredited programs.

*Exercise Physiologist. The exercise physiologist is a professional competent in graded exercise testing, exercise prescription, exercise leadership, emergency procedures, and health education for patients with cardiovascular, pulmonary, and metabolic diseases, as well as other diseases and disabilities. These positions require a minimum of a master's degree.

*Exercise Scientist. Exercise scientists work in positions where exercise is used either as a modality in rehabilitation or as a preventive measure in any number of programs intended for the development and or maintenance of physical fitness. In preparation, they have studied the basic human sciences and have had intensive clinical experiences. Positions require a degree in exercise science.

Health and Fitness Specialist. Health and fitness specialists are professionals qualified to assess, design, and implement individual and group exercise and fitness programs for healthy people and people with controlled diseases. The profession requires a minimum of an associate's degree.

Health Information Administrator. Entry-level jobs depend upon education, work experience, and place of employment. (Most health information administrators have worked as health information technicians.) Duties are related to the management of health information and systems used to collect, store, process, retrieve, analyze, disseminate, and communicate health information. A health information administrator position requires a four-year bachelor's degree. The professional certification requires successful completion of a national exam administered by the American Health Information Management Association (AHIMA).

Health Information Technician. Health information technicians must have a two-year associate's degree. Common job titles for health information technicians include coder, medical record technician, abstractor, and supervisor. The professional certification requires successful completion of a national exam administered by the American Health Information Management Association (AHIMA).

*Kinesiotherapist. Kinesiology is the study of muscles and muscle movement. Kinesiotherapists work under a physician's supervision, using therapeutic exercise and education to treat the effects of disease, injury, and congenital disorders on body movement.

Licensed Practical Nurse (LPN)/Licensed Vocational Nurse (LVN). LPNs, called LVNs in California and Texas, perform many of the same duties as registered nurses, with some exceptions, depending upon state law. LPNs and LVNs work under the supervision of physicians and registered nurses.

*Medical Assistant. Medical assistants perform administrative and clinical duties for physician/employers, usually within an ambulatory care setting, such as a medical office, clinic, or outpatient surgical center. The certified medical assistant (CMA) credential is earned through the certifying board of the American Association of Medical Assistants. The registered medical assistant (RMA) credential is obtained through the American Medical Technologists (AMT) organization. Both credentials involve specific educational requirements and require applicants to pass an examination assessing knowledge and skills. The CMA credential also requires continuing education to maintain the certification.

*Medical Illustrator. Medical illustrators create illustrations for science and medical texts and other publications, and they also function in administrative, consultative, and advisory capacities. They must be knowledgeable in the biological sciences, anatomy, physiology, pathology, general medical knowledge, and the visual arts.

Medical Laboratory Technician and Medical Technologist. Duties of medical technicians include performing simple tests in hematology, serology, blood banking, urinalysis, microbiology, and clinical chemistry. Medical technologists have completed a longer training course than laboratory technicians. They supervise technicians and assistants and perform more complicated analytical laboratory tests. Several organizations provide certification, which is often a condition of employment. In addition, many states require licensing of medical technicians and technologists.

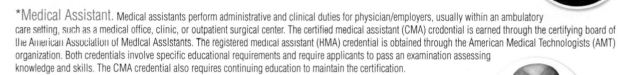

> " NOTE: A new title has recently been adopted for professionals who traditionally have been called medical technicians or medical technologists. This new title is clinical laboratory scientist. (See the U.S. Department of Labor's Bureau of Labor Statistics Web site at this address: www.bls.gov/oco/ocos096.htm.) "

Medical Massage Therapist. Massage therapists learn techniques to relieve pain from injuries, illnesses, or chronic conditions; to increase range of motion in joints; and to otherwise help patients with recovery and rehabilitation through body massage. National Certification in Therapeutic Massage and Bodywork requires at least 500 hours of formal training at an established school of massage therapy and passing the national examination offered by the National Certification Board for Therapeutic Massage and Bodywork. Medical massage therapists are supervised by physicians and employed by medical offices, hospitals, clinics, rehabilitation facilities, and other health care businesses. Licensed massage therapists may also establish their own businesses.

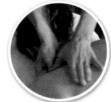

Professions marked with an asterisk are currently included in the list of CAAHEP-accredited programs.

Table 3-1 (Continued)

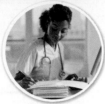

Medical Transcriptionist. Medical transcriptionists key material dictated by physicians to be placed with patients' medical records. They must have preparation in English grammar, anatomy and physiology, and pharmacology. They work in medical records departments in hospitals, managed care plan facilities, nursing homes, and ambulatory care facilities such as clinics, medical offices, and outpatient surgical centers. Transcriptionists with advanced skills may be self-employed.

Nuclear Medicine Technologist (NMT). Nuclear medicine technology programs range from one to four years, leading to a certificate, associate's degree, or bachelor's degree. Program enrollees are trained to use radionucleotides—unstable atoms that emit radiation—to diagnose and treat disease. Most NMTs work in hospitals.

Nurse Practitioner. Those individuals who have earned a registered nurse (RN) license may complete master's or doctoral degree university programs to become nurse practitioners. Nurse practitioners are skilled in physical diagnosis, psychosocial assessment, and primary health care management. They may work independently, in collaboration with a physician, or under the supervision of a physician.

Nursing Assistant. Nursing assistants provide basic patient care under the supervision of registered nurses. Routine duties include changing bed linens; taking temperature, respiratory, and blood pressure readings for patients; bathing patients and helping with personal care; helping patients with eating, walking, and exercise programs; and supporting patients when they are allowed to get out of bed. Employment opportunities exist in hospitals, long-term care facilities, and other health care institutions. In some states, the opportunity exists for nursing assistants to become certified, earning the title certified nursing assistant (CNA).

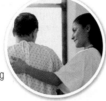

Occupational Therapist. An occupational therapist enters the field with a bachelor's, master's, or doctoral degree. Occupational therapists (OTs) work with clients who are mentally, physically, developmentally, and/or emotionally disabled to help these individuals become more independent and productive. Occupational therapists must have a license to practice in the state where they work.

Occupational Therapy Assistant. An occupational therapy assistant enters the field with a two-year associate's degree. Occupational therapy assistants work under the supervision of licensed occupational therapists.

Ophthalmic Medical Technician/Technologist. Ophthalmic medical technicians and technologists assist ophthalmologists (medical doctors who specialize in diseases and conditions of the eye) by performing such tasks as collecting data, administering diagnostic tests, and administering some treatments ordered by the supervising ophthalmologist. They may also maintain surgical instruments and office equipment. Graduates of accredited programs are eligible to take the national certifying examination at the approved levels offered by the Joint Commission on Allied Health Personnel in Ophthalmology.

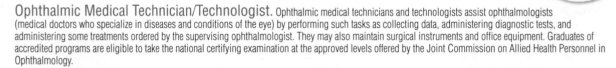

Optician. Opticians are licensed specifically to sell and/or construct optical materials.

Optometrist. Optometrists are trained and licensed to examine the eyes to determine the presence of vision problems and to prescribe and adapt lenses to preserve or restore maximum efficiency of vision.

*Orthotist and Prosthetist. Orthotists and prosthetists work directly with physicians and others to rehabilitate people with disabilities. The orthotist designs and fits devices (orthoses) for patients with disabling conditions of the limbs and spine. The prosthetist designs and fits device (prostheses) for patients who have partial or total absence of a limb.

*Perfusionist. A perfusionist operates transfusion equipment when necessary and consults with physicians in selecting the appropriate equipment, techniques, and transfusion media to be used, depending upon the patient's condition.

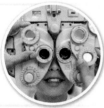

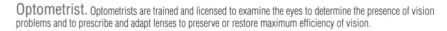

*Personal Fitness Trainer. Personal fitness trainers work with individual clients or with small groups. They help clients initiate and maintain fitness programs that maximize physical potential and health. They may become certified through the American Fitness Program Associates or through the National Federation of Professional Trainers.

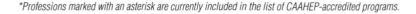

*Professions marked with an asterisk are currently included in the list of CAAHEP-accredited programs.

Phlebotomist. Phlebotomists are trained to draw blood from patients or donors for diagnostic testing or other medical purposes. They may also perform related tasks, such as preparing stains and reagents and cleaning and sterilizing equipment; taking patients' blood pressure, pulse, and respiration rates; performing ECGs; and billing, performing data entry, and answering telephones.

Physical Therapist. Physical therapists help patients restore function to muscles, nerves, joints, and bones after impairment due to illness or injury. All physical therapy programs are now at the master's or doctoral level.

Physical Therapist Assistant. Physical therapist assistants work under the supervision of licensed physical therapists in implementing treatment programs according to the patient's plan of care. Physical therapist assistants must complete a two-year program, usually offered in a community or junior college.

Physician Assistant. Physicians employ physician assistants (PAs) to perform many of the routine diagnostic and treatment procedures related to patient care. They can legally perform more procedures than registered nurses and can prescribe some medications, but they are not licensed to perform all the duties of a physician. The typical applicant for a physician assistant program already has a bachelor's degree and four years of health care practitioner experience. The average physician assistant program runs about 26 months. Graduates must then pass a national certifying examination. Once certified, PAs must complete 100 hours of continuing education every two years, and they must take the PA recertification examination every six years.

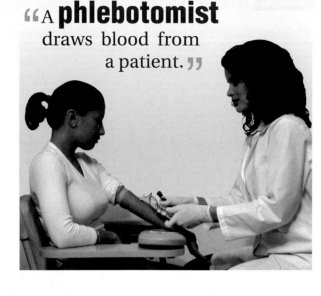

"A **phlebotomist** draws blood from a patient."

***Polysomnographic Technologist.** Polysomnographic technologists work under the supervision of physicians. They perform sleep diagnostics and provide clinical evaluations required for the diagnosis of sleep disorders. Polysomnographic technologists use such equipment as EEG, ECG, electro-oculography (EOG), and electromyography (EMG) monitors.

Radiologic or Medical Imaging Technologist. Radiologic technologists are qualified to position patients for X-rays, operate X-ray equipment, prepare X-ray films for viewing, and maintain records and images for each patient. In addition to X-ray imaging, these technologists may be trained in additional types of imaging, such as ultrasound and magnetic resonance scans. They can prepare and orally administer mixtures for contrast imaging, and in some states they are trained in venipuncture and can inject contrast mediums for imaging. They cannot interpret images. Most states require licensing of radiology technologists.

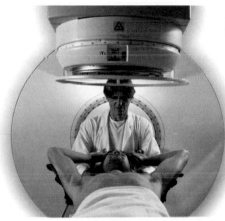

"A **radiology technologist** prepares a patient for an X-ray."

Registered Nurse. Registered nurses perform a variety of patient care duties, such as administering drugs prescribed by the supervising physician, monitoring the cardiovascular and pulmonary status of the critically ill, caring for newborns and their mothers, and assisting surgeons in the operating room. They also supervise LPNs; LVNs; nursing assistants; and other medical office, clinic, or hospital personnel. In addition, they document patient care for physicians and other health care team members. Nursing education curricula leading to the RN include two-year associate's degree and four-year baccalaureate degree programs.

Respiratory Therapist (entry level). Entry-level respiratory therapists are employed by hospitals, skilled nursing care facilities, clinics, physician offices, pulmonary function laboratories, sleep labs, and home care companies. They perform general respiratory care procedures under the supervision of an advanced-level respiratory therapist and/or a physician.

Respiratory Therapist (advanced). Advanced-level respiratory therapists assume primary responsibility for all respiratory patient care procedures to help with breathing disorders. They also supervise entry-level respiratory therapists.

***Specialist in Blood Bank Technology.** These specialists must have a bachelor's degree and certification in medical technology and must have completed the required course of study in blood bank technology. They perform both routine and specialized tests in blood bank immunohematology and perform transfusion services.

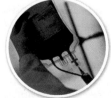

Professions marked with an asterisk are currently included in the list of CAAHEP-accredited programs.

Table 3-1 *(Continued)*

*Surgical Assistant.** As defined by the American College of Surgeons, the surgical assistant helps the surgeon carry out a safe operation with optimal results for the patient. In addition to intraoperative duties, the surgical assistant performs preoperative and postoperative duties to better facilitate proper patient care. The surgical assistant works under the direct supervision of the operating surgeon in accordance with hospital policy and appropriate laws and regulations.

*Surgical Technologist.** Surgical technologists work closely with surgeons, anesthesiologists, nurses, and other surgical personnel before, during, and after surgery. They may function as scrub, circulating, or first or second assisting surgical technologist. Duties vary according to assignment.

Professions marked with an asterisk are currently included in the list of CAAHEP-accredited programs.

than technicians or acquired qualifying experience. Since educational and credentialing requirements are subject to change, this information should be obtained from the national organization representing a profession and/or from state credentialing authorities.

The Commission on Accreditation of Allied Health Education Programs (CAAHEP) was established in 1994. CAAHEP accredits more than 2,000 programs in 22 allied health professions throughout the United States and Canada. CAAHEP provides information concerning duties, education requirements, and sources for further information about allied health professions and the location of schools offering the accredited programs. Professions marked with an asterisk in Table 3-1 are currently included in the list of CAAHEP-accredited programs.

While a variety of health care practitioners often work together as a team to provide medical care to patients, each individual is legally able to

COURT CASE

State Board of Nursing Finds Nurse Incompetent

A state board of nursing found that a nurse violated the section of the state code that regulates nursing by repeatedly failing to conform to the minimum standards of practice with regard to the proper maintenance and documentation of controlled substances. Since the finding could have led to revocation of the nurse's license, the nurse filed a petition for judicial review. The district court affirmed the board's decision, and the nurse again appealed. The state court of appeals upheld both the district court and board decisions, clearing the way for temporary or permanent revocation of the nurse's license, or other penalty. (No final decision is available, since the opinion has not yet been published.)

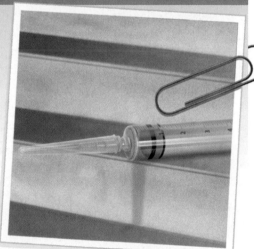

Several times while on duty, the nurse failed to properly document and account for missing controlled substances. In one instance she claimed containers of morphine and other drugs had fallen from her pocket while she was running down a stairwell. On other occasions, she claimed drug ampules had broken in her pocket, or she had misplaced syringes filled with controlled substances. Since her stories could not be corroborated, and she did not properly document losses or destruction of controlled drugs, the state court of appeals upheld the state board of nursing's finding that the nurse was incompetent in violating minimum standards of acceptable nursing practice.

Source: Matthias v. Iowa Board of Nursing, 2-153 / 01-1019, 2002 Iowa App. LEXIS 715.

perform only those duties dictated by professional and statutory guidelines. Each health care practitioner is responsible for understanding the laws and rules pertaining to his or her job and for knowing requirements concerning renewal of licenses; recertification; and payment of fees for licensure, certification, and registration.

According to many experts, drug addiction among doctors, nurses, and other health care practitioners is a problem that has not yet been addressed on a large scale. While some health care facilities do preemployment drug screening, too few do random testing for employee drug use. In your opinion, should health care practitioners be randomly tested for drug use? Why or why not?

Fraud may, in some states, be considered unprofessional conduct, or it may be separately specified as grounds for revoking a physician's license. A physician is considered guilty of fraud if "intent to deceive" can be shown. Acts generally classified as fraud include

- Falsifying medical diplomas, applications for licenses, licenses, or other credentials.
- Billing a governmental agency for services not rendered.
- Falsifying medical reports.
- Falsely advertising or misrepresenting to a patient "secret cures" or special powers to cure an ailment.

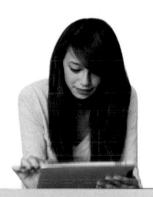

check your **progress**

9. In the United States, physicians may be licensed to practice medicine as MDs or as DOs. Distinguish between the two.

_____

_____

_____

10. Name three types of unprofessional conduct for which a physician may lose his or her license.

_____

_____

_____

Fill in the blanks or answer the following questions in the spaces provided.

11. A physician is licensed by the _____ in which he or she wishes to practice.

12. The federal government's authority regarding medical licensing extends only to

_____.

13. Revocations and suspensions of medical licenses are never _____.

14. Name four situations in which physicians do not need a valid license to practice in a specific state.

_____

_____

_____

_____

Revocations and suspensions of license are never automatic. A physician is always entitled to a written description of charges against him or her and a hearing before the appropriate state agency. If a hearing is held, the physician also has the right to counsel, the right to present evidence in his or her defense, the right to confront and question witnesses, and any other rights granted by state law. Decisions are usually subject to appeal through the state's court system.

An honest mistake or a single incident of alleged incompetence or negligence is not usually sufficient grounds for license revocation.

COURT CASE

MD's License Revocation Upheld

A New York State Appellate Court upheld a decision by the Hearing Committee of the New York State Board for Professional Medical Conduct revoking a physician's license.

The appellate court agreed that the physician had been grossly incompetent in failing to monitor the various anticoagulant medicines that a hospitalized patient was prescribed, so the patient hemorrhaged to death. In addition, the physician had altered the patient's records in an effort to blame others. Substantial evidence also supported a finding that the physician had lied by failing to disclose a criminal conviction on two applications for hospital privileges. Therefore, the revocation of the physician's license to practice medicine was upheld.

Source: Catsoulis v. New York State Department of Health et al., 2 A.D. 3d 920; 767 N.Y.S.2d 526, 2003 N.Y. App. Div.

LO 3.4

Define the major types of medical practice management systems.

Medical Practice Management Systems

There are four basic types of medical practice:

- Sole proprietorship
- Partnership
- Professional corporation
- Group practice

Laws governing the various types of practices vary, but medical office personnel should be aware of those laws that apply to their employer's practice management system.

Sole Proprietorship

In medicine's bygone days, physicians most often practiced alone, providing all patient services, from receptionist, to medical treatment, to billing, to house calls. They were engaged in a "solo practice," and they took all the profits and bore all the risks associated with the **sole proprietorship.** Today, some physicians still practice alone (with the help of employees to perform receptionist, billing, and some patient care tasks), but they are in the minority. A disadvantage to this type of practice is that the physician practicing alone has unlimited personal liability.

Two or more physicians may decide to practice individually but agree to share office space and employees. This arrangement is called an **associate practice** and allows a sharing of expenses, not a sharing of profits and liability.

sole proprietorship A form of medical practice management in which a physician practices alone, assuming all benefits and liabilities for the business.

associate practice A medical management system in which two or more physicians share office space and employees but practice individually.

Partnership

When two or more physicians decide to practice together, they may form a **partnership,** based on a legal written agreement specifying the rights, obligations, and responsibilities of each partner.

Advantages of partnerships include sharing the workload and expenses, and pooling profits and assets. A major disadvantage is that each partner has equal liability for the acts, conduct, losses, and deficits of the partnership, unless specific provisions are made for these contingencies in the initial agreement.

Professional Corporation

A **corporation** is a body formed and authorized by law to act as a single person, although constituted by one or more persons and legally endowed with various rights and duties. State law governs corporations, so requirements for incorporation may vary. The corporation may own, mortgage, or sell property; manage its own business affairs; and sue or be sued.

Physicians who form corporations are shareholders and employees of the organization. There are financial and tax advantages to forming a corporation, and fringe benefits to employees may be more generous than with a sole proprietorship or partnership. Forming a corporation also means that the incorporators and owners have limited liability in case lawsuits are filed.

Group Practice

The **group practice** may function as a corporation or as a partnership. A medical group practice is the provision of health care services by a group of three or more licensed physicians, engaged full time in a formally organized and legally recognized entity. They share the group's income and expenses in a systematic manner and also share facilities, equipment, records, and personnel involved in both patient care and business management.

Physicians in group practice may be engaged in the same specialty, calling themselves, for example, Urology Associates. They may provide care in two or three related specialties, for example, obstetrics-gynecology and pediatrics. Alternatively, they may offer a variety of services, for example, obstetrics-gynecology, pediatrics, family practice, and internal medicine.

For physicians, the advantages of group practice are much the same as those of a corporation, with the added benefit that the legal implications are not so far-reaching or complicated.

partnership A form of medical practice management system whereby two or more parties practice together under a written agreement specifying the rights, obligations, and responsibilities of each partner.

corporation A body formed and authorized by law to act as a single person.

group practice A medical management system in which three or more licensed physicians share the collective income, expenses, facilities, equipment, records, and personnel for the business.

Types of Managed Care

Managed care health plans are corporations that pay for and deliver health care to subscribers for a set fee using a network of physicians and other health care providers. The network coordinates and refers patients to its health care providers and hospitals and monitors the amount and patterns of care delivered. The plans usually limit the services subscribers may receive under the plans. Managed care plans make agreed-upon payments to providers (hospitals or physicians) for providing health care services to health care subscribers. The payment from a managed care plan to providers may be one of several types, including contracted fee schedules, percentages of billed charges, capitation, and others. (*Capitation* is a set advance payment made to providers, based on the calculated cost of medical care of a specific population of subscribers.)

LO 3.5

Define the different types of managed care health plans.

managed care A system in which financing, administration, and delivery of health care are combined to provide medical services to subscribers for a prepaid fee.

Before managed care plans, private health insurance policies were traditionally written as third-party indemnity health insurance. *Third party* means that the insurance company reimburses health care practitioners for medical care provided to policyholders. **Indemnity** is coverage of the insured person against a potential loss of money from medical expenses for an illness or accident. Indemnity insurance benefits are paid in a predetermined amount of money rather than in specific services.

In an attempt to confront increasing health care costs—due in part to increasingly large awards in litigation, an aging population that requires more health care, the expensive technology used in modern-day medicine, and the impact of third-party payers for medical care—traditional fee-for-service health insurance companies now incorporate elements of managed care into their plans. (The impact of third-party payers is that there is little incentive to keep health care costs down when health care providers and recipients know that a third party—Medicare, Medicaid, other insurance—will pay.) Consequently, virtually all insured Americans have become familiar with such cost-containment/managed care measures as coinsurance, copayment fees, deductibles, formularies, and utilization review.

indemnity A traditional form of health insurance that covers the insured against a potential loss of money from medical expenses resulting from an illness or accident.

- *Coinsurance* refers to the amount of money insurance plan members must pay out of pocket, after the insurance plan pays its share. For example, a plan may agree to pay 80 percent of the cost for a surgical procedure, and the subscriber must pay the remaining 20 percent.

- *Copayment* fees are flat fees that insurance plan subscribers pay for certain medical services. For example, a subscriber might be required to make a $20 copayment for each visit to a physician office.

- *Deductible* amounts are specified by the insurance plan for each subscriber. For instance, the deductible for a single subscriber might be $500 a calendar year. In other words, the plan does not begin to pay benefits until the $500 deductible has been satisfied.

- *Formularies* are a plan's list of approved prescription medications for which it will reimburse subscribers.

- *Utilization review* is the method used by a health plan to measure the amount and appropriateness of health services used by its members.

Health Maintenance Organizations

health maintenance organization (HMO)
A health plan that combines coverage of health care costs and delivery of health care for a prepaid premium.

Health maintenance organizations (HMOs) are one of several types of managed care organizations providing health care services to subscribers within the United States. HMOs and preferred provider organizations (PPOs) are the most common types of managed care plans. Under HMO plans, all health services are delivered and paid for through one organization. The three general types of HMOs are group model HMOs, staff model HMOs, and individual (or independent) practice associations (IPAs).

Group model HMOs contract with independent groups of physicians to provide coordinated care for large numbers of HMO patients for a fixed, per-member fee. They often provide medical care for members of several HMOs. Group model HMOs include prepaid group practices (PGPs). Physicians in PGPs are salaried employees of the HMO, usually practice in facilities provided by the HMO, and share in profits at the end of the year.

Staff model HMOs employ salaried physicians and other allied health professionals who provide care solely for members of one HMO. Subscribers to staff model HMOs can often see their doctors, get laboratory tests and X-rays, have prescriptions filled, and even order eyeglasses or contact lenses all in one location. Staff model HMOs also employ specialists or contract with outside specialists in some cases.

An **individual (or independent) practice association (IPA)** is an association of physicians, hospitals, and other health care providers that contracts with an HMO to provide medical services to subscribers. Health care practitioners who are members of an IPA may usually still see patients outside the contracting HMO. The providers who contract with an IPA practice in their own offices and receive a per-member payment, or capitation, from participating HMOs to provide a full range of health services for HMO members. These providers often care for members of several HMOs, which gives them a larger patient and income base than staff model HMOs.

Preferred Provider Organizations

Preferred provider organizations (PPOs), also called **preferred provider associations (PPAs),** are managed care plans that contract with a network of doctors, hospitals, and other health care providers who provide services for set fees. Subscribers may choose their primary health provider from an approved list and must pay higher out-of-pocket costs for care provided by health care practitioners outside the PPO group.

Physician-Hospital Organizations

Physician-hospital organizations (PHOs) are another type of managed care plan. PHOs are organizations that include physicians, hospitals, surgery centers, nursing homes, laboratories, and other medical service providers that contract with one or more HMOs, insurance plans, or directly with employers to provide health care services.

Other Variations in Managed Care Plans

Managed care plans may also include the following identifying features:

- **Gatekeeper or primary care plan.** The insured must designate a **primary care physician (PCP).** Also known as a **gatekeeper physician,** the primary care physician directs all of a patient's medical care and generates any referrals to specialists or other health care practitioners.

- **Point-of-service (POS) plan. Point-of-service plans** allow plan members to seek health care from nonnetwork physicians, but the plan pays the highest benefits for care when given by the PCP or via a referral from the PCP. When care is provided without a referral, but still within the network, the plan pays benefits at a reduced level. Members also have out-of-network benefits, but at greatly reduced payment levels.

- **Open access plan.** Under **open access plans,** subscribers may see any in-network health care provider without a referral.

Managed care plans differ from one another in some respects, but all are designed to cut the cost of health care delivery. The impact of cost-cutting measures on the quality of health care remains a major point of contention. Advocates claim that managed care plans can deliver medical services more efficiently and at much less expense than traditional fee-for-service plans. Critics argue that necessary, quality medical services are often sacrificed for profit margins. The following questions are of special concern to patients enrolled in managed care plans:

- Will the most knowledgeable and experienced physician treat my medical conditions and those of my family?

- Is my physician too concerned with saving money?

individual (or independent) practice association (IPA) A type of HMO that contracts with groups of physicians who practice in their own offices and receive a per-member payment (capitation) from participating HMOs to provide a full range of health services for members.

preferred provider organization (PPO) A network of independent physicians, hospitals, and other health care providers who contract with an insurance carrier to provide medical care at a discount rate to patients who are part of the insurer's plan. Also called **preferred provider association (PPA).**

physician-hospital organization (PHO) A health care plan in which physicians join with hospitals to provide a medical care delivery system and then contract for insurance with a commercial carrier or an HMO.

primary care physician (PCP) The physician responsible for directing all of a patient's medical care and determining whether the patient should be referred for specialty care.

gatekeeper physician The primary care physician who directs the medical care of managed care health plan members.

point-of-service (POS) plan A health care plan that allows members to seek health care from nonnetwork physicians but pays the highest benefits for care when it is given by the primary care physician (PCP) or via a referral from the PCP.

open access plan A managed care feature whereby subscribers may see any in-network health care provider without a referral.

- Must I fight to get routine procedures from my HMO?
- What if my HMO refuses to pay for a procedure I need?

In addition, physicians and other medical professionals, administrators of managed care plans, government officials, and HMO members are concerned with issues such as these:

- Do managed health care and competition actually drive down costs?
- Do regulations exist regarding patient rights in managed care plans?
- Do quality ratings for HMOs help consumers?
- Does managed health care provide higher-quality care than fee-for-service medicine?

Managed care is a fixture of modern medicine, but health care consumers and practitioners continue to debate its advantages and disadvantages, and may do so for many years to come.

LO 3.6
Discuss the federal legislation that impacts health care reimbursement and prohibits fraud and abuse in health care billing.

Legislation Affecting Health Care Plans

Patient Protection and Affordable Care Act (PPACA) A federal law enacted in 2010, to expand health insurance coverage and otherwise regulate the health insurance industry. Many provisions of the law are scheduled to take effect in 2014 and 2015.

Health Care and Education Reconciliation Act (HCERA) Also enacted in 2010, a federal law that added to regulations imposed on the insurance industry by PPACA.

When Barack Obama was elected president of the United States in 2008, he promised to initiate comprehensive changes in the American health care system. After months of heated debate, H.R. 3590, the **Patient Protection and Affordable Care Act (PPACA),** was signed into law on March 23, 2010. Additional changes to the health care system were enacted by the **Health Care and Education Reconciliation Act (HCERA),** signed into law on March 30, 2010. The two acts mandated major changes in the American health care system, which are discussed in more detail in Chapter 13. Many major provisions of the legislation are to become effective in 2014, including the formation of state-based insurance exchanges—some for small businesses to purchase coverage, and others for the uninsured and self-employed to purchase insurance. Subsidies are to be made available to individuals and families with lower incomes that fall within a specified range. The extent of the effect of the 2010 legislation on health care plans in the United States remains to be seen as all provisions are enacted over time.

Additional laws have been passed, which were intended to improve the quality of health care in the United States, to reduce fraud, and to help assure managed care and other types of health insurance subscribers

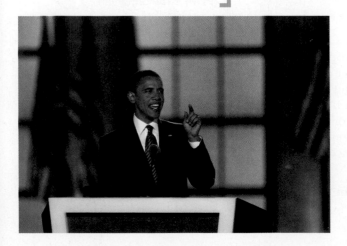

that they will not be summarily dropped or otherwise be unfairly or unlawfully discriminated against by insurance providers. Two of the most significant health care laws are the Health Insurance Portability and Accountability Act (HIPAA) of 1996, and the Health Care Quality Improvement Act (HCQIA) of 1986.

Health Insurance Portability and Accountability Act

The **Health Insurance Portability and Accountability Act (HIPAA) of 1996** was an ambitious attempt by Congress to reform the American health care system. The HIPAA helps workers keep continuous health insurance coverage for themselves and their dependents when they change jobs, but its many provisions go far beyond this mandate. The primary objectives of the law were to

1. Improve the efficiency and effectiveness of the health care industry by

   - Accelerating billing processes and reducing paperwork.
   - Reducing health care billing fraud.
   - Facilitating tracking of health information.
   - Improving accuracy and reliability of shared data.
   - Increasing access to computer networks within health care facilities.

2. Help employees keep their health insurance coverage when transferring to another job.

3. Protect confidential medical information that identifies patients from unauthorized disclosure or use.

The privacy provisions of HIPAA have had such a sweeping effect on the health care industry that the act is discussed in more detail in Chapter 8.

HIPAA also led to the creation of the **Healthcare Integrity and Protection Data Bank (HIPDB).** HIPDB is a national health care fraud and abuse data collection program for the reporting and disclosure of certain adverse actions taken against health care providers, suppliers, or practitioners. Data from HIPDB are available to federal and state government agencies and to health plans, but are not available to the general public.

Health Care Quality Improvement Act

In creating the **Health Care Quality Improvement Act (HCQIA) of 1986,** Congress found that "the increasing occurrence of medical malpractice and the need to improve the quality of medical care have become nationwide problems that warrant greater efforts than those that can be undertaken by any individual state." Accordingly, the act requires that professional peer review action be taken in some cases. It also limits the damages for professional review and protects from liability those who provide information to professional review bodies.

One of the most important provisions of the HCQIA was the establishment of the **National Practitioner Data Bank (NPDB).** Use of the NPDB was intended to improve the quality of medical care nationwide by encouraging effective professional peer review of physicians and dentists. Information that must be reported to the NPDB includes medical malpractice payments, adverse licensure actions, adverse clinical privilege actions, and

Health Insurance Portability and Accountability Act (HIPAA) of 1996 A federal statute that helps workers keep continuous health insurance coverage for themselves and their dependents when they change jobs, protects confidential medical information from unauthorized disclosure or use, and helps curb the rising cost of fraud and abuse.

Healthcare Integrity and Protection Data Bank (HIPDB) A national health care fraud and abuse data collection program established by HIPAA for the reporting and disclosure of certain adverse actions taken against health care providers, suppliers, or practitioners.

Health Care Quality Improvement Act (HCQIA) of 1986 A federal statute passed to improve the quality of medical care nationwide. One provision established the National Practitioner Data Bank.

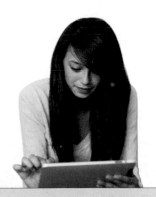

check your **progress**

15. Define *managed care*.

_____

_____

16. Name and list distinguishing characteristics of three types of managed care plans.

_____

_____

National Practitioner Data Bank (NPDB) A repository of information about health care practitioners, established by the Health Care Quality Improvement Act of 1986.

adverse professional society membership actions. The NPDB is a resource to assist state licensing boards, hospitals, and other health care entities in investigating the qualifications of physicians, dentists, and other health care practitioners.

National Practitioner Data Bank queries are mandatory for physicians when they apply for privileges at a hospital, and every two years for physicians already on the medical staff who wish to maintain their privileges. They are voluntary for hospitals conducting professional review, other health care entities with formal peer review programs, state licensing boards at any time, those who wish to self-query, and plaintiffs' attorneys under certain circumstances. The NPDB may not disclose information to a medical malpractice insurer, defense attorney, or member of the general public.

Controlling Health Care Fraud and Abuse

Partly because of the rising costs of health care, fraud and abuse within the industry have become major issues. As a result, laws have been passed to control three types of illegal conduct:

1. False claims in billing.
2. Kickbacks.
3. Self-referrals.

Several federal and state statutes prohibit false claims. HIPAA and the Federal False Claims Act are two laws that prohibit false claims and detail the penalties that can be levied against violators.

Federal False Claims Act A law that allows for individuals to bring civil actions on behalf of the U.S. government for false claims made to the federal government, under a provision of the law called *qui tam* (from Latin meaning "to bring an action for the king and for oneself").

The **Federal False Claims Act** allows for individuals to bring civil actions on behalf of the U.S. government for false claims made to the federal government, under a provision of the law called *qui tam* (from Latin meaning "to bring an action for the king and for oneself"). These individuals, commonly known as whistleblowers, are referred to as *qui tam relators* and can share in any court-awarded damages.

Suits brought under the False Claims Act are most often related to the health care and defense industries. The act prohibits

- Making a false record or statement to get a false or fraudulent claim paid by the government.
- Conspiring to have a false or fraudulent claim paid by the government.
- Withholding property of the government with the intent to defraud the government or to willfully conceal it from the government.
- Making or delivering a receipt for government property that is false or fraudulent.
- Buying government property from someone who is not authorized to sell the property.
- Making a false statement to avoid or deceive an obligation to pay money or property to the government.
- Causing someone else to submit a false claim by submitting false information.

Providing kickbacks, or giving financial incentives to a health care provider for referring patients or for recommending services or products, is prohibited under the federal Anti-Kickback Law and by state laws.

Self-referrals, or referring patients to any service or facility where the health provider has a financial interest, are prohibited by the federal Ethics in Patient Referral Act, as well as other federal and state laws.

Violations of laws against health care fraud and abuse can result in imprisonment and fines, loss of professional license, loss of health care

A registered nurse employed by a medical center from 1979 to 2002 was chair of her state nurses' association, the exclusive bargaining unit for the registered nurses at her employing medical center. In this capacity, she complained to her state Department of Public Health about the inadequacy of nurse staffing at her place of employment. The nurse alleged that staffing inadequacies were affecting patient care and delays in patient treatment. She said she had learned that delays in patient care could affect the medical center's right to participate in and receive reimbursement for Medicare- or Medicaid-related services.

Nurses at the plaintiff's medical center filed hundreds of complaints to appropriate authorities, reporting unsafe, unethical, and illegal care practices or conditions at their medical center during 2001–2002. The plaintiff and several other complaining nurses were fired in 2002. The plaintiff subsequently sued the medical center under the False Claims Act, claiming her conduct was protected under the whistleblower provisions of the act.

The court granted the medical center's motion to dismiss, stating that nothing indicated that the employee threatened a *qui tam* action, nor had she notified the employer that she was investigating fraud. Thus, the plaintiff had no grounds to sufficiently allege a retaliation claim under the FCA.

Source: Robbins v. Provena St. Joseph Medical Center (2004) U.S. Dist. LEXIS 3878.

facility staff privileges, and exclusion from participation in federal health care programs.

Patients' Bill of Rights Acts of 1999, 2001, and 2004 Concerns about the quality of medical care patients receive under managed care plans prompted Congress to first consider a Patients' Bill of Rights Act in 1999. The act contained provisions applicable to managed care plans for access to care, quality assurance, patient information and securing privacy, grievances and appeals procedures, protecting the doctor–patient relationship, and promoting good medical practice. Congress failed to act on the bill in 1999, and it was revived in 2001 as H.R. 2563, the Bipartisan Patient Protection Act of 2001. The House of Representatives passed the act in August 2001 by a narrow margin, and it was sent to the Senate. The Senate passed a revised version of the bill and sent it back to the House for reconsideration, but the bill died there. Major points of contention among lawmakers were the rights of patients to file lawsuits against managed care plans in federal or state courts and whether or not awards in such lawsuits should be limited by law to certain amounts.

The Bipartisan Patient Protection Act was revived in 2004, when S. 2083 was proposed to amend the Public Health Service Act and the Employee Retirement Income Security Act of 1974. The purpose of the bill was to protect consumers in managed care health plans and other health coverage. The bill did not become law. The American Hospital Association (AHA) adopted a patient bill of rights to be used by its member hospitals. Recently, the AHA created a document called the Patient Care Partnership to replace the bill of rights.

Patient's Bill of Rights as Defined by the Patient Protection and Affordable Care Act In June 2010, President Obama announced the Patient Protection and Affordable Care Act's Patient's Bill of Rights as outlined in the legislation. A major goal of the act, the president emphasized, is to put American consumers in charge of their health coverage and care. The new rules will

- Prevent insurance companies from limiting necessary care. For most plans, as early as July or September 2010, insurance companies could no longer refuse coverage for consumers with preexisting conditions, refuse coverage based on unintentional mistakes on applications, set lifetime limits on coverage, or set certain annual limits on coverage.

- Remove insurance company barriers between patients and doctors. Plans that are not grandfathered under the act will allow patients to choose primary care doctors from provider networks, see obstetrician-gynecologist (ob-gyn) physicians without referrals, and seek emergency care at hospitals outside a plan's network without prior approval.

- Allow young adults to be covered under parents' plans until age 26.

- Prevent arbitrary rescission (annulling or canceling) of insurance coverage.

- Review insurance premium increases and prevent unreasonable rate hikes.

LO 3.7

Define *telemedicine, cybermedicine,* and *e-health,* and discuss their roles in today's health care environment.

telemedicine Remote consultation by patients with physicians or other health professionals via telephone, closed-circuit television, or the Internet.

cybermedicine A form of telemedicine that involves direct contact between patients and physicians over the Internet, usually for a fee.

e-health Term for the use of the Internet as a source of consumer information about health and medicine.

Telemedicine

Telemedicine refers to remote consultation with physicians or other health care professionals via telephone, closed-circuit television, fax machine, or the Internet. When telemedicine was first used, it generally involved transmission of X-rays, sonograms, or other medical data between two distant points. In some cases, usually through closed-circuit television, a physician could examine a patient in a distant location, thus allowing patients in rural areas more complete access to medical care. Today, transmitted medical data includes video, audio, and written or computerized patient data. In fact, increasing use of the Internet has made telemedicine an important component of the health care system.

Two additional aspects of telemedicine are cybermedicine and e-health. **Cybermedicine** involves direct online contact between physician and patient. There are many Web sites on the Internet that allow patients to consult directly with a physician, usually for a fee. The physician may offer medical advice and even prescribe medication.

E-health is the term used for the increasing use of the Internet as a source of consumer information about health and medicine. E-health has become a popular aspect of telemedicine, as increasing numbers of patients query their doctors and other health care providers about where to find health information on the Internet and how to evaluate such information.

Health-related Internet sites included under the category "e-health" most often provide

- Consumer information services.
- Support groups.
- Prescription and nonprescription drug sales.
- Medical advice and diagnosis.
- Contract health services as part of insurance plans for covered subscribers.
- Health business support services for health professionals and health care organizations.

States are responding to the proliferation in telemedicine services with laws that address issues of reimbursement, licensure, funding, and confidentiality. Telemedicine legislation covers various health care providers, including physicians, dentists, chiropractors, nurses, and other health professionals. Since new laws regulating telemedicine are passed every year, health care practitioners who are involved in telemedicine or who plan to be involved will need to research state telemedicine laws.

Consumer Precautions regarding Telemedicine

Individuals using the Internet for health care and medical information should evaluate Web sites for reliability. Users should ask questions such as these:

- Who is sponsoring the site? Sites sponsored by or linked with major medical centers and groups, government agencies, and medical professionals or major medical publications are most likely to present reliable information.

- Are several reliable Web sites offering similar information? If so, the information is most likely to be reliable.

- Does the site tout miracle cures or peculiar therapies? Users should discuss any claims made with a trusted health care practitioner before sending for materials or "cures" or otherwise following such advice.

Advances in technology have improved our ability to record, store, transfer, and share medical data electronically. They have also magnified privacy, security, and confidentiality concerns that pertain to patient medical records. Privacy issues are discussed at length in Chapter 8.

COURT CASE

Illegal Telemedicine Drug Sale Not Deceptive Trade Practice

A Washington state medical doctor dispensed Viagra through a Web site. He did not perform physical examinations or have direct contact with any of the Web site visitors who purchased the drug. Kansas investigators conducted a "sting" operation to document that individuals, including minors, could purchase Viagra from the Web site operated by the medical doctor. The Kansas attorney general subsequently brought suit against the doctor under the Kansas Consumer Protection Act (KCPA).

The physician was barred from prescribing and dispensing drugs in Kansas via his Web site, since to do so was in violation of that state's pharmacy and medical practice acts. The state sought civil penalties under the KCPA, which resulted in the cited lawsuit. To state a claim under the KCPA, the state had to establish that the transaction was deceptive. The state claimed that since the transaction was illegal, it was necessarily deceptive. The trial court disagreed, finding that the Web site information was correct and that in order for the minor to purchase the drug, he had to falsify information on a site form. The "medical evaluation" included a specific disclaimer explaining its limitations and that it was not a substitute for a proper medical examination by a physician. The court found that the drug that was shipped was what was represented and that charges for the drug were also as represented. The trial court concluded that the transaction was not deceptive, and this ruling was affirmed by the Kansas Supreme Court. While the state was not able to impose civil penalties, the physician was no longer allowed to sell the drug in Kansas.

Source: State ex rel. Stovall v. Confimed.com, L.L.C., 38 P.3d 707 (Kansas, 2002).

CHAPTER SUMMARY

LO 3.1 How do licensure, certification, registration, and accreditation differ?

- Licensure is a mandatory credentialing process established by law, usually at the state level. Licenses to practice are required in every state for all physicians and nurses and for many other health care practitioners as well. Individuals who do not have the required license are prohibited by law from practicing certain health care professions.

- Certification is a voluntary credentialing process whereby applicants who meet specific requirements may receive a certificate.

- Registration is an entry in an official registry or record, listing the names of persons in a certain occupation who have satisfied specific requirements.

- Accreditation is the process by which health care practitioner education programs, health care facilities, and managed care plans are officially authorized.

LO 3.2 How are physicians licensed and regulated?

- Each state's medical practice acts establish procedures for licensing physicians, registered nurses, and many other health care practitioners and regulating the practice of medicine within that state.

- A physician's license can be revoked or suspended for conviction of a felony, unprofessional conduct, or personal or professional incapacity.

LO 3.3 What is the health care team?

- The health care team consists of physicians and allied health workers who generally have completed a course of study leading to licensure, certification, or registration in one of the health care professions.

LO 3.4 What are the different types of medical practice management systems?

- A physician practicing alone is a sole proprietor.

- Physicians practicing with one or more partners have a group practice, which may be a partnership or a limited liability corporation, depending upon the legal agreement the physicians sign.

LO 3.5 What is managed care, and how do the major managed care plans differ?

Managed care refers to a system that combines financing, administration, and delivery of health care to provide medical services to subscribers for a prepaid fee. Major types of managed care plans include

- Health maintenance organization (HMO): A health plan that combines coverage of health care costs and delivery of health care for a prepaid premium.

- Individual (or independent) practice association (IPA): A type of HMO that contracts with groups of physicians who practice in their own offices and receive a per-member payment from participating HMOs to provide a full range of health services for members.

- Preferred provider organization (PPO): A network of independent physicians, hospitals, and other health care providers who contract with an insurance carrier to provide medical care at a discount rate to patients who are part of the insurer's plan.

- Physician-hospital organization (PHO): A health care plan in which physicians join with hospitals to provide a medical care delivery system and then contract for insurance with a commercial carrier or an HMO.

LO 3.6 What major federal legislation has affected health care insurance and payment fraud in the United States?

- Patient Protection and Affordable Care Act (PPACA): A federal law enacted in 2010 to expand health insurance coverage and otherwise regulate the health insurance industry. Many provisions of the law are scheduled to take effect in 2014 and 2015.

- Health Care and Education Reconciliation Act: Also enacted in 2010, a federal law that added to regulations imposed on the insurance industry by PPACA.

- Health Insurance Portability and Accountability Act (HIPAA) of 1996: A federal statute that helps workers keep continuous health insurance coverage for themselves and their dependents when they change jobs, protects confidential medical information from unauthorized disclosure or use, and helps curb the rising cost of fraud and abuse.

- Health Care Quality Improvement Act (HCQIA) of 1986: A federal statute passed to improve the quality of medical care nationwide.

- Federal False Claims Act: Allows for individuals to bring civil actions on behalf of the U.S. government for false claims made to the federal government.

LO 3.7 How has telemedicine affected the delivery of health care?

- Through cybermedicine, which involves direct contact between patients and physicians over the Internet, usually for a fee.

- Through e-health, the increasing use of the Internet as a source of consumer information about health and medicine.

[ETHICS ISSUES Working in Health Care]

Ethics ISSUE 1: The "Code of Ethical Business and Professional Behavior" for the Cleveland Clinic Health System states under the heading "I. Conflicts of Interest" that "Each component of the system maintains policies that require disclosure of potential conflicts of interest to ensure that such conflict does not inappropriately influence business or professional decision-making."

Discussion Question

1. Assume you are an orthopedic surgeon working under the previously mentioned ethical guidelines. You own shares in a company called

Prosthetics, Inc., that makes prosthetic hip replacements. There are five other companies that make similar products, and you use three of the companies as providers. Can you implant a Prosthetics, Inc. device into one of your patients without disclosure of your stock ownership?

Ethics ISSUE 2: A physician who owns a health care facility is prohibited by the federal Ethics in Patient Referral Act, as well as other federal and state laws, from referring patients to his facility.

Discussion Question

1. Is the practice also unethical? Explain your answer.

Ethics ISSUE 3: By law, health care practitioners can perform only those duties that are within their *scope of practice*—that is, those duties for which they are duly licensed, certified, registered, and competent.

Discussion Question

1. Mary has been a registered nurse for 30 years. When she was 19, prior to going to nursing school, she was convicted of a felony narcotics possession and was given probation. When she received her license 30 years ago there was no background check nor was the question of a conviction on the application. She is now moving to another state and wants to get a reciprocity license. Although no background check is required, she notes that one of the rules and regulations states that "a licensee must report any misdemeanor of felony convictions." What should she do?

Ethics ISSUE 4: Joan works as a medical assistant in the Wellness Medical Practice. For two months she has been dating a colleague, Peter, who is one of the physician assistants, and Joan has now moved in with him. While going through his mail, Joan learns that Peter has just been convicted of driving while intoxicated (DWI). She looks up the state law and learns that Peter's DWI is a reportable offense.

Discussion Question

1. Should Joan confront Peter, report his DWI herself, or simply ignore the facts?

Go to **www.mhhe.com/judson6e** to practice your case review skills. Then read on for more information.

[KEY TERMS]

accreditation

allopathic

associate practice

certification

corporation

cybermedicine

e-health

endorsement

Federal False Claims Act

gatekeeper physician

group practice

Health Care and Education Reconciliation Act (HCERA)

Health Care Quality Improvement Act (HCQIA) of 1986

Healthcare Integrity and Protection Data Bank (HIPDB)

Health Insurance Portability and Accountability Act (HIPAA) of 1996

health maintenance organization (HMO)

indemnity

individual (or independent) practice association (IPA)

licensure

managed care

medical boards

medical practice acts

National Practitioner Data Bank (NPDB)

open access plan

partnership

Patient Protection and Affordable Care Act (PPACA)

physician-hospital organization (PHO)

point-of-service (POS) plan

preferred provider association (PPA)

preferred provider organization (PPO)

primary care physician (PCP)

reciprocity

registration

sole proprietorship

telemedicine

tertiary care settings

[CHAPTER 3 REVIEW]

Applying Knowledge

LO 3.1

Write "L" for licensure, "C" for certification, "R" for registration, and "A" for accreditation in the space provided to indicate which is applicable in the following descriptions.

_____ 1. Involves a mandatory credentialing process established by law, usually at the state level.

_____ 2. Involves simply paying a fee.

_____ 3. Involves a voluntary credentialing process, usually national in scope, most often sponsored by a private-sector group.

_____ 4. Required of all physicians, dentists, and nurses in every state.

_____ 5. Consists simply of an entry in an official record.

_____ 6. A process that implies that health care facilities or HMOs have met certain standards.

Circle the correct answer for each of the following questions.

7. Which of the following is mandatory for certain health professionals to practice in their field?
   a. Endorsement
   b. Reciprocity
   c. Licensure
   d. Certification

8. Licensure to practice medicine is done by
   a. Each individual state
   b. The federal government
   c. Local and state governments together
   d. The federal government and the local government

9. Which of the following statements best defines *accreditation*?
   a. It is a process that allows hospitals to license qualified employees.
   b. It is a process for licensing clinical laboratories.
   c. It is a process for officially authorizing health care education programs, facilities, and managed care plans.
   d. It is another way to become licensed as a health care practitioner.

10. Which of the following best defines the osteopathic approach to medicine?
    a. Emphasizes allopathic medicine
    b. Emphasizes the use of drugs over surgery
    c. Emphasizes surgery as the ultimate cure
    d. Emphasizes the musculoskeletal system of the body and the correction of joint and tissue problems

11. Allopathic medicine means, literally,
    a. "Different suffering"
    b. "All encompassing"
    c. "Ever enduring"
    d. "Different approach"

LO 3.3

12. Which of the following is an example of a tertiary care setting?
    a. A Catholic hospital
    b. An endoscopic center
    c. A children's hospital
    d. A free clinic for the homeless

13. Which of the following is an explanation for the increasing number of medical specialists?
    a. More women entering medicine
    b. More scholarships available for medical students
    c. Loss of prestige for generalists
    d. Forgiveness of college loans for specialists

14. A physician fails to meet continuing education requirements. He or she is guilty of
    a. Laziness
    b. Deception
    c. Unprofessional conduct
    d. Fraud

15. Which of the following is *not* a purpose of medical practice acts?
    a. To define what is meant by "practice of medicine" in each state
    b. To be sure physicians are adequately compensated for their services
    c. To explain requirements and methods for licensure
    d. To establish grounds for suspension or revocation of license

16. Each state's medical practice acts also provide for the establishment of
    a. Health care teams
    b. Hospital ethics committees
    c. Medical boards
    d. HMOs

17. Laws vary from state to state, but unprofessional conduct for medical professionals usually includes
    a. Physical abuse of a patient
    b. Inadequate record keeping
    c. Failure to meet continuing education requirements
    d. All of the above

18. Physicians' actions generally classified as fraud include
    a. Falsifying medical diplomas and other credentials
    b. Falsifying medical reports
    c. Promising a patient "secret cures" or other special ways to cure an ailment
    d. All of the above

19. The sole authority granted to the federal government in the licensing of physicians is
    a. License to practice a specialty
    b. The permit issued by the Drug Enforcement Administration for controlled substances
    c. Revocation of a physician's license for fraud
    d. An endorsement when a physician moves to a different state

LO 3.4

20. Physicians today practice primarily
    a. At the hospital
    b. In sole proprietorships
    c. In group practices
    d. In large corporations

21. When two or more physicians practice together, with a written agreement specifying the rights, obligations, and responsibilities of each partner, what is the arrangement called?
    a. A partnership
    b. A group practice
    c. A professional corporation
    d. A sole proprietorship

22. What is an advantage to forming a professional corporation to practice medicine?
    a. Physicians need just one license for the group.
    b. Fees can be higher.
    c. The incorporators and owners have limited liability in lawsuits.
    d. None of the above are true.

LO 3.5

23. Which of the following best defines a managed care health plan?
    a. Preferred provider organization
    b. A corporation that pays for and delivers care to subscribers
    c. A sole proprietorship
    d. A group practice

24. What is a copayment?
    a. A percentage of the fee for services provided
    b. A set amount that each patient pays for each office visit
    c. The portion of the fee the physician must write off
    d. The portion of the fee that the insurance company pays

25. Under this type of plan, insured patients must designate a primary care physician (PCP).
    a. Point-of-service plan
    b. Gatekeeper or primary care plan
    c. Independent practice plan
    d. Health maintenance plan

26. When physicians, hospitals, and other health care providers contract with one or more HMOs or directly with employers to provide care, what is it called?
    a. A physician-hospital organization
    b. A preferred provider plan
    c. A health maintenance organization
    d. A fee-for-service plan

27. Under this type of plan, a patient may see providers outside the plan, but the patient pays a higher portion of the fees.
    a. Health maintenance plan
    b. Independent practitioner plan
    c. Preferred provider plan
    d. Primary care plan

LO 3.6

28. The National Practitioner Data Bank
    a. Is accessible to everyone
    b. Is accessible to other providers on a routine basis
    c. Is accessible only to hospitals and health care plans
    d. Is accessible only to the government agencies monitoring health care

29. The Patients' Bill of Rights
    a. Is a state statute
    b. Is now law in 30 of the 50 states
    c. Has still not become law
    d. Is a federal law

30. What recent federal law provides for the establishment of state-run insurance exchanges?
    a. Federal False Claims Act
    b. Health Insurance Portability and Accountability Act
    c. Patient Protection and Affordable Care Act
    d. Health Care Quality Improvement Act.

31. Which of the following is *not* a stated goal of the Health Insurance Portability and Accountability Act?
    a. Ensure that every person has health insurance
    b. Improve the efficiency and effectiveness of the health care industry
    c. Help employees keep health insurance coverage when they transfer to another job
    d. Protect confidential medical information

LO 3.7

32. Which of the following statements best defines *telemedicine*?
    a. It is medicine that is practiced via telephone, closed-circuit television, fax machine, or Internet.
    b. It is medicine practiced only over the telephone.
    c. It is television programs that discuss medicine and health care.
    d. It is none of the above.

33. Cybermedicine involves
    a. Transmitting medical data over fax machines
    b. Direct online contact between physicians and patients
    c. Free medical consultations via a physician's Web site
    d. Robotic surgery

34. E-health refers to
    a. Endocrinology
    b. Consultation via e-mail from physician to patient
    c. Increasing use of the Internet for consumer health information
    d. Health business support services

CASE STUDIES

Use your critical thinking skills to answer the questions that follow each case study.

LO 3.1

Physician assistants (PAs) are employed in physician offices throughout the United States. Although the PA provides direct patient care, he or she is under the supervision of a licensed physician. Duties include taking patients' medical histories, performing physical examinations, ordering diagnostic and therapeutic procedures, providing follow-up care, and teaching and counseling patients. In most states, PAs may write prescriptions. The PA may be the only health care practitioner a patient sees during his or her visit to the physician office. Therefore, patients often refer to a PA as "the doctor." Ned, a PA for five years, says the patients he sees often address him as "doctor."

Similarly, Marie, a long-time employee of a physician in private practice, is often called "the doctor's nurse." Although Marie has never had the training necessary to become a certified medical assistant or a registered nurse, she sometimes refers to herself as the "office nurse."

35. What legal and ethical considerations are evident in these situations?

_____

_____

36. Should Ned and Marie allow patients to call them "doctor" or "nurse," respectively? Why or why not?

_____

_____

Note: A health care practitioner is held to the standard of care practiced by a reasonably competent person of the same profession. A physician assistant using the title "doctor" and a medical assistant using the title "nurse" may be held to the standard of care of a physician and a nurse, respectively, and may be accused of practicing without the appropriate license.

LO 3.2

A source of potential problems for health care practitioners is advertising. Buying print ads, creating radio spots, or sponsoring Web sites are commonplace activities for today's health care practitioners, which may subject them to a different type of lawsuit.

For example, two New Jersey patients sued their physician over the Web site ads she ran for LASIK eye surgery. The patients claimed the doctor made false or misleading statements in her ads, leading them to believe she would provide all of their treatment. Instead, the patients said a physician who was not fully licensed provided their follow-up care. (This practice is generally medically acceptable.) The two patients sued the physician under their state's Consumer Fraud Act, an area of law from which physicians have traditionally been exempt. A trial court allowed the suit to proceed, but the state supreme court reversed that decision, preventing the patients from suing the physician for advertising fraud.

37. In your opinion, should health care practitioners be protected from consumer fraud suits over advertising? Explain your answer.

_____

_____

38. As a health care practitioner, would you advertise your services? Why or why not?

_____

_____

[INTERNET ACTIVITIES LO 3.4 & LO 3.7]

Complete the activities and answer the questions that follow.

39. Conduct a Web search for "patient care partnership." This document, published by the American Hospital Association, replaces the previous Patients' Bill of Rights. What six points are listed under "What You Can Expect"?

_____

40. Visit the Web site for the National Practitioner Data Bank—Healthcare Integrity and Protection Data Bank (**www.npdb-hipdb.com**). How does one obtain information from either data bank?

_____

41. Conduct a Web search for "state telemedicine laws." Does your state have laws governing telemedicine? If so, briefly summarize them.

_____

[RESOURCES]

Joel, Lucille A. *Kelly's Dimensions of Professional Nursing*. New York: McGraw-Hill, 2011, Chap. 17.

Kubasek, Nancy, et al. *Dynamic Business Law*. New York: McGraw-Hill/ Irwin, 2009.

Liuzzo, Anthony L. *Essentials of Business Law*. New York: McGraw-Hill, 2010.

Mappes, Thomas A., and David DeGrazea. *Biomedical Ethics*. New York: McGraw-Hill, 2005, chap. 3.

Moini, Jahangir. *Medical Assisting Review*. New York: McGraw-Hill, 2008, chap. 8.

Telephone interview November 5, 2007, with Dr. Carmen Paradis, Dept. of Bioethics, Cleveland Clinic. She provided a copy of the Cleveland Clinic Health System's "Code of Ethical Business and Professional Behavior," quoted in Ethics Issue 1.

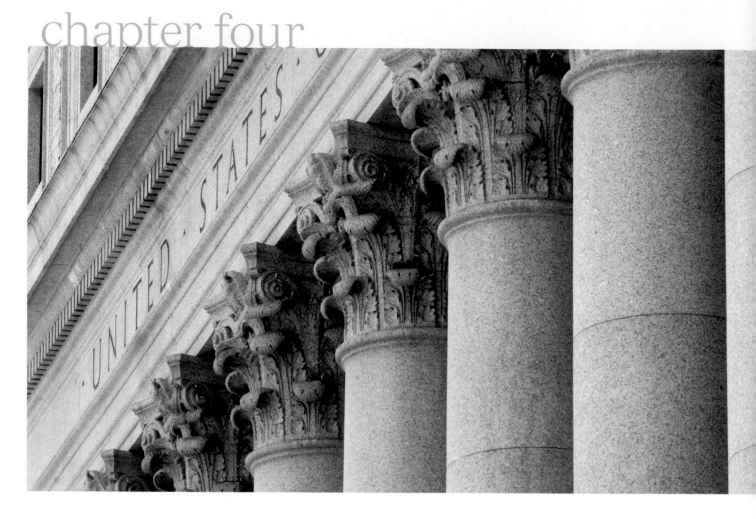

LAW, THE COURTS, AND CONTRACTS

Learning Outcomes

After studying this chapter, you should be able to:

LO 4.1 Discuss the basis of and primary sources of law.

LO 4.2 Discuss the classifications of law.

LO 4.3 Define the concept of torts and discuss how the tort of negligence affects health care.

LO 4.4 List and discuss the four essential elements of a contract.

LO 4.5 Differentiate between expressed contracts and implied contracts.

LO 4.6 Discuss the contractual rights and responsibilities of both physicians and patients.

LO 4.7 Relate how the law of agency and the doctrine of *respondeat superior* apply to health care contracts.

Cases in This Chapter

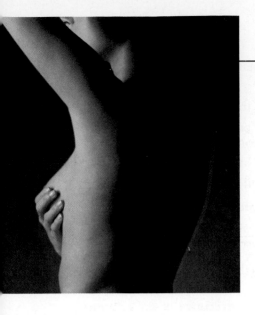

"SOMETIMES PATIENTS DON'T UNDERSTAND that what they are asking us to do is insurance fraud," says Christine, a patient billing specialist who works for a hospital in the Pacific Northwest. When Babs, a hospital patient, was treated for breast cancer, her physician obtained her informed consent to use a new treatment that he had helped develop. A drug was injected into her breast that targeted for destruction just the small malignant tumor; no healthy tissue was destroyed. Babs's medical insurance company refused to pay for the procedure, claiming it was "experimental." The procedure was new, but Babs's physician had used it many times with success. "Can't you just say I had a traditional lumpectomy," Babs asked Christine, "so my insurance company will pay for it?"

"We had to explain to Babs that this would constitute insurance fraud, and we couldn't do it," Christine explains.

From Babs's perspective, she wanted her insurance company to help pay for the expensive procedure.

From Christine's perspective, lying about the procedure performed was not only illegal but also unethical.

Why did Christine see Babs's request as insurance fraud?

What would you have recommended to Babs as a possible remedy for her dilemma over payment for the procedure?

The Basis of and Primary Sources of Law

LO 4.1

Discuss the basis of and primary sources of law.

The Federal Government

Federal laws governing the administration of health care and all other national matters derive from powers and responsibilities delegated to the three branches of government by the U.S. Constitution. As you probably recall from basic government classes, the three branches of government are legislative, executive, and judicial. Here is a quick review of the three branches' composition and responsibilities.

The two houses of Congress—the Senate and the House of Representatives—make up the *legislative branch*. Each member of Congress is elected by the people of his or her state. The House of Representatives, with membership based on state populations, has 435 seats, while the Senate, with two members from each state, has 100 seats. Members of the House of Representatives are elected for two-year terms, and senators are elected for six-year terms. The primary duty of Congress is to write, debate, and pass bills, which are then passed on to the president for approval.

Other powers of Congress include:

- Making laws controlling trade between states and between the United States and other countries.

- Making laws about taxes and borrowing money.

- Approving the printing of money.
- Declaring war on other countries.

Functions specific to the House of Representatives include the following. Members of the House can:

- Introduce legislation that compels people to pay taxes.
- Decide if a government official should be put on trial before the Senate if he or she commits a crime against the country. (Such a trial is called *impeachment*.)

Functions specific to the Senate include the following. Senators can:

- Approve and disapprove any treaties the president makes.
- Approve or disapprove any people the president recommends for jobs, such as cabinet officers, Supreme Court justices, and ambassadors.
- Hold an impeachment trial for a government official who commits a crime against the country.

The president of the United States is the chief executive of the *executive branch* of government, which is responsible for administering the law. Through his or her ability to issue **executive orders,** the president has limited legislative powers. Executive orders become law without the prior approval of Congress. They are usually issued for one of three purposes: to create administrative agencies or change the practices of an existing agency, to enforce laws passed by Congress, or to make treaties with foreign powers.

The U.S. Supreme Court heads the *judicial branch* of government, which also includes federal judges and courts in every state. The judicial branch interprets the law and oversees the enforcement of laws.

The division of powers and responsibilities among three branches of government ensures that a system of **checks and balances** will keep any one branch from assuming too much power (see Figure 4-1).

State Governments

State governments also have three branches: *legislative, executive,* and *judicial.* The number of state legislators a state may elect is based on the number of political districts in each state, since citizens elect legislators from the various districts. Therefore, the numbers of members of state legislatures are not the same as the number of members in the U.S. Congress.

State legislative branches also consist of two chambers: the Senate and the House of Representatives. In some states, the House of Representatives is called the Assembly or General Assembly. Terms served may be the same as in the federal government—six years for senators and two years for representatives or assembly members—or they may differ.

The governor is the head of the state's executive branch. Each state has its own constitution, but state constitutions cannot conflict with the U.S. Constitution. Those responsibilities not delegated by the federal constitution are left to the states (see Table 4-1).

There are four types of law, distinguished according to their origin:

1. **Constitutional law** is based on a formal document that defines broad governmental powers. Federal constitutional law is based on the U.S. Constitution (Figure 4-2). State constitutional law derives from each state's constitution.

2. **Case law** is law set by legal precedent. Case law began with **common law.** In the early days in America, laws derived from those originating in England, and they were often not written down. Matters of law

executive order A rule or regulation issued by the president of the United States that becomes law without the prior approval of Congress.

checks and balances The system established by the U.S. Constitution that keeps any one branch of government from assuming too much power over the other branches.

constitutional law Law that derives from federal and state constitutions.

case law Law established through common law and legal precedent.

common law The body of unwritten law developed in England, primarily from judicial decisions based on custom and tradition.

legal precedents Decisions made by judges in various courts that become rule of law and apply to future cases, even though they were not enacted by legislation.

statutory law Law passed by the U.S. Congress or state legislatures.

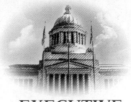

Can impeach president and remove him or her from office

Can veto congressional legislation

Can override executive's veto

Can reject judicial nominations

EXECUTIVE
Enforces Laws

LEGISLATIVE
Writes Laws

Can declare president's actions as unconstitutional

Can nominate and appoint judges

Can accept or reject judicial nominations

Can declare laws as unconstitutional

System of Checks and Balances

JUDICAL
Interprets Laws

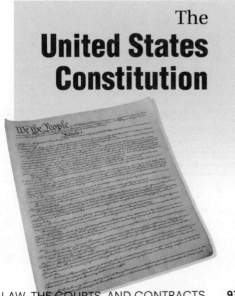

The
United States Constitution

were decided based on the customs and traditions of the people. Judges shared their decisions with other judges, and these decisions became common law.

Later, court decisions were written down, and judges could then refer to past cases to help them make current decisions. These written cases were then used as **legal precedents.** When deciding cases with similar circumstances, judges were required to follow these earlier cases or legal precedents. Today, legal precedents are the rule of law, applying to future cases, even though they were not enacted by legislation. Precedents can be changed only by the court that originally decided a case or by a higher court.

3. **Statutory law** refers to laws enacted by state or federal legislatures. Individual laws in this body of law are called statutes. (Laws passed by city governments are called municipal ordinances.) Statutes begin as bills at the federal or state levels. The bills may become laws, or the president or governors may veto

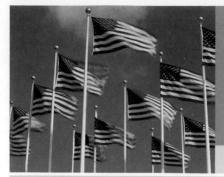

EXCLUSIVE POWERS OF THE NATIONAL GOVERNMENT AND STATE GOVERNMENTS

Table 4-1

National Government	State Governments
Print money	Issue licenses
Regulate interstate (between states) and international trade	Regulate intrastate (within the state) businesses
Make treaties and conduct foreign policy	Conduct elections
Declare war	Establish local governments
Provide an army and navy	Ratify amendments to the Constitution
Establish post offices	Take measures for public health and safety
Make laws necessary and proper to carry out the above powers	May exert powers the Constitution does not delegate to the national government or prohibit the states from using

administrative law
Enabling statutes enacted to define powers and procedures when an agency is created.

them. Once passed, the laws may be amended, repealed, revised, or superseded by legislatures. The courts can review statutes for constitutionality, application, interpretation, and other legal questions (see Figure 4-3).

4. **Administrative law** includes statutes enacted to define specific powers and procedures when agencies are created. Administrative agencies are created by Congress, by the president, or by individual state legislatures. Regulations may be passed that pertain specifically to the functions of one agency, such as the Internal Revenue Service (IRS), Social Security Administration, or Occupational Safety and Health Administration (OSHA).

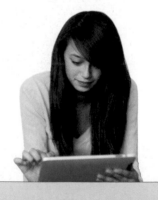

check your progress

Fill in the blanks or answer the following questions in the spaces provided.

1. Number the following two types of constitutions in the order in which they must be observed: state constitutions _____ federal constitution _____ .

2. Which branch has exclusive authority to declare war on another country?

3. Which chamber of the U.S. Congress has exclusive authority to hold an impeachment trial?

4. What are the four types of law, based on their origin?

5. Which of the above types of law began with common law?

6. Briefly define *administrative law*.

HOW A FEDERAL BILL BECOMES A LAW

CONGRESS

◄ SENATE   HOUSE ►

Subcommittee
Subcommittee performs studies, holds hearings, and makes revisions. If approved, the bill goes to the full committee.

Bill introduction
Bill is introduced by a member and assigned to a committee, which usually refers it to a subcommittee.

Bill introduction
Bill is introduced by a member and assigned to a committee, which usually refers it to a subcommittee.

Subcommittee
Subcommittee performs studies, holds hearings, and makes revisions. If approved, the bill goes to the full committee.

Committee
Full committee may amend or rewrite the bill, before deciding whether to send it to the Senate floor, recommending its approval, or to kill it. If approved, the bill is reported to the full Senate and placed on the calender.

Committee
Full Committee may amend or rewrite the bill, before deciding whether to send it to the House floor, recommending its approval, or to kill it. If approved, the bill is reported to the full House and placed on the calender.

Leadership
Senate leaders of both parties schedule Senate debate on the bill.

Full Senate
Bill is debated by full Senate, amendments are offered, and a vote is taken. If the bill passes in a different version from that passed in the House, it is sent to a conference committee.

Conference Committee
Conference committee composed of members of both House and Senate meets to iron out differences between the bills. The compromise bill is returned to both the House and Senate for a vote.

Full House
Bill is debated by full House, amendments are offered, and a vote is taken. If the bill passes in a different version from that passed in the Senate, it is sent to a conference committee.

Rules Committee
Rules committee issues a rule governing debate on the House floor and sends the bill to the full House.

Full Senate
Full Senate votes on conference committee version. If it passes, the bill is sent to the president.

Full House
Full House votes on conference committee version. If it passes, the bill is sent to the president.

President
President signs or vetoes the bill. Congress may override a veto by a two-thirds vote in both the House and Senate.

Law

- Committee action
- Bill introduction
- Floor Action
- Conference Action
- Presidential Decision

substantive law The statutory or written law that defines and regulates legal rights and obligations.

procedural law Law that defines the rules used to enforce substantive law.

criminal law Law that involves crimes against the state.

felony An offense punishable by death or by imprisonment in a state or federal prison for more than one year.

misdemeanor A crime punishable by fine or by imprisonment in a facility other than a prison for less than one year.

Classifications of Law

After laws are created through constitutional, case, statutory, or administrative law, they are classified by type. Two broad types of law are substantive and procedural. **Substantive law** is the statutory or written law that defines and regulates legal rights and obligations. It defines the legal relationships between people or between people and the state, and is further classified as criminal, civil, military, and international law. Examples of substantive laws include the criminal laws that define murder, arson, and armed robbery as crimes, and the civil laws that allow individuals to sue persons or entities.

Procedural law defines the rules used to enforce substantive law. For example, laws that require law enforcement officers to read suspects their rights (the Miranda warning), and govern the arrest and trial process are procedural laws.

Criminal and civil laws are most likely to pertain to health care practitioners.

Criminal Law

A crime is an offense against the state or sovereignty, committed or omitted, in violation of a public law forbidding or commanding it. Therefore, the body of **criminal law** involves crimes against the state. When a state or federal criminal law is violated, the government brings criminal charges against the alleged offender (for example, *New York v. John Doe*).

State criminal laws prohibit such crimes as murder, burglary, robbery, arson, rape, larceny, mayhem (needless or willful damage or violence), and practicing medicine without a license. Federal criminal offenses include matters affecting national security (treason); crimes involving the country's borders; and illegal activities that cross state lines, such as kidnapping or hijacking.

A criminal act may be classified as a felony or a misdemeanor. A **felony** is a crime punishable by death or by imprisonment in a state or federal prison for more than one year. Felonies include abuse (child abuse, elder abuse, or domestic violence), arson, burglary, conspiracy, embezzlement, fraud, illegal drug dealing, grand larceny, manslaughter, mayhem, murder or attempted murder, rape, robbery, tax evasion, and practicing medicine without a license.

Misdemeanors are less serious crimes than felonies. They are punishable by fines or by imprisonment in a facility other than a prison for one year or less. Examples of misdemeanors include some traffic violations, thefts under a certain dollar amount, attempted burglary, and disturbing the peace.

Can Knowledge of a Crime Make You Guilty? Persons who commit crimes are, of course, the principals in criminal proceedings. However, those individuals who have knowledge of a crime may, in certain circumstances, also be subject to prosecution. An *accessory* is one who contributes to or aids in the commission of a crime—by a direct act, by an indirect act (such as encouragement), by watching and not giving aid, or by concealing the criminal's crime. For example, the person in charge of billing for health care services in a medical office may be an accessory to insurance fraud if he or she takes no action, even though he or she knows that some health care practitioners are billing for services not rendered.

Civil Law

Criminal law involves crimes against the state; **civil law** does not involve crimes but instead involves wrongful acts against persons. Under civil law, a person can sue another person, a business, or the government. Civil disputes often arise over issues of contract violation, slander, libel, trespassing, product liability, or automobile accidents. Many civil suits involve family matters such as divorce, child support, and child custody. Court judgments in civil cases often require the payment of a sum of money to the injured party.

> **civil law** Law that involves wrongful acts against persons.

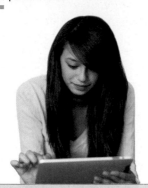

check your **progress**

Fill in the blanks or answer the following questions in the spaces provided.

7. The written law that says murder is a crime is an example of _____ law.

8. The law that says a law enforcement officer must read a prisoner his or her rights is an example of which type of law?

9. Civil law that says one person may sue another for a specific reason is broadly classified as _____ law.

10. The laws that determine the rules for one person's suing of another are broadly classified as _____ law.

11. _____ law involves crimes against the state.

12. _____ law involves wrongful acts against persons.

13. Which two types of law are most likely to affect health care providers?

14. Under criminal law, practicing medicine without a license is classified as a(n) _____ .

15. Which type of law does not involve crimes, but may involve one person suing another?

16. Court judgments in lawsuits against health care practitioners most often include what as a penalty?

Tort Liability

Civil law includes a general category of law known as torts. A **tort** is broadly defined as a civil wrong committed against a person or property, excluding breach of contract. The act, committed without just cause, may have caused physical injury, resulted in damage to someone's property, or deprived someone of his or her personal liberty and freedom. Torts may be intentional (willful) or unintentional (accidental).

Intentional Torts

Some torts involve intentional misconduct. When one person intentionally harms another, the law allows the injured party to seek a remedy in a civil

LO 4.3
Define the concept of torts and discuss how the tort of negligence affects health care.

> **tort** A civil wrong committed against a person or property, excluding breach of contract.

suit. The injured party can be financially compensated for any harm done by the **tortfeasor** (person guilty of committing a tort). If the conduct is judged to be malicious, punitive damages may also be awarded. Examples of intentional torts include the following:

Assault. The open threat of bodily harm to another, or acting in such a way as to put another in the "reasonable apprehension of bodily harm."

Battery. An action that causes bodily harm to another. It is broadly defined as any bodily contact made without permission. Battery may or may not result from the threat of assault. In health care delivery, battery may be charged for any unauthorized touching of a patient, including such actions as suturing a wound, administering an injection, or performing a physical examination.

Defamation of Character. Involves damaging a person's reputation by making public statements that are both false and malicious. Defamation can take the form of libel or slander. Libel is expressing in published print, writing, pictures, or signed statements content that injure the reputation of another. Libel also includes reading statements aloud or broadcasting for the public to hear. Slander is speaking defamatory or damaging words intended to prejudice others against an individual in a manner that jeopardizes his or her reputation or means of livelihood.

False Imprisonment. The intentional, unlawful restraint or confinement of one person by another. The offense is treated as a crime in some states. Refusing to dismiss a patient from a health care facility on his or her request, or preventing an employee or patient from leaving the facility might be seen as false imprisonment.

Fraud. Deceitful practices in depriving or attempting to deprive another of his or her rights. Health care practitioners might be accused of fraud for promising patients "miracle cures" or for accepting fees from patients for using mystical or spiritual powers to heal.

Invasion of Privacy. An intrusion into a person's seclusion or private affairs, public disclosure of private facts about a person, false publicity about a person, or use of a person's name or likeness without permission. Improper use of or breaching the confidentiality of medical records may be seen as invasion of privacy.

Intentional torts may also be crimes. Therefore, some civil wrongs may also be prosecuted as criminal acts in separate court actions. See Table 4-2 for a summary of intentional torts.

Unintentional Torts

The more common torts within the health care delivery system are those committed unintentionally. Unintentional torts are acts that are not intended to cause harm but are committed unreasonably or with a disregard for the consequences. In legal terms, this constitutes **negligence**.

Negligence is charged when a health care practitioner fails to exercise ordinary care, and a patient is injured. The accused may have performed an act or failed to perform an act that a reasonable person, in similar circumstances, would or would not have performed. "Didn't intend to do it" or "should have known better" best describe a negligent act. Under principles of negligence, civil liability exists only in cases in which the act is judicially determined to be wrongful. A health care practitioner, for example, is not necessarily liable for a poor-quality outcome in delivering health care. He or she becomes liable only when his or her conduct is determined to be malpractice, the negligent delivery of professional services.

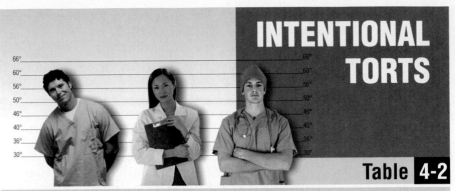

INTENTIONAL TORTS

Table 4-2

Tort	Description
Assault	Threatening to strike or harm with a weapon or physical movement, resulting in fear
Battery	Unlawful, unprivileged touching of another person
Trespass	Wrongful injury to or interference with the property of another
Nuisance	Anything that interferes with the enjoyment of life or property
Interference with contractual relations	Intentionally causing one person not to enter into or to break a contract with another
Deceit	False statement or deceptive practice done with intent to injure another
Conversion	Unauthorized taking or borrowing of personal property of another for the use of the taker
False imprisonment (false arrest)	Unlawful restraint of a person, whether in prison or otherwise
Defamation	Wrongful act of injuring another's reputation by making false statements
Invasion of privacy	Interference with a person's right to be left alone
Misuse of legal procedure	Bringing legal action with malice and without probable cause
Infliction of emotional distress	Intentionally or recklessly causing emotional or mental suffering to another
Fraud	Dishonest or deceitful practices in depriving, or attempting to deprive, another of his or her rights

Negligence and defenses to liability suits are discussed in detail in Chapter 5.

Negligence is often alleged in lawsuits against health care practitioners, as in the case, "Chiropractor's Outrageous Conduct." As illustrated in the court case on page 101, hospitals are not immune to charges of negligence.

Most times we think of medical negligence cases as those brought against doctors or medical personnel individually, but a hospital or other institution is held to the same standard of care as a doctor or a physician. So when evaluating a case for institutional negligence, the standard is, What would/should a reasonably careful hospital do under similar circumstances?

COURT CASE

Chiropractor's Outrageous Conduct Results in Trial

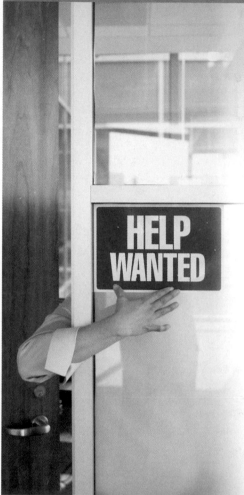

A chiropractor had two patients who became his employees. The two patients/employees sued the chiropractor for outrageous conduct and invasion of privacy, based on the fact that each plaintiff had a sexual relationship with the chiropractor, and when the two plaintiffs told the chiropractor they wanted to end their sexual relationships with him, he threatened to stop their medical treatment and to fire them. He also exposed himself to the two plaintiffs in his office, and allegedly otherwise harassed them sexually.

A trial court found for the two plaintiffs, and the chiropractor appealed. The appellate court concluded that the trial court did not err in determining that "reasonable people could find the chiropractor's conduct so outrageous in character, and so extreme in degree, as to go beyond all possible bounds of decency and be regarded as atrocious and utterly intolerable." The judgment of the trial court was affirmed.

The jury awarded Pearson $237,685 in compensatory damages on her chiropractic negligence claim, $100,000 in compensatory and punitive damages on her claim for outrageous conduct, and $200,000 in compensatory and punitive damages on her claim for invasion of privacy. The jury awarded Fahy $229,400 in compensatory damages on her chiropractic negligence claim and $100,000 in compensatory and punitive damages on her claim for outrageous conduct. The trial court entered judgment accordingly.

Note: Whether or not the chiropractor lost his license to practice was not decided by this court but was a matter for his state licensing board to decide.

Source: Pearson and Fahy v. Kancilla, 70P.3d 594 (Colo. App. 2003).

COURT CASE

Physician Sued for Negligence

A physician sterilized a female patient who had sought such a procedure to avoid having more children. The woman later became pregnant and delivered a healthy child. She sued her physician, alleging that the doctor's performance of a sterilization procedure had been negligent and seeking damages for the future expenses of raising a child. The physician filed a motion for preliminary determination. A trial court denied the motion, permitting the plaintiff to seek damages for raising the child. The physician appealed.

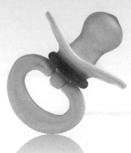

The appellate court held that the parents were not "injured" by delivering a healthy child, and, therefore, could not receive an award for damages. The court reversed the trial court's order denying the physician's motion for preliminary determination and remanded the case for "further proceedings consistent with this opinion."

Source: Chaffee v. Seslar, 786 N.E.2d 705; 2003 Ind.

Chicago Hospital's Negligence Clarified by Illinois Appellate Court

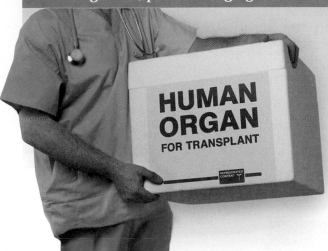

In 2008, the Illinois Appellate Court affirmed a Cook County jury's $2.7 million verdict for institutional negligence against Loyola Medical Center in a Chicago transplant error case.

The issue in *Longnecker* was whether Loyola University Medical Center was negligent when it transplanted the decedent with a severely hypertrophic replacement heart. The harvested heart was severely diseased and was considered for transplantation only because the harvesting doctors did not examine it. Despite the diseased state of the new heart, the decedent's heart surgeon went ahead with the transplant. The decedent died without ever waking up from the surgery.

Source: Longnecker v. Loyola University Medical Center, 2008 WL 2550686 (1st Dist., June 25).

There are two different ways a hospital can face liability under medical malpractice. A hospital can be held liable for the medical negligence conducted by its agents or employees, or it can be liable for its own institutional negligence. According to legal experts, a hospital owes its patients a duty to exercise a reasonable degree of care when dealing with an apparent risk.

Various types of evidence are useful in establishing a hospital's standard of care, including expert testimony, existing federal and state laws, hospital bylaws, custom and community practice, and accreditation standards. And while expert testimony is typically required in medical malpractice cases, sometimes institutional negligence can be established without expert testimony.

The Court System

The type of court that tries a case depends on the state law or federal law that was allegedly violated. The federal court system, with some exceptions, hears cases involving federal matters. State court systems are independent of one another, and each system has its own rules and regulations. Generally, state courts decide cases involving matters occurring within their own state borders.

Federal Courts **Jurisdiction** is the power of a court to hear and decide a case before it. In most common law systems, jurisdiction is conceptually divided between jurisdiction over the subject matter of a case and jurisdiction over the person of the litigants. Examples of cases over which federal courts have jurisdiction include federal crimes, federal antitrust law, bankruptcy, patents, copyrights, trademarks, suits against the United States, and areas of admiralty law (pertaining to the sea).

> **jurisdiction** The power of a court to hear and decide a case before it.

State Courts Each state has its own court system, but the general structure is the same in all states. The bottom tier consists of local courts. The next highest tier is trial courts, followed by appellate courts, and then the state supreme court. As with the federal court system, there are also special state courts with jurisdiction in certain kinds of cases.

plaintiff The person bringing charges in a lawsuit.

prosecution The government as plaintiff in a criminal case.

defendant The person or party against whom charges are brought in a criminal or civil lawsuit.

> Figure 4-4

Figure 4-4 shows the various federal and state court systems in the United States.

Players in the Court Scene

When criminal and civil cases go to court, a complaining party—the **plaintiff**—must show that he or she was wronged or injured. The government—the **prosecution**—is the plaintiff in criminal cases. A private individual is the plaintiff in civil cases. The **defendant,** who is charged with an offense, must dispute the complaint.

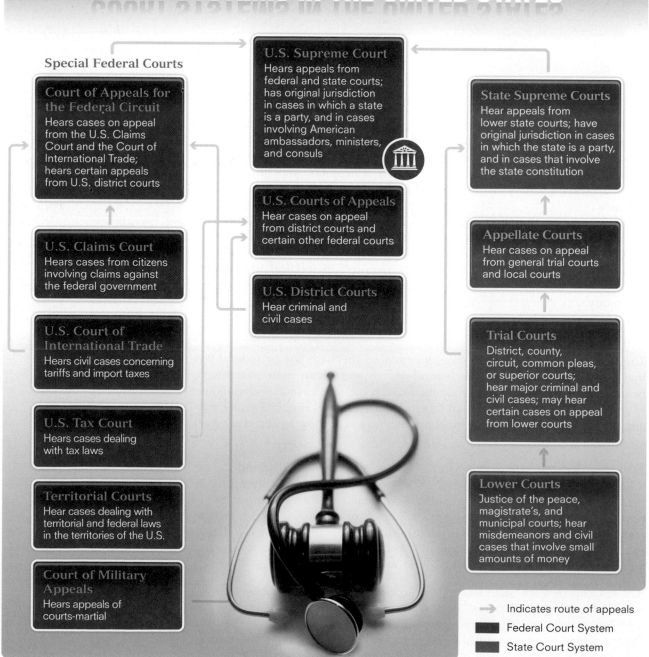

COURT SYSTEMS IN THE UNITED STATES

Special Federal Courts

Court of Appeals for the Federal Circuit
Hears cases on appeal from the U.S. Claims Court and the Court of International Trade; hears certain appeals from U.S. district courts

U.S. Claims Court
Hears cases from citizens involving claims against the federal government

U.S. Court of International Trade
Hears civil cases concerning tariffs and import taxes

U.S. Tax Court
Hears cases dealing with tax laws

Territorial Courts
Hear cases dealing with territorial and federal laws in the territories of the U.S.

Court of Military Appeals
Hears appeals of courts-martial

U.S. Supreme Court
Hears appeals from federal and state courts; has original jurisdiction in cases in which a state is a party, and in cases involving American ambassadors, ministers, and consuls

U.S. Courts of Appeals
Hear cases on appeal from district courts and certain other federal courts

U.S. District Courts
Hear criminal and civil cases

State Supreme Courts
Hear appeals from lower state courts; have original jurisdiction in cases in which the state is a party, and in cases that involve the state constitution

Appellate Courts
Hear cases on appeal from general trial courts and local courts

Trial Courts
District, county, circuit, common pleas, or superior courts; hear major criminal and civil cases; may hear certain cases on appeal from lower courts

Lower Courts
Justice of the peace, magistrate's, and municipal courts; hear misdemeanors and civil cases that involve small amounts of money

→ Indicates route of appeals
■ Federal Court System
■ State Court System

Officers of the court are responsible for carrying out courtroom duties:

- *Judges* are elected or appointed to preside over the court and in most states must be licensed attorneys. They rule on points of law about trial procedure, presentation of evidence, and all laws that apply to the case. If there is no jury, the judge determines the facts in the case. Judges hand down sentences after a verdict is rendered.

- *Attorneys* represent plaintiffs and defendants, presenting evidence so that the jury or the judge can reach a verdict.

- *Court clerks* keep court records and seals, enter court orders and judgments into the record, and keep the papers of the court.

- *Bailiffs* keep order in the courtroom and may remove disruptive persons from the court at the judge's request.

- *Court reporters* make a running account of all court proceedings, using a stenotype machine that types shorthand symbols onto a tape.

- *Juries* are most often selected from lists of registered voters. Six or 12 jurors are chosen to hear the evidence presented in court and render a verdict.

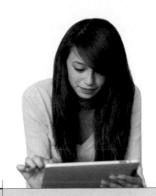

check your **progress**

Fill in the blanks to accurately complete the following statements.

17. The highest tier of federal courts consists of _____ .

18. A lawsuit brought by a patient against a health care practitioner would be heard first in a(n) _____ court.

19. Torts are wrongs committed against _____ .

20. The two broad types of torts include _____ and

_____ .

21. The type of tort most likely to concern health care practitioners is

_____ .

Contracts

A **contract** is a voluntary agreement between two parties in which specific promises are made for a consideration. The elements of a contract are important to health care practitioners because health care delivery takes place under various types of contracts. To be legally binding, four elements must be present in a contract.

1. *Agreement.* One party makes an offer, and another party accepts it. Certain conditions pertain to the offer:

   - It can relate to the present or the future.
   - It must be communicated.
   - It must be made in good faith and not under duress or as a joke.
   - It must be clear enough to be understood by both parties.
   - It must define what both parties will do if the offer is accepted.

   For example, a physician offers his or her services to the public by obtaining a license to practice medicine and opening for business. Patients accept the physician's offer by scheduling appointments,

LO 4.4

List and discuss the four essential elements of a contract.

> **contract** A voluntary agreement between two parties in which specific promises are made for a consideration.

submitting to physical examinations, and allowing the physician to prescribe or perform medical treatment. The contract is complete when the physician's fee is paid.

2. *Consideration.* Something of value is bargained for as part of the agreement. In the previous example, the physician's consideration is providing his or her services; the patient's consideration is payment of the physician's fee.

3. *Legal Subject Matter.* Contracts are not valid and enforceable in court unless they are for legal services or purposes. For example, a contract entered into by a patient to pay for services of a physician in private practice would be **void** (not legally enforceable) if the physician were not duly licensed to practice medicine. **Breach of contract** may be charged if either party fails to comply with the terms of a legally valid contract.

4. *Contractual capacity.* Parties who enter into the agreement must be capable of fully understanding all of its terms and conditions. A **mentally incompetent** person cannot enter into a legal contract. For example, persons declared legally insane, persons in a drug-altered mental state, and in some cases, persons under extreme duress are considered incapable of entering into a contract. Exceptions may be made for situations in which a contract is necessary to sustain life.

If either of the concerned parties is incompetent at the time a contract is made, the agreement may be **voidable,** that is, able to be set aside or to be validated at a later date. Say, for example, a patient enters into a contract while under the effects of a medication that can interfere with judgment. After the effects of the medication have worn off, the patient may say, "No, I don't want the contract enforced" or "Yes, I want the contract enforced."

Of special concern to health care providers is the physician–patient contract as applied to minors. Because of the risk of being accused of battery or assault, health care practitioners cannot treat a minor without the consent of a responsible parent or legal guardian, except in cases where minors suffer a life-threatening emergency, or have been legally determined to be mature. A **minor** is defined as anyone under the age of majority, which is 18 in most states, and 21 in some jurisdictions. See Chapter 11 for a more extensive discussion of minors and the administration of medical services.

Sometimes breach of contract becomes an additional issue in medical negligence lawsuits, as in the following case, "Breach of Contract Also Charged."

---

void Without legal force or effect.

breach of contract Failure of either party to comply with the terms of a legally valid contract.

mentally incompetent Unable to fully understand all the terms and conditions of a transaction, and therefore unable to enter into a legal contract.

voidable Able to be set aside or to be revalidated at a later date.

minor Anyone under the age of majority: 18 years in most states, 21 years in some jurisdictions.

COURT CASE

Breach of Contract Also Charged in Medical Negligence Lawsuit

A nurse treated an inmate at the county jail with an injection of 200 mg of Prolixin decanoate that resulted in the inmate's permanent impotence. He filed an action against the nurse, the hospital, and the health care organization for negligence and breach of contract. A jury found for the plaintiff and awarded him damages in the amount of $450,500. The defendants appealed the decision and the award. An appeals court upheld the trial court's decision and award, except for $100,000 awarded as part of the breach-of-contract claim. The appeals court held that since the plaintiff was not part of the contract between the nurse and her employer, he was not entitled to damages on that claim.

Source: Dempsey v. Pease, Mercy Health Services, St. Joseph Mercy Hospital (Court of Appeals of Michigan, 2001).

Types of Contracts

The two main types of contracts are expressed contracts and implied contracts. **Expressed contracts** are explicitly stated in written or spoken words. **Implied contracts** are unspoken. Their terms result from actions of the involved parties.

Expressed Contracts

An expressed contract may be written or oral, but all terms of the contract are explicitly stated. In the medical office, some contracts, to be legally valid, must be in writing. In each state the **Statute of Frauds,** derived from the Statute for the Prevention of Frauds and Perjuries formulated in England in 1677, states which contracts must be in writing to be enforced.

Termination of Contracts

The contract between a physician and a patient is usually terminated (ended) when all treatment has been completed and the bill has been paid. Situations may arise, however, in which premature termination of the contract takes place, as in the following situations:

> **Failure to Pay for Services.** A physician may stop treatment of a patient and end the physician–patient relationship if the patient habitually does not pay or fails to make satisfactory arrangements to pay for medical services, but only if adequate notice is given to the patient.

> **Failure to Keep Scheduled Appointments.** To protect the physician from charges of abandonment, all missed appointments should be noted on the patient's chart.

> **Failure to Follow the Physician's Instructions.** It makes no difference whether the failure is due to a patient's willfulness or negligence.

> **A Patient Seeks the Services of Another Physician.** Whenever a patient acknowledges, orally or in writing, that he or she will seek medical care from another physician, the medical office employee should document this on the patient's chart, and then send a letter to the patient verifying the termination. A copy of the letter should be filed with the patient's records. Seeking a second opinion, however, does not necessarily terminate the physician–patient relationship.

A patient may terminate a physician–patient relationship at any time. After a physician agrees to treat a patient, however, his or her responsibilities to the patient continue until the relationship is properly terminated. If a physician suddenly withdraws from treatment while the patient is still in need of medical care, fails to visit a hospitalized patient, or otherwise abandons the patient without arranging for substitute care, he or she may be charged with abandonment. Depending on the circumstances, the physician may also be charged with breach of contract and/or negligence.

To properly terminate the physician–patient relationship, the physician must give the patient formal written notice that he or she is withdrawing from the case. The physician should also note any need for the patient to receive continued medical care. In addition, the patient must be given time to find another physician. The notice of discharge of withdrawal should be sent by certified mail, return receipt requested, and a copy should be filed with the patient's records. Figure 4-5 illustrates a notice of termination.

Managed care plans *may* restrict a physician from terminating patient care without the approval of the managed care plan.

Laws Governing Payment of Fees at Fulfillment of Contracts

Certain federal and state laws govern the payment of fees when contracts

expressed contract A written or oral agreement in which all terms are explicitly stated.

implied contract An unwritten and unspoken agreement whose terms result from the actions of the parties involved.

Statute of Frauds State legislation governing written contracts.

Figure 4-5 Physician's Letter of Dismissal for Nonpayment

Health & wellness Center

Date _____

William Smith
1212 Economy Drive
Dallas, Texas
75001

Certified Mail # _____

Dear William Smith,

This letter is to inform you that I will no longer be your physician and will stop providing medical care to you effective 30 days from the date you receive this letter.

I will continue to provide routine and emergency medical care to you for 30 days while you seek another physician.

I suggest you consult the local physician referral service, your county medical society, or the yellow pages of your telephone book as soon as possible so that you may find another physician who will assume responsibility for your care.

I will be pleased to assist the physician of your choice by sending him or her a copy of your medical records.

Sincerely,

_____
(Physician Signature)

Department of _____

third-party payer contract
A written agreement signed by a party other than the patient who promises to pay the patient's bill.

have been fulfilled. For example, a type of contract often used in the medical office that falls under the Statute of Frauds, which is state law governing written contracts, is the **third-party payer contract.** Insurance policies are also third-party payer contracts, but as used here, the term means agreements by a third party to pay for services rendered to another. Such contracts must be in writing to be enforced and should be signed before health care services are rendered. For example, suppose Susan becomes ill while visiting her aunt in a distant city, and the aunt makes an appointment for Susan to see her physician. The aunt tells the medical office assistant, "I will pay Susan's bill." The medical office assistant may ask Susan's aunt to sign a third-party payer contract.

Not all financial arrangements that require written contracts fall under the Statute of Frauds. Others are governed by Regulation Z or Regulation M of the Consumer Protection Act of 1968, also known as the Truth-in-Lending

Act. Regulation Z applies to each individual or business that offers or extends consumer credit if four conditions are met:

1. The credit is offered to consumers.
2. Credit is offered on a regular basis.
3. The credit is subject to a finance charge (interest) or must be paid in more than four installments according to a written agreement.
4. The credit is primarily for personal, family, or household purposes. Regulation M applies only if credit is extended to businesses, or for commercial or agricultural purposes.

For example, Regulation Z of the Consumer Protection Act applies in a health care setting such as the following: A patient and a physician make a bilateral payment agreement (one in which both parties are mutually affected) that medical fees will be paid in four or more installments or will include finance charges. (It is legal and ethical for physicians to levy finance charges, as long as this is made clear to the patient before the charges are incurred.) This agreement must be in writing and must contain the following information:

- Fees for services.
- Amount of any down payment.
- The date each payment is due.
- The date of the final payment.
- The amount of each payment.
- Any interest charges to be made.

The patient signs the agreement and is given a copy. A second copy is filed with the patient's records.

For agreements falling under Regulation Z of the Truth-in-Lending Act, the medical office must supply the patient with a written disclosure statement (see Figure 4-6). The primary purpose of this legislation is to protect consumers from fraudulent or deceptive hidden finance charges levied by creditors, but creditors can also use it to collect outstanding debts.

The federal **Fair Debt Collection Practices Act (FDCPA)** of 1978 requires debt collectors and creditors to treat debtors fairly. It ensures fair treatment by prohibiting certain methods of debt collection. Debt collections practices prohibited by the act include harassment, misrepresentation, threats, disseminating false information about the debtor, and engaging in unfair or illegal practices in attempting to collect a debt. Personal, family, and household debts are covered under the act. This includes money owed for the purchase of an automobile, medical care, and charge accounts.

In the following court case, "No Breach of Contract," a patient sued a radiologist for breach of an expressed warranty (contract), alleging that the radiologist had told him he would not suffer any ill effects from an arteriogram procedure. What are the implications for health care practitioners who tell patients, "This procedure won't cause any damage"?

Implied Contracts

Implied contracts are those in which the conduct of the parties, rather than expressed words, creates the contract. Most contracts in the medical office are implied. For example, suppose a patient comes to a clinic complaining of a sore throat and asks to see a physician. The physician does not literally say to the patient, "I offer to treat your condition," but by making his or her services available, he or she has made an offer to treat. A patient does not state to the physician, "I accept your offer to provide medical care." Acceptance is implied by the patient's actions in allowing the physician to examine him

Fair Debt Collection Practices Act (FDCPA)
A federal statute prohibiting certain unfair and illegal practices by debt collectors and creditors. It prohibits certain methods of debt collection, including harassment, misrepresentation, threats, disseminating false information about the debtor, and engaging in unfair or illegal practices in attempting to collect a debt.

Figure 4-6 Truth-in-Lending Payment Agreement

Bruce Whiting, MD
310 Madison Avenue,
Anderson, Indiana 46027

I agree to pay $ _____ per week/month on my account balance of $_____.

Payments are due by the _____ of each_____ and will begin_____.
(week/month)   (date)

Interest will/will not be changed on the outstanding balance (see Truth-in-Lending form below for rate of interest).

I agree that if payments are not made in the full amount stated above or if payments are not received on time, the entire account balance will be considered delinquent and will be due and payable immediately.

I agree to be responsible for any reasonable collection costs or attorney fees incurred in collecting a delinquent account.

Date   Signature

This disclosure is in compliance with the Truth-in-Lending Act.

Patient's Name   Address

Responsible Party (if other than patient)   City, State, Zip Code

1. Cash price (Medical and/or Surgical Fee)
   Less cash down payment (Advance)
2. Unpaid balance of cash price
3. Amount financed
4. Finance charge
5. Total of payments (3 + 4)
6. Deferred payment price (1 + 4)
7. Annual percentage rate

The "Total of payments" shown above is payable to Bruce Whiting, MD, at the address shown above in _____ monthly installments of $_____ the first installment being payable _____ and all subsequent installments are due on the same day of each consecutive month until paid in full. (date)

Date   Signature

Figure 4-7

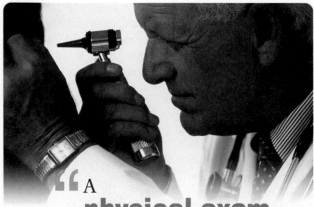

"A **physical exam** is an example of an implied contract. "

or her and prescribe treatment (see Figure 4-7). The physician's consideration is providing services. The patient's consideration is payment of the physician's fee. The contract is valid if both parties understand the offer, both are competent, and the services provided are legal.

A physician who provides emergency treatment to a patient in a situation not covered by a special arrangement, such as in an emergency room, is limited to providing treatment at the site of the emergency. In such a situation, an implied limited contract between the physician and the patient is created, based on the patient's implied request for and consent to emergency treatment. The patient's promise to pay for the physician's services is also implied. In this case, the physician's obligation for care does not extend to treatment after the emergency situation has been resolved.

Physician–Patient Contracts and Managed Care

Managed care plans have added a third element to the physician–patient contract. Physicians still have contracts with their patients, but they may also have contracted with managed care programs to deliver medical services. If a physician terminates his or her contractual relationship with a managed care plan, this does not mean he or she cannot continue to see patients insured with the plan. It simply means the managed care plan will no longer pay for the subscriber's visits to this physician.

All insurance providers, including managed care plans, have access to patients' medical records for purposes of utilization review, inpatient stay review, case management review, and quality management. Insurance providers also check enrollees' medical records to monitor care and to identify ways of preventing illness and disease.

Although the following court case, "Physician Sued for Breach," was decided in 1989, it remains relevant in today's world, where printed or electronic images of patients are likely to be widely circulated.

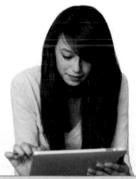

check your **progress**

22. List the four elements present in a legally valid contract, and give an example of each.

23. Tell whether each of the following examples involves an expressed or an implied contract:

    _____ A man agrees to buy his friend's car and seals the deal with a handshake.

    _____ A medical center outpatient agrees to undergo a colonoscopy.

    _____ A patient in a physician's office agrees to a physical examination.

    _____ A physician treats a patient for a broken leg in a hospital emergency room.

24. List three federal laws governing collections in the medical office.

25. Briefly explain how managed care has impacted physician–patient contracts.

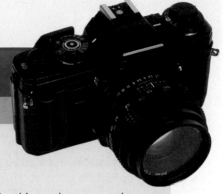

LO 4.6

Discuss the contractual rights and responsibilities of both physicians and patients.

Physicians' and Patient' Rights and Responsibilities

Physicians

A physician has the right, after agreeing to accept an individual as his or her patient, to make reasonable limitations on the relationship. The physician is under no legal obligation to treat patients who may wish to exceed those limitations. Under the provisions of the physician–patient contract, both parties have certain rights and responsibilities. A physician has the right to:

- Set up practice within the boundaries of his or her license to practice medicine. A specialist, for instance, does not have to practice outside the area of specialty and, in fact, would be severely criticized for doing so, except in an emergency in which no other physician were available.

- Set up an office wherever he or she chooses and establish office hours.

- Specialize.

- Decide which services he or she will provide and how those services will be provided.

While practicing within the context of an implied contract with the patient, the physician is not bound to:

- Treat every patient who seeks medical care. The physician is free to use his or her own discretion—with one exception. If a physician is hired specifically to treat patients in one area or locale, such as a hospital emergency room, he or she must treat every patient who comes to that locale.

- Restore the patient to his or her original state of health. The fact that a patient grows progressively worse while under a physician's care and shows improvement when care is withdrawn does not necessarily constitute liability.

- Possess the highest skills possible within the profession or the maximum education attainable.

- Effect a recovery with every patient. The physician who fails to heal a patient cannot be condemned for lack of skill.

- Be familiar with the various reactions of patients to anesthetics or drugs of any kind. However, the physician is bound to note any allergic or adverse reactions to medications reported by the patient before treatment is administered.

- Be as skilled as a specialist if he or she is a general practitioner.

- Make a correct diagnosis in every case.

- Be free from mistakes of judgment in difficult cases.

- Display infallibility of judgment.

- Continue services after being discharged by the patient or by some responsible person, even if harm should come to the patient.

- Guarantee the successful result of any treatment or operation. In fact, guarantees of "cures" may constitute fraud on the part of the physician.

Under an implied contract with the patient, the physician has the obligation to:

- Use due care, skill, judgment, and diligence in treating patients, which other physicians of the same practice usually exercise in similar locations and under similar circumstances.

- Stay informed about the best methods of diagnosis and treatment.

- Perform to the best of his or her ability, whether or not he or she is to receive a fee.

- Exercise his or her best professional judgment in all cases, particularly those in which considerable doubt is involved.

- Consider the established, customary treatment administered by members of the medical profession in similar cases.

- Abstain from performing experiments on a patient without first securing the patient's complete understanding and approval.

- Provide proper instructions for a patient's care to the person responsible for such care, so that proper treatment will be administered to the patient in the doctor's absence.

- Furnish complete information and instructions to the patient about diagnosis, options and methods of treatment, and fees for services.

- Take every precaution to prevent the spread of contagious disease.

- Advise patients against needless or unwise operations.

Patients

In the United States, patients generally have the right to choose the physician they will see, although some managed care plans may limit choices. The American Hospital Association (AHA) created a Patients' Bill of Rights in 1973, which was used extensively throughout the health care system. A variety of attempts were made to make the AHA Bill of Rights a federal law, but none succeeded. In 2008, the AHA dropped the Bill of Rights and created a brochure titled "Patient Care Partnership: Understanding

Expectations, Rights and Responsibilities" for hospitals, medical offices, and other health care facilities to use at their discretion. According to the AHA, patients should expect the following from health care providers:

- Considerate and respectful care.
- Complete current information concerning their diagnosis, treatment, and prognosis.
- Information necessary to give informed consent prior to the start of any procedure and/or treatment.
- To refuse treatment to the extent permitted by law.
- Every consideration for their privacy.
- Confidentiality.
- Reasonable responses to requests for services.
- All information about their health care.
- To know whether treatment is experimental and be free to refuse to participate in research projects.
- Reasonable continuity of care.
- To examine the bill and have it explained.
- To know which hospital rules and regulations apply to patient conduct.

Patients also have the right to terminate a physician's services if they wish. Terminating a physician's services extends to the right of hospitalized patients to leave before their physicians have discharged them, or to leave *against medical advice (AMA).*

According to a 2009 report from the Agency for Healthcare Research and Quality (AHRQ), the federal agency charged with improving the quality, safety, efficiency, and effectiveness of health care for all Americans, in 2007 (the latest year for which statistics are available) approximately 1.2 percent of all hospitalizations—368,000 hospital stays—ended when patients left against medical advice.

The AHRQ report lists three types of patients who are most likely to leave the hospital against doctors' orders:

1. Those who are worried about paying the medical bills.
2. Those with alcohol or substance abuse problems.
3. Those who have nonspecific chest pain complaints or diabetes with complications.

The best medical results depend on hospitalized patients staying until discharged by physicians, of course, but everyone who has been hospitalized knows the stay can be inconvenient and stressful. How much school work will you have to make up? Will your employer dock wages for the time missed? Who will check your house or apartment, take care of your children, water the plants, or feed the pets? And if you don't have health insurance, who will pay the medical bills?

To protect against liability for any medical consequences resulting from early discharge, the patient's insistence on leaving should be charted, and a form such as the one illustrated in Figure 4-8 should be signed and filed with the patient's medical record.

The patient also has certain implied duties to:

- Follow any instructions given by the physician and cooperate as much as possible.
- Give all relevant information to the physician to reach a correct diagnosis. If an incorrect diagnosis is made because the patient fails

Health &
wellness Center

William Smith
1212 Economy Drive
Dallas, Texas
75001

Date _____   Time _____ A.M. / P.M.

_____

Signature of Party Leaving Against Medical Advice

WITNESS: IF PARTY DEMANDING DISCHARGE IS OTHER THAN PATIENT:

_____   _____

Signature of Witness   Signature of Party

Relationship _____

INSTRUCTIONS: This demand for discharge should be signed by the patient or authorized party if he/she insists on leaving the Wellness Medical Center against medical advice. If the patient or authorized party not only demands to leave but also refuses to sign this form the following should be completed: _____
(Name of Party Demanding Discharge)
has not only demanded discharge but also has refused to sign this form documenting his/her demand.

Date _____   Time _____ A.M. / P.M.

_____

Signature of Person Receiving Demand

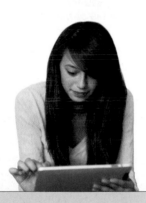

check your **progress**

Cross out the incorrect responses to complete the following statements that pertain to express or implied contracts between physicians and patients, and payment of contract fees.

26. A physician is/is not obligated to effect a recovery with every patient.

27. A physician is/is not obligated to use due care, skill, and diligence in treating each patient.

28. A physician is/is not obligated to note allergic or adverse reactions to medications reported by a specific patient.

29. A patient is/is not obligated to give all relevant information to the physician to help him or her reach a correct diagnosis.

30. A patient is/is not obligated to take part in all research relevant to his or her medical condition.

31. A patient can/cannot leave the hospital against medical advice.

32. A patient is/is not responsible for paying medical bills if the outcome of treatment is unsatisfactory.

33. A Patients' Bill of Rights was/was not enacted to give patients more rights under the law.

law of agency The law that governs the relationship between a principal and his or her agent.

to give the physician the proper information, the physician is not liable.

- Follow the physician's orders for treatment, provided the treatment is similar to that administered by members of the system or school of medicine to which the physician belongs. If a patient willfully or negligently fails to follow the physician's instructions, that patient has little legal recourse.

- Pay the fees charged for services rendered.

agent One who acts for or represents another. In performing workplace duties, the employee acts as the agent, or authorized representative, of the employer.

respondeat superior Literally, "Let the master answer." A doctrine under which an employer is legally liable for the acts of his or her employees, if such acts were performed within the scope of the employees' duties.

Law of Agency and Doctrine of *Respondeat Superior*

By law, employers are liable for the actions of their employees when employees perform said actions as part of their work under the supervision of the employer. This is called the **law of agency.** In performing workplace duties, the employee acts as the **agent** of the employer.

Agency may be expressed or implied. In the medical office, it is most often implied. Medical office employees act as the physician's agent when they schedule appointments, speak with patients and other individuals, order supplies for the office, or otherwise perform duties ordered by and supervised by the employing physician in the conduct of his or her business.

Under the doctrine of ***respondeat superior,*** or "Let the master answer," physicians are liable for the acts of their employees performed "within the course and scope" of employment if two elements are present. First, the servant (employee) must be engaged in furtherance of the master's business; and, second, he or she must be acting within the scope of the master's business. If a tortious act (implying or involving a tort) is committed not in furtherance of the employer's business, but rather for purely personal reasons disconnected from the authorized business of the master, the master is not liable under the doctrine of *respondeat superior.*

COURT CASE

Case Tried under *Respondeat Superior*

A patient underwent surgery at a hospital during which a sheath was inserted in an artery of his groin. An employee of the hospital was authorized to enter the patient's hospital room alone, check the groin area for complications, and clean the area. Following the surgery, the patient awoke to discover the employee fondling his genitals. The patient and his wife sued the hospital under the doctrine of *respondeat superior* for assault, battery, and loss of consortium.

The trial court granted summary judgment to the hospital on the grounds that an employer was not liable for the sexual misconduct of an employee. The plaintiff appealed, and the appellate court reversed because it found a question of fact existed about whether the deviation from job responsibilities was great enough to affect the hospital's liability. The hospital appealed, and the state supreme court found the hospital could not be held liable because the employee's conduct was for purely personal reasons and did nothing to further the hospital's business.

Source: Piedmont Hospital, Inc. v. Palladino, et al., 276 Ga. 612, 580 S.E.2d 215; 2003 Ga. April 29, 2003.

CHAPTER SUMMARY

LO 4.1 What is the basis of law in the United States?

- Federal statutes
- State statutes
- Municipal ordinances
- Constitutional law: Law that derives from federal and state constitutions.
- Case law: Law established through common law and legal precedent.
- Common law: The body of unwritten law developed in England, primarily from judicial decisions based on custom and tradition.

LO 4.2 How are laws classified?

- Substantive: The statutory or written law that defines and regulates legal rights and obligations.
  - Criminal law involves crimes against the state.
    - A felony is a criminal offense punishable by death or by imprisonment in a state or federal prison for more than one year.
    - A misdemeanor is a crime punishable by fine or imprisonment in a facility other than a prison for less than one year.
  - Civil law does not involve crimes, but instead involves wrongful acts against persons. Under civil law, a person can sue another person, a business, or the government.
- Procedural: Law that defines the rules used to enforce substantive law.

LO 4.3 What are torts, and how do they affect health care practitioners?

- A tort is a civil wrong committed against a person or property, excluding breach of contract.
  - Intentional torts involve intentional misconduct.
  - Unintentional torts are acts that are not intended to cause harm but are committed unreasonably or with a disregard for the consequences. In legal terms, this constitutes negligence, a charge most often alleged against health care practitioners.

LO 4.4 What is a contract, and what are its essential elements?

- A contract is a voluntary agreement between two parties in which specific promises are made for a consideration. It includes:
  - The agreement: One party makes an offer, and another party accepts it.
  - The consideration: Something of value is bargained for as part of the agreement.

- Legal subject matter: Contracts are not valid and enforceable in court unless they are for legal services or purposes.
- Contractual capacity: Parties who enter into the agreement must be capable of fully understanding all of its terms and conditions.

LO 4.5 How do expressed contracts differ from implied contracts?

- Expressed contracts are spoken or written in precise terms.
- Unexpressed contracts are not spoken or written in precise terms, but are understood.

LO 4.6 What are the contractual rights and responsibilities of both physicians and patients?

A physician has the right to:

- Set up practice within the boundaries of his or her license to practice medicine. A specialist, for instance, does not have to practice outside the area of specialty and, in fact, would be severely criticized for doing so, except in an emergency in which no other physician were available.
- Set up an office wherever he or she chooses and establish office hours.
- Specialize.
- Decide which services he or she will provide and how those services will be provided.

The physician has the obligation to:

- Use due care, skill, judgment, and diligence in treating patients.
- Stay informed about the best methods of diagnosis and treatment.
- Perform to the best of his or her ability.
- Exercise his or her best professional judgment in all cases.
- Consider the established, customary treatment administered by members of the medical profession in similar cases.
- Abstain from performing experiments on a patient without first securing the patient's complete understanding and approval.
- Provide proper instructions for a patient's care to the person responsible for such care.
- Furnish complete information and instructions to the patient about diagnosis, options and methods of treatment, and fees for services.
- Take every precaution to prevent the spread of contagious disease.
- Advise patients against needless or unwise operations.

Patients have the right to:

- Receive considerate and respectful care.
- Receive complete current information concerning his or her diagnosis, treatment, and prognosis.
- Receive information necessary to give informed consent prior to the start of any procedure and/or treatment.
- Refuse treatment to the extent permitted by law.
- Receive every consideration of his or her privacy.
- Be assured of confidentiality.

- Obtain reasonable responses to requests for services.
- Obtain information about his or her health care.
- Know whether treatment is experimental and be free to refuse to participate in research projects.
- Expect reasonable continuity of care.
- Examine his or her bill and have it explained.
- Know which hospital rules and regulations apply to patient conduct.
- Terminate the physician–patient contract, which includes leaving a hospital/treatment against medical advice.

Patients are obligated to:

- Follow any instructions given by the physician and cooperate as much as possible.
- Give all relevant information to the physician to reach a correct diagnosis. If an incorrect diagnosis is made because the patient fails to give the physician the proper information, the physician is not liable.
- Follow the physician's orders for treatment, provided the treatment is similar to that administered by members of the system or school of medicine to which the physician belongs. If a patient willfully or negligently fails to follow the physician's instructions, that patient has little legal recourse.
- Pay the fees charged for services rendered.

LO 4.7 What is the law of agency, and how does the doctrine of *respondeat superior* apply to health care contracts?

- The law of agency governs the relationship between a principal and his or her agent. An agent is one who acts for or represents another. In performing workplace duties, for example, the employee acts as the agent, or authorized representative, of the employer.
- *Respondeat superior* is Latin for "Let the master answer." Under this doctrine an employer is legally liable for the acts of his or her employees, if such acts were performed within the scope of the employees' duties.

[ETHICS ISSUES Law, the Courts, and Contracts]

Ethics ISSUE 1: Advertising by health care providers used to be considered inappropriate and unprofessional. However, now advertising by health care providers is commonplace and accepted by the various professional organizations, as long as there are no false or misleading statements.

Discussion Questions

1. A dentist advertises that he specializes in creating "dazzling smiles." In your opinion, is this an ethical advertisement? Explain your answer.

2. A chiropractor advertises "miracle" treatments to alleviate back pain. In your opinion, is this an ethical advertisement? Explain your answer.

_____

_____

3. Check your local newspaper for advertising by health care providers. Listen carefully to television ads by health care providers. Bring to class at least two ads from the newspaper and notes from the ads you listened to on television. Be sure to sort out ads that are for providers and those that are for prescription or nonprescription drugs. Are those ads misleading? Do they make promises that cannot be kept? Explain your answer.

_____

_____

4. Study the print ads and notes from television ads you collected for the previous exercise. Choose two as examples. What advantages and disadvantages for consumers can you see to the ads?

_____

_____

5. What advantages and disadvantages for health care practitioners can you see to the ads?

_____

_____

Ethics ISSUE 2: The patient–physician relationship is contractual in nature. That means that either the physician or the patient may terminate the relationship. The physician must abide by certain rules when terminating an established relationship, but the patient is free to terminate the relationship at any time. Physicians may decline to undertake the care of a patient whose medical condition is not within the physician's current competence. Physicians may not decline to accept patients because of race, color, religion, national origin, or sexual orientation, or on any other basis that would constitute individual discrimination.

Discussion Question

1. A dental hygienist refuses to work on a patient because he has revealed that he is HIV positive. Is her decision ethical? Explain your answer.

_____

_____

Ethics ISSUE 3: While in private practice, physicians may determine that they will not accept certain new patients because of their inability to pay or because they have an insurance plan with a poor reimbursement policy.

Discussion Question

1. Should all physicians be required to accept a certain number of patients who cannot pay their bills? In other words, should physicians be required to do a certain amount of charity care? Explain your answer.

_____

_____

Ethics ISSUE 4: The first objective and the primary goal of every code of ethics and ethics guideline for health care practitioners is the *welfare of the patient.*

Discussion Question

1. A nursing assistant working under the supervision of a registered nurse in a hospital has witnessed several occasions when the RN behaves abusively to elderly patients. What should the nursing assistant do?

_____

_____

Go to **www.mhhe.com/judson6e** to practice your case review skills. Then read on for more information.

KEY TERMS

administrative law

agent

breach of contract

case law

checks and balances

civil law

common law

constitutional law

contract

criminal law

defendant

executive order

expressed contract

Fair Debt Collection Practices Act (FDCPA)

felony

implied contract

jurisdiction

law of agency

legal precedents

mentally incompetent

minor

misdemeanor

negligence

plaintiff

procedural law

prosecution

respondeat superior

Statute of Frauds

statutory law

substantive law

third-party payer contract

tort

tortfeasor

void

voidable

CHAPTER 4 REVIEW

Applying Knowledge

Answer the following questions in the spaces provided.

LO 4.1

1. List and define three functions a state government *can* assume.

_____

_____

_____

_____

2. Which governmental functions are reserved strictly for the federal government?

_____

_____

_____

_____

3. Define *common law.*

_____

_____

_____

_____

4. Define *administrative law.*

_____

_____

_____

_____

5. Decisions made by judges in the various courts and used as a guide for future decisions are called what?

_____

_____

_____

_____

Circle the correct answer for each of the following questions.

LO 4.2

6. Substantive law
  a. Defines the legal relationships between people or between people and the state
  b. Is never written down
  c. Is a type of common law
  d. Is created solely by executive order

7. Procedural law
  a. Is the same as substantive law
  b. Defines the rules used to enforce substantive law
  c. Applies only to criminal law
  d. Does not involve penalties for violations

8. Criminal law
  a. Includes financial payment for violations, but never jail time
  b. Never involves health care practitioners
  c. Involves crimes against the state
  d. Allows violators to be tried in civil court

9. Civil law
  a. Includes felonies and misdemeanors
  b. Is the area of law most likely to affect health care practitioners
  c. Does not involve court cases
  d. Involves crimes against the state

10. A civil offense
    a. Is never unethical
    b. Never involves lawsuits
    c. May involve a family matter
    d. Never applies to health care practitioners

11. *Jurisdiction* refers to
    a. The city where a felony occurs
    b. The fines levied for civil offenses
    c. Crimes against people
    d. The court that has the authority to hear and decide a case

LO 4.3

12. Define *tort*.
    a. A tort is a specific type of felony.
    b. A tort is a civil wrong committed against a person or property.
    c. *Tort* is another term for breach of contract.
    d. A tort is none of the above.

13. What is a tortfeasor?
    a. It is the attorney who represents a client in civil court.
    b. It is a person who commits a felony.
    c. It is the person who commits a tort.
    d. It refers to a court's specific jurisdiction.

14. Negligence is
    a. An intentional tort
    b. The same as assault
    c. A criminal matter
    d. An unintentional tort

15. Intentional torts
    a. Include negligence
    b. Always involve jail time when successfully prosecuted
    c. Include assault, battery, and defamation
    d. Are always felonies

16. If a physician examines a patient without consent, he or she could be charged with which of the following offenses?
    a. Breach of contract
    b. Kidnapping
    c. Battery
    d. Defamation of character

LO 4.4

17. A contract
    a. Is breached only if all parties agree
    b. Is valid only if parties on both sides are competent
    c. Can never be broken
    d. Is valid if an illegal act is involved

18. For what are health care practitioners legally liable?
    a. For all unsatisfactory medical outcomes
    b. For actions of their employees, performed in the course of employment
    c. For actions of their employees away from work
    d. For actions of their coworkers, performed on the job

19. What is the *consideration* of a contract?
    a. The fee, if any, that will be charged
    b. Something of value bargained for
    c. The terms of the agreement
    d. None of the above

20. A contract may be voidable if
    a. One party leaves town
    b. One party decides to cancel the contract
    c. One party is a minor
    d. One party engages in an illegal act

21. Under what circumstances may breach of contract be charged?
    a. If either party fails to fulfill the terms of a valid contract
    b. If one party becomes angry with the other
    c. If the contract was invalid from the beginning
    d. None of the above

LO 4.5

22. The Statute of Frauds
    a. Is federal legislation governing health practitioners accused of fraud
    b. Covers both expressed and implied contracts
    c. Is state legislation governing written contracts
    d. Must be revised every 10 years.

23. Third-party payer contracts
    a. May be implied
    b. Are legally invalid
    c. Promise, in writing, that a third party will pay a patient's medical bill
    d. Are never used in the medical office

24. Regulation Z of the Consumer Protection Act of 1968 requires that certain financial arrangements be in writing and include
    a. Proof of ability to pay a debt
    b. A finance charge
    c. A minimum of 10 installment payments
    d. Proof that the arrangement is for business purposes

25. Which of the following is an example of an implied limited contract?
    a. A physician in a medical clinic examines a new patient.
    b. A physical therapist meets regularly with a patient and administers range of motion exercises.
    c. A dental hygienist cleans a patient's teeth.
    d. A physician at the scene provides emergency care to a car accident victim.

LO 4.6

26. List 10 items to which a physician is *not* bound contractually in the context of an implied physician–patient contract.

_____   _____

_____   _____

_____   _____

_____   _____

_____   _____

27. List 10 items to which a physician is obligated in an implied physician–patient contract.

_____   _____

_____   _____

_____   _____

_____   _____

_____   _____

28. List five responsibilities borne by the patient in an implied contract.

_____

_____

29. Name four situations in which premature termination of the physician–patient contract may occur.

_____

_____

30. Why must a physician give the patient ample notice when withdrawing from a case?

_____

_____

LO 4.7

31. Briefly explain how the law of agency applies to health care practitioners.

_____

_____

32. How does the doctrine of _respondeat superior_ relate to the law of agency?

_____

_____

[CASE STUDIES]

Use your critical thinking skills to answer the questions that follow each case study.

LO 4.3 and LO 4.6

An internist had a 54-year-old obese patient who smoked and had a stressful job. After he died of a heart attack, an autopsy revealed that the overweight man had coronary artery disease. The patient's family sued the physician for negligence and won a $3.5 million judgment against the internist. During jury deliberations, some jurors who heard testimony in the case argued that the physician did everything possible to try to help the patient, but others maintained that he could have done more.

33. In your opinion, was the internist negligent for not referring this patient to a cardiologist, as the patient's wife claimed in court? Why or why not?

_____

_____

34. In your opinion, does this case show that people need to take more personal responsibility for what they do to their bodies? Explain your answer.

_____

_____

LO 4.4

Dan, a medical office assistant in a busy clinic, is a sympathetic and understanding employee. Therefore, when an elderly patient complained to him that she "felt terrible most of the time," Dan consoled her. "Don't worry, Mrs. Smith," he told the woman. "Dr. Jones will make you feel better in no time."

35. Has Dan, acting as Dr. Jones's agent, created an implied contract with Mrs. Smith? Explain your answer.

_____

_____

36. If so, can Mrs. Smith sue Dr. Jones if he fails to fulfill the "terms" of the contract? Explain your answer.

_____

_____

37. How might you respond to a patient under similar circumstances?

_____

_____

LO 4.6

38. Does a patient have the legal right to leave the hospital, even though his or her physician believes treatment is incomplete? What procedure should be followed if a patient leaves a hospital against medical advice?

_____

_____

39. Does a patient have the right to know if medical treatment is experimental and to refuse to participate in such treatment? Explain your answer.

_____

_____

INTERNET ACTIVITIES LO 4.1 and LO 4.2

Complete the activities and answer the questions that follow.

40 Find a Web site that defines the term *affidavit*. Briefly explain the term, and describe a situation in which a health care professional may have to give an affidavit.

_____

_____

41. Visit the Web site for the U.S. House of Representatives. List any health care legislation currently pending before the House that you believe is relevant to the health care profession you will practice.

_____

_____

42. List two additional Web sites where information about health care legislation can be found.

_____

_____

[RESOURCES]

Hwang, Stephen W. "Discharge against Medical Advice" (May 2005). U.S. Department of Health and Human Services Web site: **www.webmm. ahrq.gov/case**.

Kubasek, Nancy, et al. _Dynamic Business Law_. New York: McGraw-Hill, 2009.

Liuzzo, Anthony L. _Essentials of Business Law_. New York: McGraw-Hill, 2010.

Mitchell, Joyce, and Lee Haroun. _Introduction to Health Care_. New York: Delmar, 2002.

Payne, January W. "Why People Leave the Hospital against Medical Advice." _U.S. News and World Report_ (August 27, 2009). **http://health. usnews.com**.

Prickett-Ramutkowski, Barbara, et al. _Medical Assisting: A Patient-Centered Approach to Administrative and Clinical Competencies_. New York: McGraw-Hill, 1999.

part two

Legal Issues for Working Health Care Practitioners

chapter five

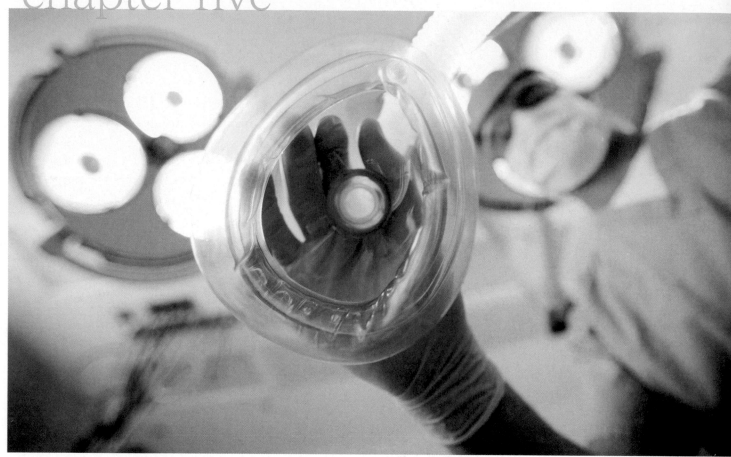

PROFESSIONAL LIABILITY AND MEDICAL MALPRACTICE

Learning Outcomes

After studying this chapter, you should be able to:

LO 5.1 Identify three areas of general liability for which a physician/employer is responsible.

LO 5.2 Describe the reasonable person standard, standard of care, and duty of care.

LO 5.3 Briefly outline the responsibilities of health care practitioners concerning privacy, confidentiality, and privileged communication.

LO 5.4 Explain the four elements necessary to prove negligence (the four Ds).

LO 5.5 Outline the phases of a lawsuit.

LO 5.6 Name two advantages to alternative dispute resolution.

Cases in This Chapter

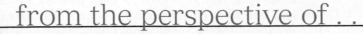

from the perspective of . . .

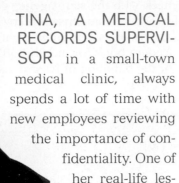

TINA, A MEDICAL RECORDS SUPERVISOR in a small-town medical clinic, always spends a lot of time with new employees reviewing the importance of confidentiality. One of her real-life lessons is about the new employee, Samantha, who accidentally and innocently violated confidentiality, causing the clinic where she worked to be sued.

Samantha saw one of her high school friends in the hallway of the clinic. The friend told Samantha that she was pregnant. A week later, Samantha saw her friend's mother in the local grocery store and congratulated her on becoming a grandmother. What Samantha did not know was that her friend

was not planning to continue the pregnancy and had told no one that she was pregnant. The clinic was sued for violating confidentiality. Tina's strong advice to all employees has since become: "What you learn in this clinic *stays* in this clinic."

From Tina's perspective, even remarks that seem innocent and harmless, if spoken outside the health care workplace, can violate privacy and create liability for employers and employees.

From the perspective of new employees, Samantha's experience is a lesson well-learned.

From the perspective of Samantha, who did not think twice before she spoke, what she thought were innocent remarks created a distressing and damaging situation. Samantha's career in health care was over before it had begun.

How can Tina impress on employees under her supervision the importance of maintaining patient privacy?

What course of action should Samantha have taken after her friend told her she was pregnant?

Liability

All competent adults are **liable,** or legally responsible, for their own acts, both on the job and in their private lives. As homeowners and operators of automobiles, we carry liability insurance in case someone is injured in our homes or we are involved in a car accident. In the workplace, employers carry liability insurance to cover situations in which employees, or anyone else on the premises, may be injured or harmed.

As employers, physicians have general liability for

The Practice's Building and Grounds. Adequate upkeep will help ensure that employees and patients are not injured on the premises. Employers must provide protection against theft, fire, and burglary in the building and must take all precautions to ensure that patients' records are protected. Theft, fire, and liability insurance to cover the workplace is a must for the physician/employer.

Automobiles. If employees must use their own or the physician's automobile in the performance of their daily work (for example, to drop off or pick up mail or supplies), the employer must be adequately insured for liability in the event of an accident.

LO 5.1
Identify three areas of general liability for which a physician/employer is responsible.

[**liable** Legally responsible or obligated.

Employee Safety. Employers must provide a reasonably comfortable and safe work environment for employees. State (and, in some instances, federal) regulations apply, but they vary from state to state. Employers should check with the state agency governing safety in the workplace, with workers' compensation laws, and with state medical societies to determine safety rules, rights, and responsibilities. A general safety procedure book for medical office workers should include guidelines for the handling of hazardous laboratory wastes and materials.

COURT CASE

Hospital Liable for Surgeon's Injuries

In November 1998, Dr. Loomis, a neurosurgeon in private practice, was visiting his patients in Evansville Hospital, where he had surgery privileges, when he stopped at the coffee-break pantry to pour himself a cup of coffee. As he walked to pick up the coffee pot, he slipped in a puddle of water on the floor. Dr. Loomis fell backward onto his left side, landing on the region of his left kidney, and injuring his left elbow.

After the accident, Dr. Loomis developed severe pain in his left elbow. The pain kept him from sleeping at night. While Dr. Loomis usually performed about 250 surgeries per year, after his fall he could perform only three, and those with great difficulty.

Dr. Loomis's condition worsened. He developed an arm tremor. The hair on his arm fell out, and the skin underneath became shiny. His arm would occasionally turn purple, and his arm muscles atrophied. He began to compensate by using his right arm, but the overuse he placed on the right arm produced carpal tunnel syndrome and arthritis in that arm.

In December 1998, Dr. Loomis's physician diagnosed reflex sympathetic dystrophy (RSD), a syndrome where the body's repair mechanisms are activated in response to a normal injury "but never get turned off." In April 1999, Dr. Loomis stopped seeing patients because of the pain in his arm, and he sold his practice. Shortly thereafter, Loomis's physician told him that it was unlikely he would ever be able to practice neurosurgery again.

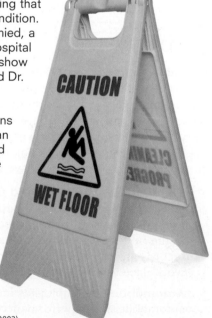

In December 1999, Dr. Loomis filed a complaint against the hospital, alleging that the hospital negligently failed to maintain its floor in a reasonably safe condition. After motions for partial summary judgment filed by both parties were denied, a jury trial began on July 24, 2001. When Dr. Loomis rested his case, the hospital moved for judgment on the evidence, alleging that no evidence existed to show that the coffee-break pantry was in a dangerous condition, and that it owed Dr. Loomis no duty. The trial court denied the hospital's motion.

Both parties submitted final jury instructions. One of the hospital's instructions defined the term "licensee" and outlined the duty owed to a licensee by an occupier of land. The trial court refused the hospital's instructions and instead instructed the jury that Dr. Loomis was an invitee to whom the hospital owed a duty of reasonable care.

In July 2001, the jury returned a verdict for Dr. Loomis. The jury assessed 100 percent of the fault to the hospital and none against Dr. Loomis. The jury awarded Dr. Loomis $16,950,000 that constituted damages for loss of income, pain and suffering, and medical expenses.

The hospital appealed the verdict and the size of the award, but the appellate court affirmed the trial court's judgment.

Source: St. Mary's Medical Center of Evansville, Inc. v. Gregory J. Loomis, M.D., 783 N.E.2d 274 (Ind. App. 2002).

Standard of Care and Duty of Care

Standard of care refers to the level of performance expected of a health care practitioner in carrying out his or her professional duties. **Duty of care** is the obligation of health care workers to patients and, in some case, nonpatients. Physicians have a duty of care to patients with whom they have established a doctor–patient relationship, but they may also be held to a duty of care toward people who are not patients, such as the patient's family members, former patients, and even office personnel. Generally, if actions or omissions within the scope of a health care practitioner's job could cause harm to someone, that person is owed a duty of care.

For example, medical facility custodians are nonpatients to whom a duty of care is owed. Various drugs, equipment, and supplies are used and discarded daily in a medical facility. Procedures for the proper disposal of drugs and potentially hazardous materials should be detailed in a facility's safety manual (Figure 5-1), so that employees who handle these materials do not accidentally prick themselves with used needles or otherwise injure themselves.

In some instances, depending on the situation and state law, physicians may have a duty under standard of care to warn nonpatients of danger, as in the case of a psychiatric patient who threatens harm to others or in the case of a patient with a communicable disease.

Two court cases, "Therapists Found Guilty of Failure to Warn" (p. 132) and "Sharing a Prescription Drug Proves Costly" (p. 133), show that courts vary widely in establishing a duty of care, according to the laws in the states where lawsuits are adjudicated. In "Sharing a Prescription Drug Proves Costly," wrongful death was also charged, which is discussed in further detail as you progress through this chapter.

As mentioned in Chapter 4, we are responsible for our actions (or our failure to act) under the **reasonable person standard.** That is, we may be charged with negligence if someone is injured because we failed to perform an act that a reasonable person, in similar circumstances, would perform or if we committed an act that a reasonable person would not commit. Professionals—individuals who are specially trained to perform specific tasks—are held to a higher standard of care than nonprofessionals (laypersons). If a patient is injured because a health care professional failed to exercise the care and expertise that under the circumstances could reasonably be expected of a professional with similar experience and training, then that professional may be liable for negligence.

Physicians

A physician in general practice is expected to conform to the standards of other general practitioners in his or her own or a comparable community. A specialist is held to a higher standard of care than that expected of a general practitioner. The standard of care for a specialist is generally the same as that for like specialists, wherever they practice. Similarly, any health care practitioner—nurse, phlebotomist, dental

LO 5.2

Describe the reasonable person standard, standard of care, and duty of care.

standard of care The level of performance expected of a health care practitioner in carrying out his or her professional duties.

duty of care The legal obligation of health care workers to patients and, sometimes, nonpatients.

reasonable person standard That standard of behavior that judges a person's actions in a situation according to what a reasonable person would or would not do under similar circumstances.

> **Figure 5-1**

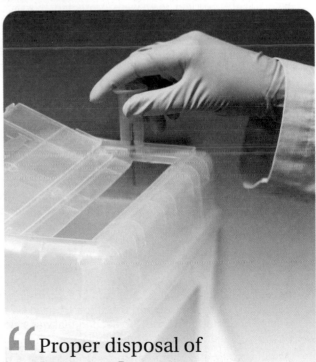

"" Proper disposal of **hazardous** and **medical wastes** helps protect all medical facility employees. ""

LANDMARK COURT CASE

Therapists Found Guilty of Failure to Warn

In October 1969, Prosenjit Poddar, a foreign student from Bengal, India, killed Tatiana Tarasoff. Two months before, Poddar had confided his intention to kill Tarasoff to Dr. Lawrence Moore, a psychologist employed by the Cowell Memorial Hospital at the University of California at Berkeley. Poddar told Moore he would kill Tarasoff after she returned from spending the summer in Brazil.

Acting on this information, Moore notified the campus police, who briefly detained Poddar, but determined that Poddar was rational and released him. Upon Poddar's release, Moore's superior, Dr. Harvey Powelson, directed that all of the letters and notes Moore had written while counseling Poddar be destroyed and no further action be taken to detain Poddar in the future.

Soon thereafter, Poddar convinced Tarasoff's brother to share an apartment with him near Tarasoff's residence. When she returned from Brazil, Poddar went to Tarsoff's home and killed her. Tarasoff had not been warned of the possible danger Poddar posed.

Tarasoff's parents sued, arguing that the psychologist had a duty to warn them of Poddar's danger to their daughter, and that the campus police negligently released Poddar without notifying them of their daughter's grave danger. They also argued that the police failed to confine Poddar, under the Lanterman-Petris-Short Act, a California law designed to protect mentally ill and mentally disabled persons from certain abuses, and to guarantee and protect the public interest.

The defendants argued that there was no duty of care toward Tatiana Tarasoff, and that, as employees of the state, they had governmental immunity. The trial court granted the defendants' motion to dismiss. On the plaintiffs' appeal, the court affirmed dismissals against defendant police on all claims, stating there was no duty to plaintiffs. Dismissals against the defendant therapists were also upheld, holding they were protected by governmental immunity. Plaintiffs appealed to the Supreme Court of California.

The Supreme Court allowed plaintiffs to amend their appeal to state that the therapists failed to warn Tatiana (rather than her parents, as in the original complaint).

The Supreme Court of California heard the case, based on the question, did defendant therapists have a duty to warn Tatiana Tarasoff?

Yes, the court determined. It was found that defendant therapists should have determined that Poddar presented a serious danger to Tarasoff, and they failed to exercise reasonable care to protect her from that danger (i.e., when a therapist determines that a patient poses a danger to another individual, he or she is obligated to use reasonable care to protect that individual). Therefore, defendant therapists breached their duty of care to Tatiana Tarasoff and were negligent by not warning her of the possible danger posed by Poddar.

Source: Tarasoff v. Regents of University of California, 17 Cal.3d 425, 131 Cal. Rptr. 14, 551 P.2d 334 (1976).

Prosenjit Poddar was later convicted of second-degree murder, but the conviction was appealed and overturned, based on the decision that the jury was inadequately informed. No second trial was held, and Poddar was released on the condition that he return to India.

Would you have expected state law to establish a psychiatrist's duty to warn third parties about a dangerous patient? Why or why not?

A restaurant worker, Kasey, attended an employee holiday party held at his workplace. Also present were a coworker and her boyfriend, Followill. Kasey brought a narcotic drug to the party, which his doctor had prescribed for his back pain. He gave his coworker eight of the pain pills, who, in turn, gave them to her boyfriend, Followill. Followill died in his sleep that evening, due to a combination of the prescription drug and alcohol in his system. Plaintiff Gipson, Followill's mother, sued defendant, Kasey, for wrongful death.

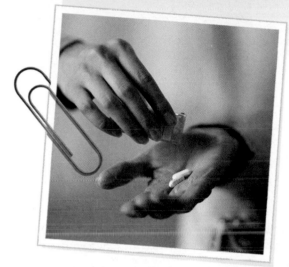

The issue presented in court was whether persons who were prescribed drugs owed a duty of care, making them potentially liable for negligence, when they improperly give their drugs to others. The defendant contended that because Arizona law does not impose a duty on social hosts who serve alcohol to adults, there should similarly be no duty here.

The supreme court in this case ruled that such a duty was owed, extending not from the relationship between the two workers, but from state statutes that prohibited distributing prescription drugs to persons not covered by the prescription. The Arizona Supreme Court referred the case back to the superior court for further proceedings consistent with the opinion regarding duty of care.

Source: Gipson v. Kasey, 214 Ariz. 141, 150 P.3d 228 (Ariz. 2007).

Does the verdict in this case surprise you?

As illustrated in the court case, what risks does one assume when he or she shares personal prescription drugs with others?

---

assistant, physician assistant—is expected to conform to the standards of like practitioners in his or her own or a comparable community.

Direct patient contact is not always necessary for establishing a duty, as the following case, "Hospital and Surgeon Also Liable," illustrates.

Courts have generally held that informal consultations among physicians do not create a doctor–patient relationship and thus do not create a duty of care, as discussed in the following classic case, "Consultation Did Not Establish a Duty of Care."

Guidelines for Physicians and Other Health Care Practitioners

The following guidelines can help all health care practitioners stay within the scope of their practices and operate within the law and the policy of any employing health care facility. All are addressed at length throughout the text.

- Practice within the scope of your training and capabilities.
- Use the professional title commensurate with your education and experience.
- Maintain confidentiality.
- Prepare and maintain health records.
- Document accurately.
- Use appropriate legal and ethical guidelines when releasing information.

COURT CASE

Hospital and Surgeon Also Liable

When a couple's two-month-old baby experienced respiratory distress, they took him to the hospital. The baby had a heart murmur, and surgery was recommended. During surgery, the perfusionist, a technician responsible for oxygenation of the patient's blood, made critical mistakes while operating a heart-lung machine. As a result, the flow of oxygen to the patient's brain was stopped, causing brain damage. The child, six years old when this case was finally settled, suffered from cerebral palsy, clinical blindness, loss of speech, and mental retardation. A trial court ruled that although the perfusionist was the employee of a subcontractor at the time of the child's injuries, the hospital was not absolved of vicarious liability for the technician's negligence.

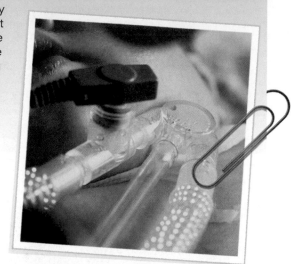

The case concerned liability of the hospital, which had an admission form that the parents signed, acknowledging that they had been advised that "[A]ll physicians, residents and students who provide services in Shands . . . are employees, agents or servants of the University of Florida, Board of Regents, and are not employees, agents or students of Shands" [and] "that the law limits the liability for acts or omissions of employees, agents or servants of the State of Florida, including the Board of Regents, to $100,000 per claim and $200,000 per incident."

The Florida Supreme Court eventually heard the case, and upheld the premise that a hospital and a surgeon may both be liable for a perfusionist's negligence in certain circumstances, and also upheld the jury-awarded damages of $9,138,848.03.

Source: Shands Teaching Hospital and Clinic, Inc. v. Juliana, 863 So.2d 343 (Fla. App. 1 Dist. 2003).

In your opinion, should a hospital be able to avoid liability for employee negligence by hiring individuals as "independent contractors"?

COURT CASE

Duty Established by Referral

A plastic surgeon examined a patient in a hospital emergency department. An X-ray of the patient's knee revealed a possible malignant neoplasm, so the plastic surgeon referred the patient to an orthopedist, but did not tell the patient why. The patient did not keep any of the three appointments he scheduled with the orthopedist, and the orthopedist refused to reschedule him.

The patient died of cancer, and his estate sued the two physicians. A lower court granted summary judgment to the orthopedist, but an appeals court reversed, holding that a doctor–patient relationship began when the orthopedist accepted the referral and scheduled the patient for an appointment. The court also said that "a letter to plaintiff advising him of his condition and to consult with another physician without delay might well have been sufficient" to discharge the duty to the patient.

Source: Davis v. Weiskopf, 108 Ill. App. 3d 505, 439 N.E.2d 60 (Ill. App. 2 Dist. 1982).

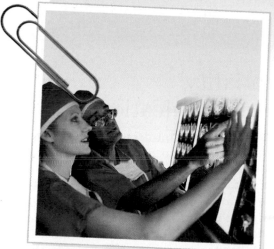
- Follow an employer's established policies dealing with the health care contract.
- Follow legal guidelines and maintain awareness of health care legislation and regulations.
- Maintain and dispose of regulated substances in compliance with government guidelines.
- Follow established risk management and safety procedures.
- Meet the requirements for professional credentialing.
- Help develop and maintain personnel, policy, and procedure manuals.

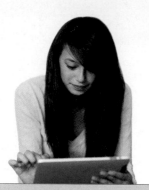

Laws clearly dictate what a member of a health care profession can and cannot do on the job. However, in addition to knowing the law, a health care practitioner should know what policies and procedures apply specifically to his or her place of employment. Policy and procedure manuals that clearly define a health care practitioner's responsibilities can serve as a valuable guide and as evidence that policies and procedures are in writing if legal suits should arise.

check your **progress**

1. As employers, physicians have general liability for _____.

Write "T" or "F" in the blank to indicate whether you think the statement is true or false.

_____ 2. *Standard of care* refers to the level of performance expected of a health care practitioner in carrying out his or her professional duties.

_____ 3. *Duty of care* is the obligation of health care practitioners to patients but never applies to nonpatients.

_____ 4. An obstetrician who helps deliver a baby to a woman who happens to be riding with him in a taxicab would be held to the reasonable person standard.

_____ 5. Policies and procedures of the employing medical facility, as well as the law, should be considered when a health care practitioner performs his or her duties.

LO 5.3

Briefly outline the responsibilities of health care practitioners concerning privacy, confidentiality, and privileged communication.

confidentiality The act of holding information in confidence, not to be released to unauthorized individuals.

privileged communication Information held confidential within a protected relationship.

Privacy, Confidentiality, and Privileged Communication

Not only do physicians and other health care professionals owe a duty of care to patients, but it is also their ethical and legal duty to safeguard a patient's privacy and maintain **confidentiality.**

Privileged communication refers to information held confidential within a protected relationship. Attorney–client and physician–patient are examples of relationships in which the law, under certain circumstances, protects the holder of information from forced disclosure on the witness stand. Privileged communication statutes vary from state to state, but in most states, patients may sue a physician or any other health care practitioner for breach of confidence if the holder released protected information and damage to the patient resulted. In many states, breach of confidence is grounds for revocation of a physician's license.

Since health care procedures and facilities present numerous opportunities for a breach of confidentiality (as was the case with Samantha in the chapter's opening scenario), health care practitioners must make every effort to safeguard each patient's privacy. Privacy, confidentiality, and privileged communication are such important subjects for health care practitioners that they are discussed separately in Chapter 8. Chapter 8 also includes a discussion of the many requirements of the Health Insurance Portability and Accountability Act (HIPAA).

The following suggestions for maintaining confidentiality of patient health care records can serve as a guide for all health care practitioners who may be asked to provide or release patient information:

- Do not disclose any information about a patient to a third party without signed consent. This extends to insurance companies, attorneys, and curious neighbors, and it includes acknowledging whether or not the person in question is a patient.

- Do not decide confidentiality on the basis of whether or not you approve of or agree with the views or morals of the patient.

- Do not reveal financial information about a patient, since this is also confidential. For instance, be discreet when revealing a patient's account balance so that others in the vicinity do not overhear.

- When talking on the telephone with a patient, do not use the patient's name if others in the room might overhear.

- Use caution in giving the results of medical tests to patients over the telephone to prevent others in the medical office from overhearing. Furthermore, when leaving a message on a home answering machine or at a patient's place of employment, simply ask the patient to return a call regarding a recent visit or appointment on a specific date. No mention should be made of the nature of the call. It is inadvisable to leave a message with a receptionist or coworker on an answering machine for the patient to call an oncologist, an obstetrician-gynecologist, and so

COURT CASE

Newspaper Cannot Get Autopsy Photos

On February 18, 2001, while he was driving the last lap of the Daytona 500 race at the Daytona International Speedway, NASCAR driver Dale Earnhardt's car struck the wall, and he was killed instantly. An autopsy was performed the following day.

Since the *Orlando Sentinel* had been running a series of articles about NASCAR safety, the newspaper requested copies of Earnhardt's autopsy photos so that a medical examiner it had hired could determine if wearing the HANS device for head stabilization might have saved the race car driver's life. Upon learning of the *Sentinel's* request, Dale Earnhardt's widow, Teresa, filed suit in Volusia County Circuit Court seeking an injunction to prevent the *Sentinel's* representa-

tive from examining the photos. Mrs. Earnhardt claimed that releasing the photos would violate the Earnhardt family's privacy. The Circuit Court judge granted a temporary injunction, stating that the family's privacy interest outweighed the public interest in seeing the photographs.

Before the case was settled, the Florida legislature passed a law, known as the Earnhardt Family Protection Act, that allows autopsy photographs or recordings of the autopsy to be examined only by a surviving spouse, parent, or child. Anyone else must obtain a court order and examine the materials under the "direct supervision of the custodian." Exceptions were made for some service providers, such as the medical examiner and state or

federal agencies performing official duties. The law restricted access to such information by journalists and others.

Mrs. Earnhardt settled her suit against the *Orlando Sentinel* on March 16, 2001. An independent medical expert could examine Earnhardt's autopsy photos; then the photos would be permanently sealed.

Several news organizations challenged the constitutionality of the Earnhardt Family Protection Act, but the law has been upheld in Florida as constitutional.

Source: Campus Communications, Inc. v. Earnhardt, 27 Fla. L. Weekly D1595, 821 So.2d 388 (Fla. App. 5 Dist. 2002).

forth. If test results are abnormal, usually the physician speaks directly to the patient, and an appointment is made to discuss the results.

- Do not leave medical charts or insurance reports where patients or office visitors can see them. See that confidentiality protocol is duly noted in the office procedures manual, and make sure new employees learn it.

- If a patient is unwilling to release privileged information, the information should not be released. Exceptions include legally required disclosures, such as those ordered by subpoena; those dictated by statute to protect public health or welfare; or those considered necessary to protect the welfare of a patient or a third party.

COURT CASE

Forensic Photos Displayed on the Internet

On October 31, 2006, Nicole Catsouras, 18, the daughter of Christos and Lesli Catsouras and the sister of Danielle, Christina, and Kira Catsouras, was decapitated in an automobile accident. California Highway Patrol officers arrived at the scene, cordoned off the area where the accident occurred, and took control of the decedent's remains. The CHP officers took multiple photographs of Nicole's decapitated corpse. The photographs were downloaded or otherwise transmitted to one or more CHP computers, but they also reached 2,500 Internet Web sites in the United States and the United Kingdom that were not involved in the official investigation of the car crash. Nicole's family members were subjected to malicious taunting by persons making use of the graphic and horrific photographs. For example, Nicole's father received e-mails containing the photographs, including one titled "Woo Hoo Daddy" that said "Hey, Daddy I'm still alive." Some Web sites painted the decedent's life in a false light, including one that described her as "stupid" and a "swinger." As a proximate result of the acts of defendants, plaintiffs suffered severe emotional and mental distress.

Nicole's surviving family members filed suit against the CHP. A California appeals court eventually heard the case, deciding that family members have a common law privacy right in the death images of a decedent, subject to certain limitations. The court also held: "We conclude that the CHP and its officers owed plaintiffs a duty of care not to place decedent's death images on the Internet for the purposes of vulgar spectacle." The court found three factors important in the case (freedom of the press was not at issue):

"foreseeability, moral blame, and the prevention of future harm. It was perfectly foreseeable that the public dissemination, via the Internet, of photographs of the decapitated remains of a teenage girl would cause devastating trauma to the parents and siblings of that girl. Moreover, the alleged acts were morally deficient. We rely upon the CHP to protect and serve the public. It is antithetical to that expectation for the CHP to inflict harm upon us by making the ravaged remains of our loved ones the subjects of Internet sensationalism. It is important to prevent future harm to other families by encouraging the CHP to establish and enforce policies to preclude its officers from engaging in such acts ever again."

Accordingly, the court found that the Catsouras family could bring an action for invasion of privacy against the California Highway Patrol.

Source: *Catsouras v. Department of California Highway Patrol,* 181 Cal. App. 4th 856 — Cal: Court of Appeals, 4th Appellate Dist., 3rd Div. 2010.

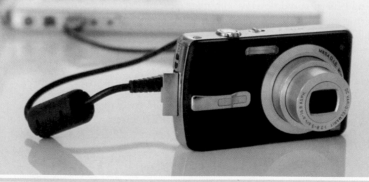

Confidentiality may be waived under the following circumstances:

- Sometimes when a third party requests a medical examination, such as for employment, and that party pays the physician's fee.

- Generally when a patient sues a physician for malpractice and patient records are subpoenaed.

- When a waiver has been signed by the patient allowing the release of information (see Figure 5-2).

The issue of confidentiality is not always clear-cut. For example, are autopsy records protected as medical records, or are they considered public record and, therefore, subject to release on demand? The court case, "Newspaper Cannot Get Autopsy Photos," shows how one court decision answered that question.

A more recent court case, "Forensic Photos Displayed on the Internet," made headlines in the matter of the unauthorized release of forensic photos to the media, and the right to privacy of family members of a decedent.

> **Figure 5-2** Consent to Release Information

I authorize:

Name of person or institution _____
(Provider of information)

Street address _____

City, state, Zip code _____

To release medical information to:

Name of person or institution _____
(Recipient of information)

Street address _____

City, state, Zip code _____

Attention _____

Nature of information to be disclosed:

☐ Clinical notes pertaining to evaluation and treatment _____

☐ Other, please specify _____

Purpose of disclosure:

☐ Continuing medical care _____

☐ Second opinion _____

☐ Other, please specify _____

This authorization will automatically expire one year from the date of signature, unless specified otherwise _____

This consent may be revoked at any time by sending written notice to the above-named provider of information. Any release of information made prior to the revocation of this complaint, authorization is not a breach of confidentiality. Disclosed information may be reviewed by contacting the provider of information.

Patient's name _____

Signature of patient or legal guardian _____ Date _____

Complete address _____

Relationship, if not the patient _____ Patient's date of birth _____

Specific consent for release of information protected by state or federal law

Iowa law (and in some cases federal law) provides special confidentiality protection to information relating to substance abuse, mental health, and HIV-related testing. In order for information to be released on this subject matter, this specific authorization and the above authorization must be signed:

I authorize release of information relating to:

☐ Substance abuse (alcohol/drug abuse)
Signature of patient or legal guardian _____ Date _____

☐ Mental health (includes psychological testing and mental health counseling)
Signature of patient or legal guardian _____ Date _____

☐ HIV-related information (AIDS-related testing)
Signature of patient or legal guardian _____ Date _____

Date Information is sent _____

Sent by (name) _____

To the recipient of this information: This information has been disclosed to you from records protected by federal confidentiality rules. The federal rules prohibit you from making further disclosure without additional consent.

LO 5.4

Explain the four elements necessary to prove negligence (the four Ds).

The Tort of Negligence

The unintentional tort of negligence is the basis for professional malpractice claims and is the most common liability in medicine. When health care practitioners are sued for medical malpractice, the term generally means any deviation from the accepted medical standard of care that causes injury to a patient.

In a court case decided in 1965 (see the classic court case, "Hospital Found Negligent"), for the first time a hospital was found guilty of negligence. Since then, under the theory of corporate liability hospitals have been found to have an independent duty to patients, including a duty to grant privileges only to competent doctors, to supervise the overall medical treatment of patients, and to review the competence of staff physicians.

All medical professional liability claims are classified in one of three ways, based on the root word *feasance,* which means "the performance of an act."

malfeasance The performance of a totally wrongful and unlawful act.

Malfeasance. The performance of a totally wrongful and unlawful act. For example, in the absence of the employing physician, a medical assistant determines that a patient needs a prescription drug and dispenses the wrong drug from the physician's supply. Medical assistants are not licensed to practice medicine, and the wrong drug was dispensed, so the act was totally wrongful and unlawful and could be called malfeasance.

misfeasance The performance of a lawful act in an illegal or improper manner.

Misfeasance. The performance of a lawful act in an illegal or improper manner. Suppose a physician orders his or her nurse-employee to change a sterile dressing on a patient's burned hand. The nurse changes the dressing but does not use sterile technique, and the patient's burn becomes infected. The nurse is legally authorized to carry out the physician's instructions in dressing the patient's hand, but violated proper procedure in carrying out the physician's order.

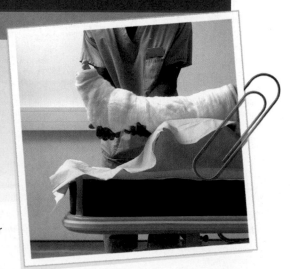

COURT CASE

Hospital Found Negligent

A patient was admitted to a small hospital's emergency room in southern Illinois with a broken leg. The treating doctor was not an orthopedic specialist, and complications developed. The patient developed gangrene in the injured leg, and it was amputated.

In a lawsuit the patient brought against the hospital, the hospital was required to pay damages when the court decided that the facility was negligent in permitting the treating doctor to do orthopedic work and in not requiring him to review his operative procedures to be sure they were current. The hospital was also found negligent in failing to exercise adequate supervision in the case and in not requiring consultation, especially after complications developed.

Source: Darling v. Charleston Community Memorial Hospital,
33 Ill.2d 326, 211 N.E.2d 253 (Ill. 1965).

Physician Tried for Negligence

In March, 2002, Margarita Munoz, who had been suffering from breakthrough bleeding daily for two months, asked her primary care doctor to remove an intrauterine device (IUD). Her physician tried but was unable to remove the IUD. Munoz's primary care doctor referred her to Dr. Gordon B. Clark, who performed a physical exam. At that time, Munoz was mostly asymptomatic, except for dysmenorrhea—painful cramping during menstruation—and abnormal uterine bleeding. Dr. Clark advised Munoz that her pelvic sonogram showed a complex adnexal mass arising from her right ovary, which could be a cyst or could be cancerous. Because of her history of ovarian cysts, Clark said that one alternative treatment for Munoz was the removal of her ovaries through laparoscopic surgery. Munoz chose that alternative.

In August 2002, Clark performed the laparoscopic surgery and thought he had removed Munoz's ovaries, fallopian tubes, and IUD. Clark sent the removed tissues to a pathologist for examination. From the tissue samples, the pathologist determined that Clark had removed mostly uterine tubes, but had only grazed the ovarian surface. Dr. Clark did not contact the pathologist to discuss her findings or conduct any tests that might explain the discrepancy. Instead, he chose to believe he had successfully removed Munoz's ovaries, and he told the patient that he had removed her ovaries, fallopian tubes, and IUD. He started Munoz on hormone replacement therapy to ward off surgically induced menopause.

Unaware of the discrepancy between the pathologist's report and Dr. Clark's remarks to her, Munoz continued her life as usual. During this time, she experienced severe abdominal pain, breakthrough bleeding, and premenstrual headaches. In April 2004, Munoz visited a hospital emergency room. Doctors there conducted an ultrasound exam of her pelvis and ordered a CT scan. Test results showed a large lobulated multicystic mass in Munoz's pelvis, suggestive of an "ovarian neoplasm" (tumor of the ovary).

Munoz consulted an obstetrician-gynecologist, who found that her ovaries contained endometrial tissue. The specialist removed Munoz's uterus and ovaries and sent the removed tissues to a pathologist, who confirmed the removal of those organs and tissues.

In March 2006, Munoz sued Dr. Clark for medical malpractice. The trial court found for Munoz and awarded damages. Dr. Clark appealed, but the trial court's verdict for the plaintiff was upheld. Justice Hill of the appellate court wrote:

Medical malpractice is negligence of a health care professional in the diagnosis, care, and treatment of a patient.

In a medical malpractice case, the plaintiff must prove the following elements: (1) The physician owes the owes the patient a duty of care and was required to meet or exceed a certain standard of care to protect the patient from injury; (2) the physician breached this duty or deviated from the applicable standard of care; and (3) the patient was injured and the injury proximately resulted from the physician's breach of the standard of care.

The elements of negligence are never presumed. Therefore, expert testimony is generally required to establish the appropriate standard of care and causation because such matters are outside the knowledge of the average person without specialized training. In certain medical malpractice claims, expert testimony is not required because the standard of care and causation are within the common knowledge of a layperson. But, the application of the common knowledge exception is extremely limited.

Source: *Munoz v. Clark*, 2009 Kan. App.; 199 P.3d 1283.

Consult the explanation of the 4 Ds of negligence on p. 142 and identify them in this case.

Nonfeasance. The failure to act when one should. For example, a newly certified emergency medical technician is first on the scene of a traffic accident. An injured motorist stops breathing and appears to be in cardiac arrest. The EMT, though trained in cardiopulmonary resuscitation, "freezes" and does nothing. The patient dies. In failing to act, the EMT could be guilty of nonfeasance.

There are four elements that must be present in a given situation to prove that a health care professional is guilty of negligence. Sometimes called the "four Ds of negligence," these elements include

- *Duty*—The person charged with negligence owed a duty of care to the accuser.

- *Dereliction*—The health care provider breached the duty of care to the patient.

- *Direct Cause*—The breach of the duty of care to the patient was a direct cause of the patient's injury.

- *Damages*—There is a legally recognizable injury to the patient.

In this chapter's opening scenario, how does Samantha's act illustrate the four Ds? In your opinion, does her act illustrate malfeasance, misfeasance, or nonfeasance?

When a plaintiff sues a health care practitioner (defendant) for negligence, the burden of proof is on the plaintiff. That is, it is up to the accuser's attorney to present evidence of the four Ds.

State statutes must be consulted for restrictions that apply to actions against health care providers. Some states limit damage awards or mandate procedural rules that must be followed in medical malpractice claims. In some states, for example, medical review panels must screen claims before they are brought to court. The panel examines the facts and then issues a finding of "malpractice" or "no malpractice." Such panels are generally composed of physicians with expertise in the medical specialty in question and sometimes include a neutral attorney.

The Joint Commission (TJC—formerly the Joint Commission on Accreditation of Hospital Organizations, or JCAHO) Standards on Medical Mistakes and Patient Safety

Avoiding medical mistakes and safeguarding patients while they are being examined or treated are vital issues for health care practitioners, both to ensure excellent patient care and to avoid issues of medical malpractice liability.

While conscientious health care practitioners do their best to avoid making mistakes, they are human, and mistakes do occur. The legal and ethical response when health care mistakes are made is to report the mistake to attending physicians and supervisors and on the patient's medical record, and to tell the patient he or she has been harmed. In fact, health care practitioners and health care facilities that try to cover up mistakes are most likely to be sued, and hospitals and other facilities that fail to disclose mistakes could lose their Joint Commission accreditation.

To further address patient safety, as of January 1, 2004, all TJC-accredited health care organizations are surveyed for implementation of the following requirements:

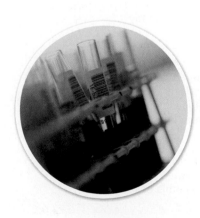

1. Improve the accuracy of patient identification.

- Use at least two patient identifiers whenever taking blood samples or administering medications or blood products. Do not use a hospital patient's room number as an identifier.

- Prior to the start of any surgical or invasive procedure, confirm the correct patient, procedure and site, using active—not passive—communication.

2. Improve the effectiveness of communication among caregivers (Figure 5-3).

   - Use a process for taking verbal or telephone orders or critical test results that requires a verification read-back by the person receiving the information.

   - Standardize abbreviations, acronyms, and symbols used throughout the organization, including a list of all such terms that are *not* to be used.

3. Improve the safety of using high-alert medications.

   - Remove concentrated electrolytes (including, but not limited to, potassium chloride, potassium phosphate, and sodium chloride) from patient care units.

   - Standardize and limit the number of drug concentrations available in the organization.

4. Eliminate wrong-site, wrong-patient, wrong-procedure surgery.

   - Create and use a preoperative verification process, such as a checklist, to confirm that appropriate documents, such as medical records and imaging studies, are available.

   - Use procedures to mark the surgical site and involve the patient in the marking process.

5. Improve the safety of using infusion pumps.

   - Ensure free-flow protection on all general-use and patient-controlled analgesia intravenous infusion pumps.

6. Improve the effectiveness of clinical alarm systems.

   - Use regular preventative maintenance and testing of alarm systems.

   - Be sure that alarms are activated with appropriate settings and can be heard over distances and competing noise within a care unit.

7. Reduce the risk of health care–acquired infections.

   - Comply with current Centers for Disease Control and Prevention (CDC) hand hygiene guidelines.

   - Manage as sentinel events all identified cases of unanticipated death or major permanent loss of function associated with a health care–acquired infection.

TJC established these requirements to help accredited health care organizations address issues of patient safety that can lead to adverse events that, in turn, can result in lawsuits.

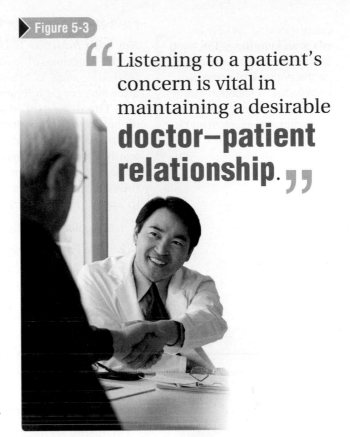

Figure 5-3

"Listening to a patient's concern is vital in maintaining a desirable **doctor–patient relationship**."

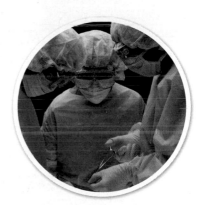

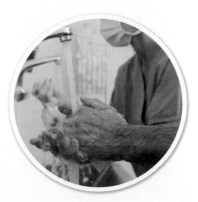

Res Ipsa Loquitur

res ipsa loquitur "The thing speaks for itself"; also known as the doctrine of common knowledge. A situation that is so obviously negligent that no expert witnesses need be called.

Res ipsa loquitur is Latin for "the thing speaks for itself." It is also known as the doctrine of common knowledge. It means that the mistake is so obvious—such as leaving a sponge or surgical instrument inside a patient after surgery or operating on the wrong body part—that negligence is obvious. The defendant in such a case may argue that the event was an inevitable accident and had nothing to do with his or her responsibility of control or supervision. Traditionally, expert witnesses did not have to be called to testify in a medical malpractice lawsuit alleging *res ipsa loquitur*, but courts have made exceptions in many cases and allowed expert witness testimony. Judicial consideration of this doctrine varies. Generally, for *res ipsa loquitur* to apply, three conditions must exist:

1. The act of negligence must obviously be under the defendant's control.
2. The patient must not have contributed to the act.
3. It must be apparent that the patient would not have been injured if reasonable care had been used.

Cases that fall under the doctrine of *res ipsa loquitur* include

- Unintentionally leaving foreign bodies, such as sponges or instruments, inside a patient's body during surgery.
- Accidentally burning or otherwise injuring a patient while he or she is anesthetized.
- Damaging healthy tissue during an operation.
- Causing an infection by the use of unsterilized instruments.

check your **progress**

6. Define *privileged communication*.

_____

_____

7. Is a breach of confidentiality an offense for which a health care practitioner can be sued? Explain your answer.

_____

_____

8. Distinguish among *malfeasance, misfeasance,* and *nonfeasance.*

_____

_____

_____

_____

_____

9 Name the four Ds of negligence.

_____

_____

Damage Awards and Medical Malpractice Insurance

When a defendant is found guilty of a tort—such as negligence, breach of contract, libel, or slander—the plaintiff is awarded compensation based on the extent of his or her injuries, loss of income, damage to reputation, or other harm that can be proved. This monetary compensation is called **damages.** Table 5-1 explains the various types of damages and how the court determines them.

damages Monetary awards sought by plaintiffs in lawsuits.

Physicians and many other professional health care providers carry liability insurance, which pays damage awards in the event of a negligence or malpractice suit up to the limits of the policy.

Medical groups maintain that high damage awards in tort cases have led to a malpractice insurance crisis for physicians, especially those in high-risk specialties, such as obstetrics-gynecology, orthopedic surgery, and general surgery. Recent studies and news articles have reported that doctors in some states are participating in walkouts and demonstrations, relocating to states where caps have been legislated on medical malpractice damage awards, limiting procedures, performing additional patient tests to cover all liability bases, and even leaving the profession. Furthermore, some hospitals have shut down or threatened to shut down trauma centers, and long-term care facilities have closed.

In an attempt to address rapidly rising premiums for medical malpractice insurance, some states have placed caps on damage awards in medical malpractice cases. Attorney organizations, however, insist that damage caps are unfair to injured patients.

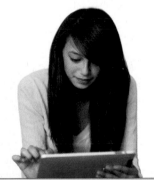

check your **progress**

10. *Res ipsa loquitur* means _____.

11. *Res ipsa loquitur* is also known as the doctrine of _____.

12. Name two types of cases that fall under the doctrine of *res ipsa loquitur*.

_____

_____

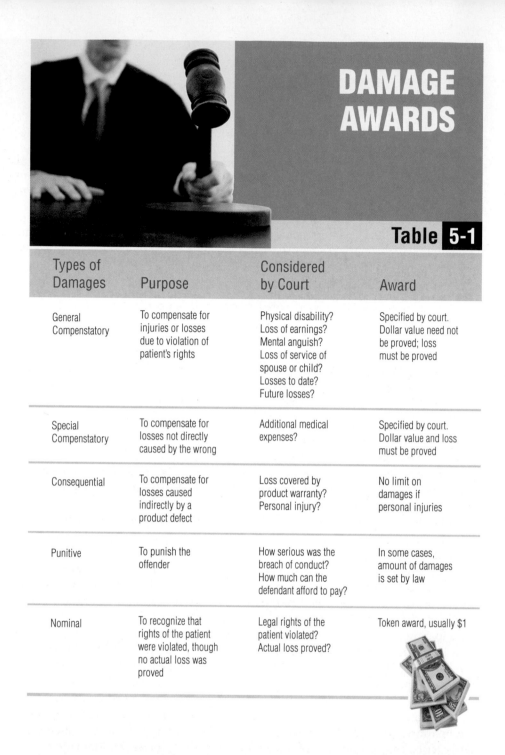

DAMAGE AWARDS

Table 5-1

Types of Damages	Purpose	Considered by Court	Award
General Compenstatory	To compensate for injuries or losses due to violation of patient's rights	Physical disability? Loss of earnings? Mental anguish? Loss of service of spouse or child? Losses to date? Future losses?	Specified by court. Dollar value need not be proved; loss must be proved
Special Compenstatory	To compensate for losses not directly caused by the wrong	Additional medical expenses?	Specified by court. Dollar value and loss must be proved
Consequential	To compensate for losses caused indirectly by a product defect	Loss covered by product warranty? Personal injury?	No limit on damages if personal injuries
Punitive	To punish the offender	How serious was the breach of conduct? How much can the defendant afford to pay?	In some cases, amount of damages is set by law
Nominal	To recognize that rights of the patient were violated, though no actual loss was proved	Legal rights of the patient violated? Actual loss proved?	Token award, usually $1

The issue is an important one for both health care practitioners and patients and is not likely to be settled uniformly across the country. As a future or present health care practitioner, you should stay informed on the issues of medical malpractice insurance and tort reform and form your own opinion.

Wrongful Death Statutes

wrongful death statutes
State statutes that allow a person's beneficiaries to collect for loss to the estate of the deceased for future earnings when a death is judged to have been due to negligence.

Most states have enacted **wrongful death statutes** which allow a patient's beneficiaries to collect from a health care practitioner for loss to the patient's estate of future earnings when a patient's death is judged to have been due to negligence of health care practitioners. In most states, a cap has been placed on the amount of damages that can be recovered in a civil action for wrongful death.

The state may also prosecute a health care practitioner under criminal statutes for the wrongful death of a patient. The following court cases illustrate wrongful death actions.

COURT CASE

Hospital Sued in Wrongful Death Case

A wrongful death suit was brought by a woman's husband against a Randolph County, Illinois, hospital following her death. The plaintiff alleged that during the course of treatment for his wife's back pain, the defendant doctor had prescribed too many medications, which led to her wrongful death.

The defendant doctor testified at the Illinois trial that he had in fact prescribed her numerous medications during the two and a half years he treated her. The decedent had previously been diagnosed with a bulging disc in her back and had a history of pain in her back, leg, and abdomen since 1992. However, despite the numerous narcotic medications the doctor prescribed, she continued to suffer pain in her back, abdomen, hip, and knees. The doctor's testimony stated that during the several years he treated the decedent that he never saw any sign of overmedication.

However, the plaintiff's expert's testimony refuted the doctor's claim that the plaintiff could not have been overmedicated and stated that on autopsy it was discovered that she had significantly elevated levels of Percocet and Demerol, both narcotic pain medications, in her system. The expert also testified that these elevated levels of medications contributed to the plaintiff's death.

The Illinois jury returned a verdict in favor of the plaintiff in the amount of $100,000 which was reduced by 50 persent on the basis of the decedent's contributory negligence. That is, even though the jury found the defendant doctor contributed to the plaintiff's death, it also found the decedent contributed to her own death by taking the prescribed medications. (In contributory negligence situations, the verdict amount is reduced by whatever degree the jury finds the plaintiff contributed to his or her own negligence. So in this case, the plaintiff was essentially awarded $50,000 by the jury.)

Even though the plaintiff won in this case, he brought an appeal to a higher court, alleging that the lower court erred by refusing to add to the verdict. The basis of his appeal rested on a claim that the jury award "was manifestly inadequate and contrary to the evidence" (i.e., that the jury award was too little, given the plaintiff's loss and the overwhelming evidence against the defendant doctor). The plaintiff's argument quoted the defendant doctor's attorney, who stated in his closing argument that if there were liability against the doctor, "a fair verdict on damages would be $1 million."

The appellate court rejected the plaintiff's argument, and affirmed the lower court's refusal to add to the verdict award. The appellate court cited the Illinois Wrongful Death Act, stating that under the act it was impossible to measure the propriety of damage awards by comparing the present case with other Illinois wrongful death cases. The appellate court also explained that it did not see any evidence in the court record referring to a specific loss of money or economic loss as a result of the decedent's death. Because the appellate court did not see any clear evidence to demonstrate that the jury or lower court erred in regard to the amount, it deferred to the jury: "It is not within our province to substitute our judgment for that of the jury to determine the monetary value of the loss of society in this case." The appeals court also rejected that part of the plaintiff's argument that was based on the defendant doctor's attorney's closing statements, stating that the commentary by the defense counsel was an opinion and should not be considered a binding judicial admission.

Source: Dobyns v. Chung,
399 Ill. App.3d 272, 926 N.E.2d 847 (Ill. App. 5 Dist. 2010).

Medical wrongful death cases do not always involve physicians, as in the following case.

COURT CASE

EMTs Follow Protocol

A woman suffered chest pains and the county's fire rescue team was dispatched to her home, where a team member determined she had sustained a heart attack. The patient's daughter asked that she be transported to a hospital where her doctor was waiting for her. However, the rescue team said that because the patient was "critical" and "unstable," written protocol dictated that she be transported to the closest appropriate facility. The patient died shortly after arriving at that hospital.

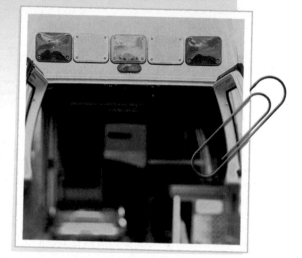

The patient's estate representative sued for wrongful death, but the suit was dismissed. The plaintiff appealed, and the appeals court determined that there was no breach of duty of care, and that the fire rescue team performed in a reasonably prudent manner. The appeals court affirmed the lower court's decision to dismiss.

Source: Franco v. Miami-Dade County, 32 Fla. L. Weekly D21, 947 So.2d 512 (Fla. App. 3 Dist. 2006).

LO 5.5

Outline the phases of a lawsuit.

Elements of a Lawsuit

As indicated in Chapter 4, the type of court that hears a case depends on the offense or complaint. In civil malpractice or negligence cases, the party bringing the action (plaintiff) must prove the case by presenting to a judge or jury evidence that is more convincing than that of the opposing side (defendant).

Phases of a Lawsuit

The typical malpractice or negligence lawsuit proceeds as follows:

1. A patient feels he or she has been injured.

2. The patient seeks the advice of an attorney.

3. If the attorney believes the case has merit, he or she then requests copies of the patient's medical records. The attorney reviews the medical records and the appropriate standard of care to ascertain merits of the case. In some states, before proceeding to a lawsuit, the attorney must obtain an expert witness report stating that the standard of care has been violated. An affidavit to that effect must then be submitted. An affidavit is a sworn statement in writing made under oath. It may also be a declaration before an authorized officer of the court.

Pleading Phase

4. The plaintiff's (injured patient's) attorney files a complaint with the clerk of the court. In this document, the plaintiff states his or her version of the situation and the amount of money sought from the defendant (the practitioner being sued) for the plaintiff's injury.

5. A **summons** is issued by the clerk of the court and is delivered with a copy of the complaint to the defendant, directing him or her to respond to the charges. If the defendant does not respond within the specified time limit, he or she can lose the case by default.

6. The defendant's attorney files an answer to the summons, and a copy of it is sent to the plaintiff. In this document, the defendant presents his or her version of the case, either admitting or denying the charges. The defendant may also file a counterclaim or a cross-complaint.

7. If a cross-complaint is made, the plaintiff files a reply.

Interrogatory or Pretrial Discovery Phase

8. The court sets a trial date.

9. Pretrial motions may be made and decided. For example, the defendant may request that the lawsuit be dismissed, the plaintiff may amend the original complaint, or either side may request a change of venue (ask that the trial be held in another place).

10. Discovery procedures may be used to uncover evidence that will support the charges when the case comes to court. A court order called a **subpoena** may be issued commanding the presence of the physician or a medical facility employee in court or requiring that a **deposition** be taken. A deposition is sworn testimony given and recorded outside the courtroom during the pretrial phase of a case. (See the following section entitled "Witness Testimony.")

    An **interrogatory** may be requested instead of or in addition to a deposition. This is a written set of questions requiring written answers from a plaintiff or defendant under oath.

    The subpoena commanding a witness to appear in court and to bring certain medical records is called a **subpoena** *duces tecum*. Failure to obey a subpoena may result in contempt-of-court charges. Contempt of court is willful disobedience to or open disrespect of a court, judge, or legislative body. It is punishable by fines or imprisonment.

11. A pretrial conference may be called by the judge scheduled to hear the case. During this conference, the judge discusses the issues in the case with the opposing attorneys. This helps avoid surprises and delays after the trial starts and may lead to an out-of-court settlement. (*Note:* At any point after the complaint is filed before the case comes to trial, an out-of-court settlement may be reached.)

Trial Phase

12. The jury is selected (if one is to be used), and the trial begins.

13. Opening *statements* are made by the lawyers for the plaintiff and the defendant, summarizing what each will prove during the trial.

14. Witnesses are called to testify for both sides. They may be cross-examined by opposing attorneys.

15. Each attorney makes closing *arguments* that the evidence presented supports his or her version of the case. No new evidence may be presented during summation.

16. The judge gives instructions to the jury (if one was chosen), and the jury retires to deliberate.

17. The jury reaches a verdict.

18. The final judgment is handed down by the court. The judge bases his or her decision for judgment on the jury's verdict.

summons A written notification issued by the clerk of the court and delivered with a copy of the complaint to the defendant in a lawsuit, directing him or her to respond to the charges brought in a court of law.

subpoena A legal document requiring the recipient to appear as a witness in court or to give a deposition.

deposition Sworn testimony given and recorded outside the courtroom during the pretrial phase of a case.

interrogatory A written set of questions requiring written answers from a plaintiff or defendant under oath.

subpoena *duces tecum* A legal document requiring the recipient to bring certain written records to court to be used as evidence in a lawsuit.

Appeals Phase

19. Posttrial motions may be filed.

20. An appeal may be made for the case to be reviewed by a higher court if the evidence indicates that errors may have been made or if there was injustice or impropriety in the trial court proceedings. During an appeal, the judge has the option of affirming, reversing, or modifying a decision. A judgment is final only when all options for appeal have been exercised.

Witness Testimony

An estimated 9 out of 10 lawsuits are settled out of court, but health care practitioners are often asked to give testimony. Testimony may be given in court on the witness stand, or it may be given in an attorney's conference room in a pretrial proceeding called a deposition. (See the earlier section entitled "Interrogatory or Pretrial Discovery Phase.") Depositions are of two types:

1. Discovery depositions.

2. Depositions in lieu of trial.

Discovery depositions cover material that will most likely be examined again when the witness testifies in court. Since there will be an opportunity for the opposing attorney to question the witness a second time in court, the deposition need not cover every possible question.

Both before a deposition and before in-court testimony, the witness is sworn to tell the truth and then is questioned by attorneys representing both sides. During courtroom testimony, however, a judge is present to rule on objections raised by the attorneys. When an objection is raised, the witness should stop speaking until the judge either *sustains* or *overrules* the objection. If the objection is sustained, the witness need not answer the question. If the objection is overruled, the witness must answer. If in doubt about whether an objection to a question was sustained or overruled, the witness may ask the judge whether a question should be answered. During a deposition, witnesses should take the attorney's advice regarding questions that should be answered.

Depositions in lieu of trial are used instead of the witness's in-person testimony in court. Since the opposing attorney has one opportunity to question the witness, questions are thorough, and the witness should carefully consider his or her answers.

Sometimes depositions in lieu of trial are videotaped, to be played in the courtroom during the trial. Witnesses whose depositions will be videotaped should be informed in advance, so they can dress as though they were appearing in court in person.

testimony Statements sworn to under oath by witnesses testifying in court and giving depositions.

Witnesses may offer two kinds of **testimony:** fact and expert. Health care practitioners or laypersons may offer *fact testimony,* and this type of testimony concerns only those facts the witness has observed. For example, regarding testimony in a medical malpractice case, medical assistants, LPNs/LVNs, and registered nurses may testify about how many times a patient saw the physician, the patient's appearance during a particular visit, or similar observations. If asked to give fact testimony, a health care practitioner's powers of observation and memory are more important than his or her professional qualifications. A health care practitioner giving fact testimony is not allowed to give his or her opinion on the facts.

Only experts in a particular field have the education, skills, knowledge, and experience to give *expert testimony.* In medical negligence lawsuits, physicians are usually called as expert witnesses to testify to the standard of care regarding the matter in question. Expert witnesses may, and usually do, give their opinions on the facts. If the defendant/physician is a specialist, the expert witness generally practices or teaches in the same specialty. Acceptable expert witnesses are not coworkers, friends, or acquaintances of the defendant. It is ethical and acceptable for expert witnesses to set and accept a fee commensurate with time taken from regular employment and time spent preparing their expert testimony.

Courtroom Conduct

Most health care practitioners will never have to appear in court. If you should be asked to appear, however, the following suggestions can help:

- Attend court proceedings as required. If you were subpoenaed but fail to appear, you could be charged with contempt of court. (If either the plaintiff or the defendant fails to appear, that person forfeits the case.)

- Find out in advance when and where you are to appear, and do not be late for scheduled hearings.

- Bring the required documents to court, and present them only when requested to do so.

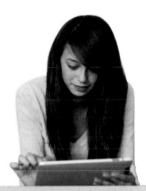

check your **progress**

13. Name the four phases of a typical medical professional liability lawsuit, and describe how a medical assistant might be involved in each trial phase.

_____

_____

14. A subpoena *duces tecum* is issued during which trial phase?

_____

15. The complaint is filed during which trial phase?

_____

16. During which trial phase is the court's judgment handed down?

_____

_____

17. A judgment is final only when

_____

_____

18. Distinguish between *deposition* and *interrogatory*.

_____

_____

- Before testifying, refresh your memory concerning all the facts observed about the matter in question, such as dates, times, words spoken, and circumstances.

- When testifying, speak slowly, use layperson's terms instead of medical terms whenever possible, and do not lose your temper or attempt to be humorous.

- Answer all questions in a straightforward manner, even if the answers appear to help the opposing side.

- Answer only the question asked, no more and no less.

- Because you are testifying about what you recall, be careful of broad generalizations, such as "That is all that took place." A better answer might be, "As I recall, that is what took place."

- Your attorney may help you prepare your testimony, but do not discuss your testimony with other witnesses or others outside the courtroom. Answer truthfully if asked whether you discussed your testimony with counsel.

- Appear well groomed, and dress in clean, conservative clothing.

LO 5.6
Name two advantages to alternative dispute resolution.

alternative dispute resolution (ADR) Settlement of civil disputes between parties using neutral mediators or arbitrators without going to court.

Alternative Dispute Resolution

Alternative dispute resolution (ADR), also known as appropriate dispute resolution, consists of techniques for resolving civil disputes without going to court. As court calendars have become overcrowded in recent years, ADR has become increasingly popular. Several alternative methods of settling legal disputes are possible, including mediation, arbitration, and a combination of the two methods called med-arb.

Some states require mediation and/or arbitration for certain civil cases, while in other states alternative dispute resolution methods are voluntary. *Mediation* is an ADR method in which a neutral third party listens to both sides of the argument and then helps resolve the dispute. The mediator does not have the authority to impose a solution on the parties involved.

Arbitration is a method of settling disputes in which the opposing parties agree to abide by the decision of an arbitrator. An arbitrator is either selected directly by the disputing parties or chosen in one of the following two ways:

1. Under the terms of a written contract, an arbitrator is chosen by the court or by the American Arbitration Association.

2. If no contract exists, each of the two involved parties selects an arbitrator, and the two arbitrators select a third.

In an informal proceeding, each side presents evidence and witnesses. In the alternative dispute resolution method called med-arb, the mediator resolves the dispute if the two parties are unable to reach agreement after mediation.

Advocates of alternative dispute resolution claim that these methods are faster and less costly than court adjudication. Critics claim that medical malpractice cases are best decided when all the factual information is brought out, as in pretrial judicial discovery procedures. Critics also argue that selecting arbitrators acceptable to both parties can take weeks, months, even years, and that attorneys' fees and damage awards can be as costly as in court-tried cases. Figure 5-4 illustrates a sample arbitration agreement to be signed by the patient and physician involved in a dispute.

Figure 5-4 Sample Patient–Physician Arbitration Agreement

Article 1: It is understood that any dispute as to medical malpractice, that is as to whether any medical services rendered under this contract were unnecessary or unauthorized or were improperly, negligently, or incompetently rendered, will be determined by submission to arbitration as provided by California law, and not by a lawsuit or resort to court process except as California law provides for judicial review of arbitration proceedings. Both parties to this contract, by entering into, are giving up their constitutional right to have such dispute decided in a court of law before a jury, and instead are accepting the use of arbitration.

Article 2: I understand and agree that this arbitration agreement binds me and anyone else who may have a claim arising out of or related to all treatment or services provided by the physician, including any spouse or heirs of the patient and any children, whether born or unborn at the time of the occurrence giving rise to any claim. This includes, but is not limited to, all claims for monetary damages exceeding the jurisdictional limit of the small claims court, including, without limitation, suits for loss of consortium, wrongful deaths, emotional distress or punitive damages. I further understand and agree that if i sign this agreement on behalf of some other person for whom I have responsibility, then, in addition to myself, such person(s) will also be bound, along with anyone else who may have a claim arising out of the treatment or services rendered to that person. I also understand agree that this agreement relates to claims against the physician and any consenting substitute physician, as well as the physician's partners, associates, association, corporation or partnership, and the employees, agents, and estates of any of them. I also hereby consent to the intervention or joinder in the arbitration proceeding of all parties relevant to a full and complete settlement of any dispute arbitrated under this Agreement, as ser forth in the CA/HHS/CMA Medical Arbitration Rules.

Article 3: I understand and agree that I will be bound by this arbitration agreement and that this agreement will be valid and enforceable for any and all treatment provided by the physician in the future regardless of the length of time since my last visit to this physician, and regardless of the fact that the patient -physician relationship between myself and the physician may be interrupted for any reason and then recommenced.

Article 4: I understand that i do not have to sign this agreement to receive the physician's services, and that if i do sign the agreement and change my mind within 30 days of today, then i may cancel this agreement by giving written notice to the undersigned physician within that time stating that i want to withdraw from this arbitration agreement.

Article 5: On behalf of myself and all others bound by this agreement as set forth in Article 2, agreement is hereby given to be bound by the Medical Arbitration Rules of the California Association of Hospitals and Health Systems (CAHHS) and the California Medical Association (CMA), as they may be amended from time to time, which are hereby incorporated into this agreement, A copy of these rules is included in the pamphlet in which this agreement is found. Additional copies of the Rules are available from the California Medical Association, P.O. Box 7690, San Francisco, Ca. 94120-7690, Attention: Arbitration Rules, I understand that disputes covered by this Agreement will be covered by California law applicable to actions against health care providers, including the Medical Injury Compensation Reform Act of 1975 (including any amendments thereto).

Article 6: Optional: retroactive effect
If I intend this agreement to cover services rendered before the date it is signed (for example, emergency treatment), I have indicated the earlier date I intend this agreement to be effective from and initialed below.

Earlier effective date: _____   Patient's initials: _____

Article 7: I have read and understood all the information in this pamphlet, including the explanation of the Patient-Physician Arbitration Agreement, this Agreement, and the rules. I understand that In the case of any pregnant woman, the term "patient" as used herein means both the mother and the mother's expected child or children.

If any provision of this arbitration agreement is held invalid or unenforceable, the remaining provisions shall remain in full force and shall not be affected by the invalidity of any other provision.

Notice: By signing this contract you are agreeing to have any issue of medical malpractice decided by neutral arbitration and you are giving up your right to a jury or court trial. See article 1 of this contract.

_____   Dated: _____
(Patient, Parent, Guardian or Legally Authorized Representative of Patient)

If signed by other than patient, indicate relationship: _____

Physician's agreement to arbitrate:

In consideration of the foregoing execution of this Patient-Physician Arbitration Agreement, I likewise agree to be bound by the terms set forth in this agreement and In the rules specified in Article 5 above.

_____   Date:_____
(Physician or Duly-Authorized Representative)

_____
Title—e.g., Partner, President, etc.   Print name of Physician, Medical Group, Partnership or Association

© California Medical Association, 1996.

CHAPTER SUMMARY

LO 5.1 What are the three areas of general liability for which a physician/employer is responsible?

- The practice's building and grounds.
- Automobiles used as part of employees' duties.
- Employee safety.

LO 5.2 What are the differences among the reasonable person standard, standard of care, and duty of care?

- Under the reasonable person standard, individuals may be charged with negligence if someone is injured because he or she failed to perform an act that a reasonable person, in similar circumstances, would perform or if he or she committed an act that a reasonable person would not commit.

- Standard of care is the level of performance expected of a health care practitioner in carrying out his or her professional duties.

- Duty of care is the legal obligation of health care workers to patients and, sometimes, nonpatients.

LO 5.3 What are the responsibilities of health care practitioners concerning privacy, confidentiality, and privileged communication?

- Health care practitioners have a legal and ethical obligation to safeguard a patient's privacy and maintain confidentiality, which is the act of holding information in confidence, not to be released to unauthorized individuals.

- Privileged communication refers to information held confidential within a protected relationship, such as the physician–patient relationship, and patients may sue for breach of confidence if protected information is released and results in damage to the patient.

LO 5.4 What are the four Ds of negligence?

- *Duty*—The person charged with negligence owed a duty of care to the accuser.

- *Dereliction*—The health care provider breached the duty of care to the patient.

- *Direct Cause*—The breach of the duty of care to the patient was a direct cause of the patient's injury.

- *Damages*—There is a legally recognizable injury to the patient.

LO 5.5 What are the phases of a lawsuit?

- Pleading phase.
- Interrogatory or pretrial discovery phase.
- Trial phase.
- Appeals phase.

What is the difference between testimony by deposition and interrogatory testimony?

- A deposition is sworn testimony given and recorded outside the courtroom during the pretrial phase of a case. An interrogatory is a written set of questions requiring written answers from a plaintiff or defendant under oath.

LO 5.6 What is alternative dispute resolution?

- Settlement of civil disputes between parties using neutral mediators or arbitrators without going to court.

ETHICS ISSUES Professional Liability and Medical Malpractice

Ethics ISSUE 1: As citizens and as professionals with special training and experience, health care practitioners are ethically obligated to assist in the administration of justice. If a patient who has a legal claim requests a health care practitioner's assistance, he or she should furnish medical evidence, with the patient's consent, to secure the patient's legal rights.

Medical experts should have recent and substantive experience in the area in which they testify and should limit testimony to their sphere of medical expertise.

Discussion Questions

1. An orthopedic surgeon who has been retired from practice for 15 years and is a friend of the plaintiff's has been called to testify in the plaintiff's suit alleging damage to his hip joint sustained in a car accident. In your opinion, is it ethical for the physician described previously to testify? Explain your answer.

_____

_____

2. In your opinion, is it ever ethical for a health care practitioner to testify against another health care practitioner in a medical malpractice law suit? Explain your answer.

_____

_____

3. As a health care practitioner, do you consider it ethical to charge for your services to testify as an expert witness? Explain your answer.

_____

_____

4. Are there circumstances when you might consider it unethical to charge for your services as an expert witness? Explain your answer.

_____

_____

Ethics ISSUE 2: Health care practitioners are ethically bound to respect the patient's dignity and to make a positive effort to secure a comfortable and considerate atmosphere for the patient, in such ways as providing appropriate gowns and drapes, private facilities for undressing, and clear explanations for procedures.

Discussion Questions

1. An adolescent male patient is visibly uncomfortable as a female physician begins a physical examination. What actions might the physician and/or her attending certified medical assistant take to make the patient more comfortable?

_____

_____

2. A hospital patient who is mentally disabled becomes extremely agitated and violent. She disrobes and runs through the hallways. Nurses and other employees are unable to calm the woman, and security officers arrive. Other patients and employees in the area stand around watching the woman as the officers attempt to subdue her. As a health care practitioner in the immediate vicinity, what, if anything, might you do to protect the woman's privacy?

_____

_____

3. A woman requests a breast exam when, on self-examination, she detects a small lump. Her male family physician performs the breast examination without a chaperone, and begins massaging the patient's nipple in a suggestive manner. What should the patient do?

_____

_____

4. Are there legal implications in the previous example? Explain your answer, detailing any preventative measures that could have been taken to avoid them.

_____

_____

Go to **www.mhhe.com/judson6e** to practice your case review skills. Then read on for more information.

[KEY TERMS]

alternative dispute resolution (ADR)	malfeasance	standard of care
confidentiality	misfeasance	subpoena
damages	nonfeasance	subpoena *duces tecum*
deposition	privileged communication	summons
duty of care	reasonable person standard	testimony
interrogatory	*res ipsa loquitur*	wrongful death statutes
liable		

[CHAPTER 5 REVIEW]

Applying Knowledge

Circle the correct answer for each of the following questions.

LO 5.1

1. As employers, physicians have *general* liability in what three areas?
   a. Hospitals, medical offices, and clinics
   b. The practice's buildings and grounds, automobiles, and employee safety

c. Telephone consultations, house calls, and office calls
d. None of the above

2. According to the reasonable person standard as discussed in this chapter, in which of the following situations might a person be charged with negligence?
   a. A woman is injured when she steps in front of a car and no one prevents the accident.
   b. A bystander does not intervene when a man with a gun robs another person on the street.
   c. A nurse fails to document her administration of a patient's medicine, and another nurse unknowingly administers a second dose, which constitutes an injurious overdose for the patient.
   d. A motorist stops to aid victims of a car accident

3. An off-duty certified medical assistant helps a pregnant woman deliver in a movie theater restroom. To what standard of care could the CMA be held?
   a. Any reasonable person
   b. A nurse
   c. Any CMA
   d. A physician

4. In the previous situation, to whom is a duty of care owed?
   a. No duty of care is owed because no health care relationship was established.
   b. A duty of care is owed to the CMA.
   c. A duty of care is owed to the woman and her baby.
   d. None of the above is true.

5. Which of the following statements is true of standard of care?
   a. Titles are not important, if appropriate care is administered.
   b. If a certified nursing assistant is able to perform the duties of a nurse, he or she should be legally and ethically be allowed to use the title "nurse."
   c. If one uses the title "nurse," one can be held to the standard of care of a nurse.
   d. Standard of care has no legal implications.

6. If a custodian sues an employing physician for ordering her to lift a heavy bookcase that injures her back, what is the issue of liability?
   a. Reasonable person standard
   b. Standard of care
   c. Privacy standard
   d. Duty of care

7. To establish a standard of care in a trial, _____ is (are) required.
   a. Deposition
   b. Subpoena
   c. Expert testimony
   d. Interrogatories

8. In which of the following situations has patient privacy been violated?
   a. A female patient is ushered into a medical clinic examination room, and a male phlebotomist draws a blood sample.
   b. A CMA knocks, then enters an exam room to take a patient's blood pressure.
   c. A physician performs a physical examination.
   d. In the presence of other patients in a clinic waiting room, a CMA tells a patient that her pregnancy test was positive.

9. What is the basis for most medical malpractice claims?
   a. Practicing medicine without a license
   b. Missed diagnoses

   c. Negligence

   d. Assault

10. A patient falls on a hospital's slippery tile floor and injures herself. Assuming that patient safety procedures were lax, what undesirable occurrence could result for the hospital?
   a. The patient could leave without paying his or her bill.
   b. The patient could become angry and refuse further treatment.
   c. The patient could sue the hospital.
   d. The patient could decide never to use the hospital's services again.

11. Which of the following is *not* one of the four Ds of negligence?
   a. Damages
   b. Dereliction
   c. Duty
   d. Desertion

12. The performance of a totally wrongful and unlawful act is a
   a. Malfeasance
   b. Nonfeasance
   c. Misfeasance
   d. Tortfeasor

13. The failure to act when one should is called
   a. Malfeasance
   b. Nonfeasance
   c. Misfeasance
   d. Tortfeasor

14. *Res ipsa loquitur* is the doctrine of
   a. Common sense
   b. Common damages
   c. Common knowledge
   d. Common belief

15. When a patient sues a physician for negligence, who has the burden of proof in court?
   a. The plaintiff
   b. The defendant
   c. The judge
   d. The jury

16. What purpose do expert witnesses serve in a medical negligence lawsuit?
   a. They testify that the person accused is of good character.
   b. They testify about the medical care given to the patient.
   c. They testify that the accuser is of good character.
   d. None of the above.

17. The doctrine of *res ipsa loquitur* might be applied in which of the following?
   a. A surgeon operates on a patient's foot, but it is the wrong foot.
   b. A woman's front teeth are knocked out while she is under anesthesia for surgery on her toe.
   c. A woman is anesthetized for a tubal ligation, but receives a hysterectomy.
   d. All of the above.

18. Monetary compensation awarded by a court of law is called
   a. Damages
   b. Subpoena
   c. Affidavit
   d. None of the above

19. Damages awarded by the court so that the defendant pays for violation of rights where the dollar value need not be proved are called
   a. General compensatory
   b. Punitive

    c. Nominal

    d. Special compensatory

20. Damages awarded by the court where the dollar value need not be proved but the loss must be proved are called

    a. General compensatory

    b. Punitive

    c. Nominal

    d. Special compensatory

21. Damages that recognize the wrong but award only a token amount are called

    a. General compensatory

    b. Punitive

    c. Nominal

    d. Special compensatory

22. Damages awarded by the court to punish the defendant are called

    a. General compensatory

    b. Punitive

    c. Nominal

    d. Special compensatory

LO 5.5

23. A written notification to appear in court to defend against a lawsuit is called a(n)

    a. Interrogatory

    b. Summons

    c. Deposition

    d. Subpoena

24. A court order for an individual to appear in court is called a(n)

    a. Interrogatory

    b. Deposition

    c. Subpoena

    d. Summons

25. An order to bring certain records to court is called a(n)

    a. Interrogatory

    b. Summons

    c. Subpoena

    d. Subpoena *duces tecum*

26. Which of the following best defines the term *deposition?*

    a. A written notification to appear in court

    b. Sworn testimony given and recorded outside the courtroom during the pretrial phase of a case

    c. A written notification to bring certain records to court

    d. A written list of questions and answers

27. Who is most likely to give factual testimony in a trial?

    a. A person who was present during certain events, and can tell what happened

    b. A expert who knows how certain medical treatments should be performed

    c. A witness who was not present during disputed events, but can determine if they might have occurred as indicated by other testimony

    d. None of the above

28. Which of the following legal actions may be taken if you are subpoenaed to appear in court as a witness or to give a deposition and you fail to appear?

    a. You can immediately be jailed.

    b. No action will be taken.

    c. You may be charged with contempt of court.

    d. You are asked to come in at a more convenient time.

29. What is the result if you are the plaintiff or the defendant in a lawsuit and you fail to appear in court?
   a. The case can be lost by default.
   b. No action is taken.
   c. You can immediately be jailed.
   d. You are asked to reschedule a court date.

30. A jury is selected in the _____ phase of a lawsuit.
   a. Appeals
   b. Pleadings
   c. Trial
   d. Pretrial discovery

31. A plea is made for the case to be reviewed by the higher court in the _____ phase of a lawsuit.
   a. Appeals
   b. Pleadings
   c. Trial
   d. Pretrial discovery

32. In the _____ phase of a lawsuit, subpoenas are issued.
   a. Trial
   b. Appeals
   c. Pretrial discovery
   d. Pleadings

33. A jury is selected in the _____ phase of a lawsuit
   a. Trial
   b. Appeals
   c. Pretrial discovery
   d. Pleadings

34. Attorneys make opening and closing statements in the _____ phase of a lawsuit.
   a. Trial
   b. Appeals
   c. Pretrial discovery
   d. Pleadings

35. Witnesses are called to testify in the _____ phase of a lawsuit.
   a. Trial
   b. Appeals
   c. Pretrial discovery
   d. Pleadings

36. A deposition is taken in the _____ phase of a lawsuit.
   a. Trial
   b. Appeals
   c. Pretrial discovery
   d. Pleadings

LO 5.6

37. Which of the following statements best defines *alternative dispute resolution?*
   a. A specific type of court case
   b. Dismissal of a court case
   c. Refusal to allow expert witnesses in a court case
   d. Settlement of civil disputes between parties using neutral mediators or arbitrators without going to court

38. How is *mediation* best defined?
   a. Attorneys on opposing sides reach a decision out of court.
   b. A suit is dismissed for lack of grounds.
   c. A neutral third party listens to both sides of the argument and then helps resolve the dispute.
   d. None of the above.

CASE STUDIES

Use your critical thinking skills to answer the questions that follow each case study.

LO 5.1 and LO 5.2

A 33-year-old male swallows 30 antidepressants and tells his wife, "I want to die." She takes him to the local hospital's emergency department where he is treated and released that same evening. In the hospital parking lot he pushes a security guard and is arrested and taken into custody. In the county jail a nurse places the man on suicide watch. The following evening, while still in custody, a psychologist speaks to the man for five minutes, then releases him from suicide watch. The man is returned to his cell, and two hours later he hangs himself.

39. Does the emergency department have liability for discharging a suicidal patient without further treatment?

_____

_____

40. Does the psychologist have liability for releasing the patient from suicide watch after a five-minute consult?

_____

_____

41. The psychologist is an "independent contractor" of the jail. Is the county liable for his actions?

_____

_____

LO 5.2

A woman gave birth in the back seat of a taxicab while en route to the hospital. To what standard of care would each of the following individuals be held?

42. The taxicab driver who comforted the mother.

_____

_____

43. A registered nurse, also a passenger in the cab, who assisted the mother.

_____

_____

44. A physician in general practice who was a passenger in the cab with the expectant mother and assisted the birth taking place in the cab.

_____

_____

45. A police officer who stopped the cab for speeding, observed the situation, and assisted the birth.

A woman trained in cardiopulmonary resuscitation (CPR) worked as the office manager for an insurance business. When her coworker at the next desk had a heart attack and fell to the floor, the office manager began CPR and shouted for others in the room to dial 911. The department supervisor came running and told the office manager to stop CPR. She reluctantly obeyed. Emergency medical technicians arrived, but the heart attack victim died.

46. The victim's husband sued the supervisor, the office manager, and the employees' parent organization for failure to render medical assistance. In a finding for the defendants, an appeals court ruled there was "no duty of care" for the employees to render assistance. Despite this court's ruling, in a similar situation, would you have acted as the CPR-trained office manager did? Explain your answer.

LO 5.4

During an endoscopic retrograde cholangiopancreatography (ERCP) (a gallbladder X-ray that requires injection of a dye), an inexperienced nurse injected the dye too forcefully and caused the patient to develop pancreatitis (inflammation of the pancreas) and suffer other debilitating injuries.

47. The patient sued and won. Refer to the four Ds of negligence to explain the court's decision.

An on-call ophthalmologist, without seeing the patient, diagnosed his eye pain, sensitivity to light, and nausea as sinusitis. In fact, the patient had acute angle closure glaucoma and lost sight in the eye.

48. When this case came to trial, the court found in favor of the patient/plaintiff. Explain the court's decision based on the four Ds of negligence.

INTERNET ACTIVITIES LO 5.1 and LO 5.6

Complete the activities and answer the questions that follow.

49. Visit the Web site of the American Arbitration Association. Click on "AAA University," then on "View Laws and Statutes." Name one national law governing arbitration.

50. Find the Web site for The Joint Commission (TJC)—formerly the Joint Commission on Accreditation of Healthcare Organizations (JCAHO). Briefly summarize what you see under "Joint Commission Vision." Conduct two Web searches: one for "medical malpractice insurance" and a second for "tort reform." Briefly summarize how the two relate. Do all reliable sources advocate tort reform as one solution to high medical malpractice insurance rates? Explain your answer.

RESOURCES

The Free Dictionary Web site: **http://legal-dictionary.thefreediction-ary.com/duty+of+care.**

Joel, Lucille A. *Kelly's Dimensions of Professional Nursing*. New York: McGraw-Hill, 2011.

The Joint Commission Web site: **www.jointcommission.org/.**

Kubasek, Nancy, et al. *Dynamic Business Law*. New York: McGraw-Hill, 2011.

The 'Lectric Law Library Web site: **www.lectlaw.com/files/exp24.htm.**

Mallor, Jane P., et al. *Business Law and the Legal Environment*. New York: McGraw-Hill, 2002.

Melvin, Sean. *The Legal Environment of Business*. New York: McGraw-Hill, 2010.

DEFENSES TO LIABILITY SUITS

Learning Outcomes

After studying this chapter, you should be able to:

LO 6.1 List and define the four Cs of medical malpractice prevention.

LO 6.2 Describe the various defenses to professional liability suits.

LO 6.3 Explain the purpose of quality improvement and risk management within a health care facility.

LO 6.4 Discuss five different types of medical liability insurance.

Cases in This Chapter

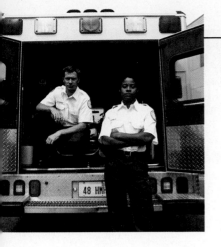

AS AN EMERGENCY MEDICAL TECHNICIAN (EMT), Daryl has encountered a number of "difficult" patients. For example, called to a residence by a man who had accidentally cut his wrist while slicing bread, he and his new partner, Joann, found the man bleeding profusely, and nearly hysterical.

"Don't touch me!" he screamed when the two EMTs began their assessment of his injuries.

Joann, startled, pulled back and removed her hand from the man's uninjured wrist. Daryl, however, proceeded calmly and carefully, but with determination.

"We're here to help you," Daryl replied in a level voice, making eye contact with the man. "We need to get that bleeding stopped; then we can get you the help you need." As he spoke, Daryl gently applied pressure to the man's bleeding wound and motioned for Joann to begin the assessment of the injured man's vital signs.

The man, agitated and sweating, continued to rant, but as Daryl spoke to him calmly, explaining each action he and Joann performed, he finally quieted enough to cooperate. By the time the EMTs transported the man to the hospital emergency room for treatment, he was able to calmly recount his accident to the physician on duty.

"When people are injured they're in pain and usually scared," Daryl explained to a shaken Joann later. "We have to stay calm, and just talk to them until they understand we're only there to help them, and we will be as gentle as possible. If we get in their face, and try to force them to do what we want, it's only going to make matters worse. And since people who are angry and upset are most likely to sue, we can also help prevent complaints later by staying calm and professional."

From Daryl's perspective, he needed to calm the patient before he could effectively assess his injuries.

From Joann's perspective, the "difficult" patient prevented her from thinking first of her training and staying calm.

From the patient's perspective, the profuse bleeding from his wound frightened him, and he was probably going into shock, as well.

Because the man was bleeding profusely, should Daryl and Joann have ignored his state of mind and forcibly restrained the man to begin treatment immediately?

Communicating effectively with patients or clients is often the most difficult aspect of a health care practitioner's job, but it is also one of the most vital. How could Joann have helped Daryl calm the patient?

Preventing Liability Suits

Malpractice litigation not only adds to the cost of health care, it also takes a psychological toll on both patients and health care practitioners. Both sides would probably agree that prevention is preferable to litigating a malpractice claim. Health care practitioners who use reasonable care in preventing professional liability claims are least likely to be faced with defending themselves against such claims. Figure 6-1 shows the four Cs of medical malpractice prevention.

LO 6.1

List and define the four Cs of medical malpractice prevention.

Figure 6-1

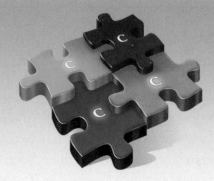

THE FOUR Cs OF MEDICAL MALPRACTICE PREVENTION

How can you protect yourself from a medical malpractice lawsuit?
By following the four Cs of medical malpractice prevention.

Caring

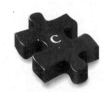

- There are two important benefits to showing your patients that you care. First is improvement in their medical condition. A secondary benefit is the decreased likelihood that your patients will feel the need to sue if treatment has unsatisfactory results, or if adverse events occur. Of course it is important that you be sincere in your concern, because others often quickly sense insincerity and may distrust you.

- Avoid destructive and unethical criticism of the work of other physicians and/or other health care practitioners. Do not discuss with a patient his or her former physician. Listen carefully to each patient's complaints and remarks about dissatisfaction with treatment, and see that the comments reach the treating physician.

Communication

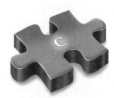

- If you communicate clearly and ask for confirmation that you have been understood, you will be more likely to earn your patients' and your colleagues' trust and respect. If your duties include taking telephone messages, relate them accurately.

- Offer to make appointments when appropriate. Remember that when health care practitioners other than physicians, or in some instances physician assistants, diagnose or prescribe, they may be charged with practicing medicine without a license. When adverse events occur, use correct procedures in reporting the event, and never avoid or ignore any patients involved.

Competence

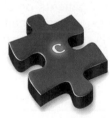

- Know your professional area well, including your limitations. Follow standards of care and appropriate procedures for medical practitioners in similar practices and in similar communities. Avoid any action that you are not fully trained or equipped to handle.

- Maintain and constantly update your knowledge and skills.

- Consult with other health care practitioners appropriately, early, and often.

- Know the requirements of good medical practice in caring for each patient.

- If you prepare or administer medications, check each drug three times: once when taking it from the supply cabinet, again when preparing the dosage, and a third time when returning the container to the shelf. All outdated medications should be discarded and promptly replaced. Prescription blanks should not be left on desktops or work areas.

- Stay informed about general medical and scientific progress by reading professional journals, attending seminars and professional association meetings, and fulfilling continuing study requirements.

Charting

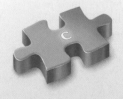

- Documentation is proof. For legal purposes, if it isn't in writing and explained completely and accurately, it wasn't done. Medical records should include X-rays, test results, progress notes, and anything else related to the patient's medical treatment.

- Document as though the patient will read his or her medical record. Never write something you would not want the patient to see.

Physician/Employers and Medical Facilities

The following guidelines for physician/employers and/or medical facilities can help you evaluate the quality of care offered by your physician/employer or medical facility and make appropriate suggestions for improving patient care and reducing liability risks in the workplace environment.

- Physician/employers should carefully select and supervise all employees and should be careful in delegating duties to them, expecting them to perform only those duties they may reasonably be expected to perform, based on their qualifications, credentials, training, and experience.

- Physicians should exhaust all reasonable methods of securing a diagnosis before embarking on a therapeutic course.

- Physicians should use conservative and the least dangerous methods of diagnosis and treatment whenever possible, rather than those that involve highly toxic agents or risky surgical procedures.

- As telemedicine has become more commonplace, physicians often diagnose and prescribe medication for new patients and for established patients over the Internet. Physicians also prescribe medication for established patients over the telephone. To avoid malpractice claims, any communication with the patient, whether over the Internet or by telephone, should be properly documented in the patient's medical record. Health care practitioners who communicate with patients over the Internet should know and conform to state and federal laws regarding the practice of telemedicine.

- Except in emergencies, male physicians should not examine female patients and female physicians should not examine male patients unless an assistant, a nurse, or a member of the patient's family is present. In ideal situations, a female medical assistant or female nurse should be present when a male physician examines a female patient, and when a female physician examines a male patient, a male medical assistant or male nurse should be present. Due to shortages of male nurses and male medical assistants, however, this may be impossible. In any case, physicians can protect themselves from unfounded patient charges by having a nurse, physician assistant, or medical assistant of either sex present during examinations.

- Physician/employers should check equipment and facilities frequently for safety, including the reception area. All employees should know safe procedures for operating equipment and should remind physician/employers when repair or replacement of equipment is necessary for continued safe operation. Employees should be alert to all hazards in the medical office that might cause injury, such as slippery floors, electric cords in unsafe places, tables with sharp edges, and so forth. The reception area at the health care facility should include a safe area for children, perhaps including such items as child-sized tables and chairs and picture books.

- When using toxic agents for diagnosis or treatment, physicians should know customary dosages or usage for such substances, any possible

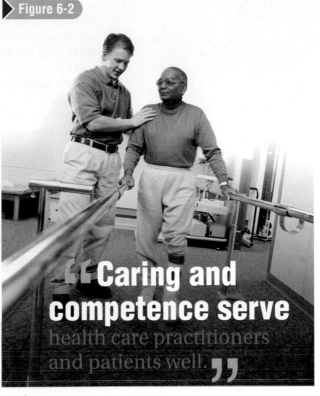

> Figure 6-2

"Caring and competence serve health care practitioners and patients well."

side effects or known toxic reactions, and the proper methods for treating reactions. Medical assistants and other medical office employees should ensure that when supplies are received, they are handled according to office policy and that all relevant literature is readily accessible to physicians. As required by the Occupational Safety and Health Administration (OSHA), employees should have access to Material Safety Data Sheets (MSDS) for each hazardous chemical in use in the medical facility. (See Chapter 10 for more information about OSHA medical workplace requirements.)

Why Do Patients Sue?

From a medical/legal standpoint, in an article in the March 2003 issue of *Family Practice Management*, Dr. R. J. Roberts of the University of Wisconsin Medical School identified seven common reasons for medical malpractice lawsuits:

1. Cancer misdiagnosis, failure to diagnose, or a delay in diagnosis.
2. Birth injury or negligent maternity care.
3. Wrong diagnosis and misdiagnosis of negligent fracture or trauma.
4. Delay in diagnosis or failure to consult in a timely manner.
5. Medication errors or medication malpractice resulting from negligent drug treatment.
6. Malpractice resulting from a physician's negligent procedures or surgical errors.
7. Failure to obtain informed consent.

Other studies have found additional reasons when patients were asked directly why they sued physicians. The first major study to determine why patients sue hospitals and health care practitioners and what might prevent an injured patient or his or her family members from filing a lawsuit was conducted in 1992 by Gerald B. Hickson and others. This study looked at factors that prompted parents to file medical malpractice suits after a perinatal injury. (*Perinatal* refers to the period immediately before and after a child's birth.)

According to Hickson and his colleagues, there are six common reasons for patients suing for medical malpractice, as shown in Table 6-1.

In a separate, equally well-known study, Charles Vincent and others examined why patients and their relatives sue physicians, and also investigated which actions might have prevented litigation. Study participants were given a list of 13 statements and asked whether they agreed or disagreed with each one. Table 6-2 lists the results.

Just over 41 percent of the respondents in the Vincent study said that certain actions after their injuries might have prevented litigation. In order of frequency, such actions included:

1. An explanation and apology.
2. Correction of the mistake.
3. Financial compensation.
4. Correct treatment at the time.
5. An admission of negligence.
6. Listening to the patient.
7. Disciplinary action against medical personnel involved.
8. Honesty.
9. Investigation by the hospital.

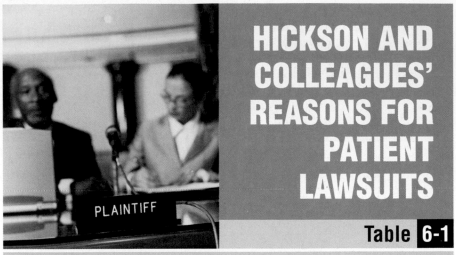

HICKSON AND COLLEAGUES' REASONS FOR PATIENT LAWSUITS

Table 6-1

Reason	Percentage of Respondents
Plaintiffs advised by knowledgeable acquaintances to sue	33
Recognized a coverup	24
Needed money	24
Recognized that the child would have no future	23
Needed information about what had happened	20
Wanted revenge or to protect others from harm	19

Source: Adapted from Gerald B. Hickson et al., "Factors That Prompted Families to File Medical Malpractice Claims Following Perinatal Injuries," *Journal of the American Medical Association* 267 (1992), p. 1359.

Another report by the American Society of Anesthesiologists Committee on Professional Liability stated that one of the most common reasons patients start legal proceedings is due to communication failures between physicians and patients. The report quoted Dale Ann Micalizzi, who lost her son Justin, a healthy 11-year-old, in 2001 when he died suddenly during surgery for osteomyelitis of his ankle. Micalizzi spent years trying to learn what had happened to her son, and although she did eventually receive an apology from the hospital where his surgery was performed, she was never allowed to see the results of investigations into the matter.

"Almost no one wants to sue their doctors, especially following the death of a child," Micalizzi told Ronald S. Litman in an article published online (http://depts.washington.edu/asaccp/prof/asa73_12_20_21.pdf). "We love docs for caring for our children. But the stonewalling and the lack of responsibility and accountability that can occur after a complication infuriates patients and families. They want answers and a discussion even if nothing was intentionally or accidentally done wrong. Patients and families feel that the medical community owes them this. When they don't receive it, their own community pushes them into doing something, and litigation is the last straw."

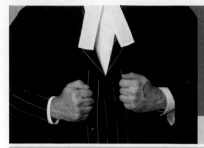

VINCENT AND COLLEAGUES' FINDINGS ON WHY PATIENTS SUE

Table 6-2

Why Injured Patients Sued	Percentage Who Agreed with Statement
Prevent injury from happening to anyone else	91
To receive an explanation	91
Wanted the doctors to realize what they had done	90
To get an admission of negligence	87
To make the doctor realize how I felt	68
My feelings were ignored	67
Wanted financial compensation	66
I was angry	65
Didn't want the doctor to get away with it	54
Wanted the doctor to be disciplined	48
Allowed me to cope with my feelings	46
Because of the staff's attitude afterward	43
To get back at the doctor	23

Source: Adapted from Charles Vincent et al., "Why Do People Sue Doctors? A Study of Patients and Relatives Taking Legal Action," *The Lancet* 343 (1994), pp. 1609, 1611.

Micalizzi has become a patient advocate since her son's death. Table 6-3 shows her recommendations for physicians when a complication occurs.

In short, few patients sue health care practitioners they like and trust (see Figure 6-3). If patients perceive health care providers as cold, uncaring, or rude, however, they may be more inclined to sue if something goes wrong, and patients who feel ignored, deserted, or who suspect that there is a medical "coverup" may also be more inclined to sue.

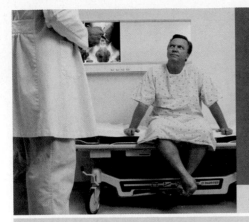

MICALIZZI'S SUGGESTIONS FOR THINGS NOT TO SAY AFTER MEDICAL COMPLICATIONS

Table 6-3

Things physicians should not say:

YOU signed the consents for surgery and anesthesia.

Are you receiving counseling? You need to get over it.

These things happen and you may never know what went wrong.

I have no idea what happened—go ask a specialist.

I guess I can squeeze you in for a meeting, but I'm very busy.

I don't have to share [certain] investigations with you.

I didn't tell the resident to begin surgery alone.

Medicine is an imperfect science—I did nothing wrong.

Things patients and families want and need following an adverse event:

Immediate unbiased investigation with complete disclosure.

To be listened to and taken seriously. Don't protect us. Don't lie to us. Don't diminish our need to know.

Practices and systems changed to prevent a similar event.

Standards of care mandated with regulatory systems in place and someone put in charge.

Respect, empathy, apology.

Medical bills dismissed.

Justice.

Source: Adapted from Ronald S. Litman, "Physician Communication Skills Decrease Malpractice Claims." **http://depts.washington.edu/asaccp/prof/asa73_12_20_21.shtml.**

Figure 6-3

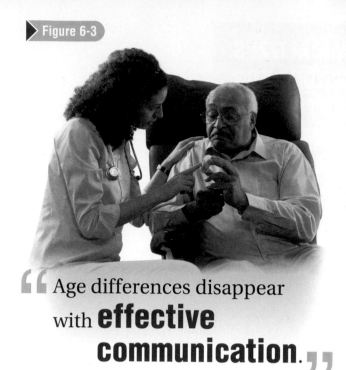

"Age differences disappear with **effective communication**."

Communicating with Patients

Patients who see the medical office as a friendly place are generally less likely to sue. As a health care practitioner and/or a medical facility employee, you can help prevent medical malpractice lawsuits by:

- Developing good listening skills and nonverbal communication techniques so that patients feel the time spent with them is not rushed. For example, patients will see a health care practitioner as caring and interested if he or she sits rather than stands while interviewing or conversing with the patient. Conversely, lack of eye contact and defensive body postures convey disinterest to a patient. In short, obey the Golden Rule when communicating with patients.

- Setting aside a certain time period during the day for returning patients' telephone calls and advising patients over the phone. Medical facility staff members responsible for answering the telephone should learn to recognize when patients' reported symptoms require the physician's immediate attention and when patients should be advised to seek emergency care.

- Reminding physicians to thoroughly explain illnesses and treatment options, including risks and possible complications, in terms the patient can understand. Patients should be encouraged to ask questions and to participate in the decision-making process. The best way to keep patients' expectations in line is through education. When dealing with accidents and bad results, a straightforward approach is desirable.

- Checking to be sure that all patients or their authorized representatives sign informed-consent forms before they undergo medical and surgical procedures. Next of kin or designated representatives must also sign informed-consent forms to authorize autopsies.

- Avoiding statements that could be construed as an admission of fault on the physician's part. If a lawsuit is filed against a physician, his or her employees should say nothing to anyone except as required by the physician's attorney or the court. However, an employee may be held liable if he or she knowingly remains silent to protect a physician who has performed an illegal act.

- Using tact, good judgment, and professionalism in handling patients. Physicians should insist on a professional consultation if the patient is not doing well, if he or she is unhappy and complaining, or if the patient's family expresses dissatisfaction.

- Refraining from making overly optimistic statements about recovery or prognoses. Health care practitioners who are not physicians or physician assistants generally do not diagnose or prescribe, but their responsibilities may include patient education. For example, nurses and medical assistants often discuss the patient's problems and review treatment options, and this is entirely appropriate. However, such health care practitioners should not make promises on the physician's behalf, such as "The doctor will have you feeling better soon."

- Advising patients when their physicians intend to be gone for long periods of time and reminding physicians to recommend or make available qualified substitutes. The patient must not be abandoned. If a physician is retiring, moving to another location, leaving the practice of medicine, or otherwise becoming unavailable, patients should be informed, and a copy of a letter of referral, notice of a physician's intended absence from practice, or letter of dismissal should be placed in the patient's record. Notices placed in local newspapers are also appropriate if a physician retires, moves, dies, or leaves the practice of medicine. The name and telephone number of the covering physician should be available for those patients requesting care in the absence of their regular physician.

- Making every effort to reach an understanding about fees with the patient before treatment so that billing does not become a point of contention. When handling fees for the physician, employees should explain all charges to patients, detailing those that are not included in regular fees. They should also follow legal collection procedures.

Documentation

Patient records are often used as evidence in medical malpractice cases, and improper documentation can lose a case (see Chapter 7). In some situations that may arise in medical practice, such as drug testing or the examination of a rape victim, evidence may need to be collected in a certain manner to be admissible in court. When in doubt about what documentation to make, you should contact legal authorities for advice.

Physicians should keep records that clearly show what treatment was done and when it was done. It is important that they be able to demonstrate that nothing was neglected and that the care given fully met the standards demanded by law. Physicians should also document all referrals to other physicians, withdrawals from cases, and cases in which patients refuse to follow their advice. Today's health care environment requires complete documentation of actions taken and, in many cases, actions not taken. Medical facility employees should pay particular attention to the following:

Referrals. Make sure the patient understands whether the referring physician's staff will make the appointment and notify the patient or whether the patient must call to set up the appointment. Make notations that the patient has been referred, and follow up with telephone calls to verify that an appointment was scheduled and kept. Note whether or not reports of the consultation were received in your office, and document all recommendations from the referring physician concerning further care of the patient.

Missed Appointments. At the end of each day, a designated person in the medical office should gather all patient records of those who missed or canceled appointments without rescheduling. Charts and electronic or handwritten schedule books should be dated, stamped, and documented "no show" or "canceled, no reschedule," respectively. The treating physician should review these records and note whether or not follow-up is indicated. If follow-up occurs, it should be documented as completed.

Dismissals. To avoid charges of abandonment, the physician must formally withdraw from a case or formally dismiss the patient. Be sure that a letter of withdrawal or dismissal has been filed in the patient's records.

Treatment Refusals. A patient's decision to decline treatment, evaluation, or testing should be documented in the patient record. "Informed refusal" should be obtained with respect to any treatment or procedure which could have either diagnostic or therapeutic consequences. "Informed refusal" should be obtained in writing or, at the very least, noted in the patient's medical record.

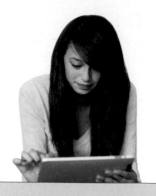

All Other Patient Contact. Patients' records should include reports of all tests, procedures, and medications prescribed, including refills. Make sure all necessary informed-consent papers have been duly signed and filed in a patient's record. Keep a record of all telephone conversations with the patient. Remember that correct documentation requires the initials or signature of the person making a notation on the patient's medical record, as well as the date and time. Remember the rule, "If it wasn't documented, it wasn't done."

check your **progress**

1. Name and briefly define the four Cs of medical malpractice prevention.

2. Briefly describe how practicing effective communication skills can help prevent a medical malpractice lawsuit.

3. If a patient refuses treatment, what legal options remain for the health care practitioner in charge?

4. Name five reasons often cited for the suing of health care practitioners by patients and their families.

COURT CASE

Physician Sued for Malpractice

A gynecologist treated a woman for pelvic pain. The physician eventually performed a hysterectomy, which was successful and relieved the woman's pain. Later, the woman complained of mild incontinence. The woman's physician found that she had a cystocele (herniation of part of the bladder through the wall of her vagina), and this condition progressed to a rectocele, when the rectum also herniated through the wall of the patient's vagina. Since the patient's stress incontinence had also progressed, the gynecologist recommended surgery, but she did not discuss Kegel exercises with the patient. (Kegel exercises are designed to strengthen muscles in a woman's pelvic floor and muscles supporting the urethra.)

Surgery was performed, and it corrected the patient's incontinence and the anatomical defects that caused it. However, shortly after surgery, the patient developed pain in her right leg. A second surgery was performed to release two sutures that the gynecologist believed might be impinging on the patient's obturator nerve and causing the pain. The pain persisted, and a third surgery on the patient's leg was performed. The third surgery and follow-up did not alleviate the patient's pain, despite referrals to and treatments by specialists in physical medicine, pain management, and neurosurgery. The pain and impairment in the patient's right leg was finally diagnosed as due to nerve damage as a result of the hysterectomy.

The patient filed suit alleging the following:

1. The gynecologist negligently failed to offer the nonsurgical option of Kegel exercises.

2. The patient would have chosen and performed the nonsurgical option had it been offered.

3. The Kegel exercises probably would have corrected the patient's incontinence without surgery.

4. The patient's nerve damage would have been avoided if the surgery had not been done.

The trial court found for the patient and named an award. The gynecologist appealed. The court of appeals held that (1) evidence was legally sufficient to show that patient would have opted for nonsurgery Kegel exercises had they been offered to her, but that (2) evidence was legally insufficient to show that patient's SUI would have been cured or sufficiently improved to avoid surgery.

The trial court's decision was reversed.

Source: Archer v. Warren, 118 S.W.3d 779, 2003 Tex. App.

How does this court action illustrate the importance of effective communication between health care practitioners and patients?

Types of Defenses

When, in spite of all best efforts to avoid litigation, a medical malpractice lawsuit is filed, the physician or other health care professional must defend himself or herself against the charges.

Denial

Denial of wrongdoing, or the assertion of innocence, may be used as a defense in professional liability suits. If some of the alleged facts are true, defendants may not claim innocence. Instead, they should claim that the charge or charges do not meet all of the elements of the theory of recovery. In other words, the charge may be missing one of the four Ds of negligence.

Affirmative Defenses

Affirmative defenses that may be used by the defendant in a medical professional liability suit allow the accused to present factual evidence that the patient's condition was caused by some factor other than the defendant's negligence.

Contributory Negligence When the defense claims **contributory negligence,** this alleges that the patient or complaining party, through a "want of ordinary care," caused or contributed to his or her own injury. The physician may deny that he or she committed a negligent act and claim the

LO 6.2
Describe the various defenses to professional liability suits.

> **denial** A defense that claims innocence of the charges or that one or more of the four Ds of negligence are lacking.

> **affirmative defenses** Defenses used by defendants in medical professional liability suits that allow the accused to present factual evidence that the patient's condition was caused by some factor other than the defendant's negligence.

COURT CASE

Patient Can Contribute to Negligence

A man who was a detainee at a county jail was taken to a county hospital emergency room when he complained of pain in his lower abdomen, nausea, and vomiting of blood for two weeks. An RN took the man's vital signs, finding his blood pressure to be 159/106 and his pulse to be fast. The nurse also drew blood and ordered initial lab work. A physician saw the patient and ordered that a nasogastric tube be inserted to check for blood in the stomach. The nurse tried to insert the tube, but the patient complained that it was extremely painful and said he did not want the tube inserted. The nurse explained why the tube was necessary, but the patient declined, insisting that his problems were due to his appendix. He signed a form indicating that he was refusing medical treatment against medical advice. The man was returned to the jail, where he died one week later of gastrointestinal hemorrhaging.

Blood test results that came back after the patient left the hospital were abnormal, indicating a life-threatening condition. Since the patient had signed himself out of the hospital, and the hospital claimed it no longer had a duty to him, his test results were not forwarded to the physician who examined the patient or to the patient.

The administrator of the patient's estate filed a malpractice suit against the nurse and the hospital. A trial jury found for the defendants, under the defense of contributory negligence. The administrator appealed, but the appellate court affirmed the lower court's judgment.

Source: Margaret Lyons as the administratrix of the estate of Kenneth Cook, deceased, v. Walker Regional Medical Center, Inc., and Laurie Hunter, 868 So.2d 1071 Supreme Court of Alabama, 2003.

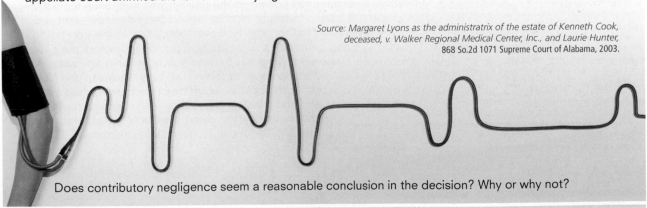

Does contributory negligence seem a reasonable conclusion in the decision? Why or why not?

contributory negligence
An affirmative defense that alleges that the plaintiff, through a lack of care, caused or contributed to his or her own injury.

comparative negligence
An affirmative defense claimed by the defendant, alleging that the plaintiff contributed to the injury by a certain degree.

assumption of risk A legal defense that holds that the defendant is not guilty of a negligent act because the plaintiff knew of and accepted beforehand any risks involved.

patient was totally responsible for the damage or injury. Alternatively, the physician may admit negligence but claim that the patient was also somehow at fault and so contributed to the injury.

In some states, damages are apportioned according to the degree to which a plaintiff contributed to the injury. This is called **comparative negligence.** For instance, if the court decides that a patient, through his or her own negligence, contributed 20 percent toward the injury and the physician contributed 80 percent, the patient's damage award may be reduced by 20 percent.

In hearing cases alleging contributory negligence, the court will consider the patient's ability to comprehend and carry out the physician's instructions. Minors or adults who are unconscious, mentally disabled, insane, or otherwise incompetent may be judged unable to have contributed to a negligent act.

Assumption of Risk **Assumption of risk** is a defense based on the contention that the patient knew of the inherent risks before treatment was performed and agreed to those risks. Informed consent (see Chapter 7) is vital to this defense, since the defendant must show that the patient was fully informed of the risks prior to treatment and that the risks inherent in the treatment were the cause of the patient's injury.

For example, in one lawsuit in which the defendant used the assumption of risk defense, it was held that a physician was not liable for injuries suffered by a chronically ill woman when she fell in the examining room while attempting to undress without assistance. Because she had refused assistance, the woman had assumed the risk of injury.

COURT CASE

Court Finds It Improper to Blame Patient

A patient went to his doctor complaining of loss of equilibrium, unsteady gait, vomiting, and weight loss. He admitted drinking six cans of beer every day up to the day before. He had had lung cancer surgery six months earlier. His physician admitted him to the hospital with diagnoses of alcoholic cerebellar degeneration, cirrhosis of the liver, and metastasized brain cancer. The physician wrote an order for Valium prn (as necessary) if the patient showed signs of acute alcohol withdrawal such as hallucinations, delirium tremens, or disorientation. The nurses gave the Valium starting the second hospital day until the physician stopped it on the fourth. The nurses gave the Valium even though the patient never showed signs of acute alcohol withdrawal. According to the record in the Appellate Court of Illinois, the patient always appeared alert, oriented, and coherent. The court said that made it inappropriate and negligent for the nurses to give the prn Valium.

On the fourth day the patient fell trying to return to bed from his bathroom. He got out of bed and got to the bathroom without a problem, but then he apparently leaned on the inside of the door. It opened and did not support him. He fell and broke his hip. That required surgery. He spent his last few months in pain hobbling with a walker and a cane.

Postmortem examination confirmed the patient died from brain tumors. He did not have cirrhosis or alcohol-related brain damage—that was a medical misdiagnosis. However, according to the court, it was negligent for the nurses to give prn Valium without the patient showing signs of the medical condition for which the medication was ordered. The court believed the Valium produced sedation which caused a patient who was fully alert and oriented when assessed to become disoriented and unsteady. This ruling gave the widow grounds to sue the hospital for the deceased's fractured hip.

Source: Brady v. McNamara, 724 N.E.2d 949 (311 Ill. App. 3rd 1999).

COURT CASE

Assumption of Risk Defense Denied

A physician treated a patient for Crohn's disease (a painful inflammation of the small intestine of indeterminate cause). To treat the patient's pain, the physician prescribed Percocet and Tylenol #3 with codeine. The patient developed an addiction to the drugs and was forced to undergo extensive drug rehabilitation. The plaintiff patient sued the physician, alleging that he negligently prescribed dangerous and addictive narcotic drugs and failed to recognize her addiction to them. A trial court granted a directed verdict to the physician on the basis of the plaintiff's assumption of risk. The patient appealed.

The appellate court agreed that the doctor was negligent in failing to fully consider the possibility that the patient could become addicted to the drugs he prescribed. Testimony indicated that errors in the patient's medical record could have interfered with the physician's ability to effectively monitor the patient's drug use. The appellate court found that the patient's classic drug-addicted behavior, in attempting to acquire additional narcotics, did not automatically relieve the physician from his duty to monitor her for signs of abuse or relieve the doctor from any liability for continuing to prescribe narcotics. Insofar as addiction is a compulsive behavior, the court could not find that the patient voluntarily acquiesced to the risks involved with taking excessive medication.

The judgment of the trial court was reversed, and the case was returned to the trial court for a new trial.

Source: Conrad-Hutsell v. Colturi, 2002 Ohio 2032; 2002 Ohio App.

From the standpoint of assumption of risk by patients who take drugs for pain relief, does the court decision make sense? Why or why not?

In other cases it has been held that individuals submitting to X-ray treatment assume the risk of burns from a proper exposure to X-rays but not the risk of negligence in the application of the treatment.

Emergency If services were provided during an **emergency,** this may also be used as an affirmative defense. The health care practitioner who comes to the aid of a victim in an emergency would not be held liable under common law if the defense established that

1. A true emergency situation existed and was not caused by the defendant.
2. The appropriate standard of care was met, given the emergency situation.

> **emergency** A type of affirmative defense in which the person who comes to the aid of a victim in an emergency is not held liable under certain circumstances.

Health care professionals who provide assistance in emergencies may also be protected from liability under Good Samaritan Acts, which are discussed in Chapter 7.

While the court case, "Emergency Defense Established," dates from 1970, the trial court's opinion clearly illustrates the elements required for a health care practitioner to establish an emergency defense. Since using an emergency defense is possible in defending a medical malpractice suit, should Daryl in the chapter's opening scenario have worried about calming his patient? Explain your answer.

Technical Defenses

When defenses to liability suits are based on legal technicalities, instead of on factual evidence, they are called **technical defenses.** Technical defenses include those that claim the statute of limitations has run out, there is insufficient evidence to support the plaintiff's claim of negligence, and the assertion that the plaintiff has no standing to sue.

> **technical defenses** Defenses used in a lawsuit that are based on legal technicalities.

Emergency Defense Established

The father of a minor plaintiff sought consequential damages in a malpractice suit against an anesthesiologist. The patient suffered cardiac arrest during a tonsillectomy. Resuscitation was performed, and the patient's heartbeat was restored, but she was left with severe and extensive brain damage.

The defendants used an emergency defense. The plaintiff alleged that cardiac arrest is a complication that is a constant possibility in surgery and, therefore, not to be considered "an emergency within the meaning of the emergency doctrine."

A trial court found for the defendants. The court held that

1. In an emergency a person does not have the time to think in the way that he or she would in ordinary circumstances.

2. When a layperson or a professional is confronted with an emergency, conduct is to be judged according to his or her skill, care, and due diligence with respect to the emergency.

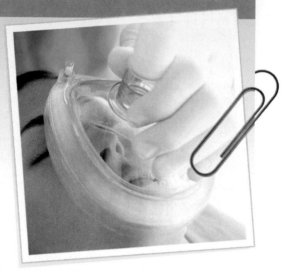

Source: Linhares v. Hall, 357 Mass. 209, 257 N.E.2d 429 Mass. 1970.

release of tortfeasor
A technical defense that prohibits a lawsuit against the person who caused an injury (the tortfeasor) if he or she was expressly released from further liability in the settlement of a suit.

res judicata "The thing has been decided." Legal principle that a claim cannot be retried between the same parties if it has already been legally resolved.

Release of Tortfeasor A tortfeasor is one who is guilty of committing a tort. Suppose a third party causes injury to a person as in an automobile accident, and a physician treats the injured person. In most states, the party who caused the accident (the tortfeasor) is liable both for the victim's injury and for any medical negligence by the physician who treats the injured victim. This is the basis for the **release of tortfeasor** defense.

If the injured party sues the tortfeasor, settles the case, and then releases the tortfeasor from further liability, the injured party cannot also sue the physician unless the victim expressly reserved that right in the release. If the victim's settlement with the tortfeasor provided compensation for all medical expenses, the release of tortfeasor is usually an absolute defense.

Laws governing release of tortfeasor contain many modifiers, which must be applied in individual cases.

Res Judicata Under the doctrine of *res judicata,* "The thing has been decided," a claim cannot be retried between the same parties if it has already been legally resolved. For example, if a patient sues a physician for negligence and loses, the patient cannot then sue the physician for breach of contract based on evidence presented in the trial for negligence. If a patient refuses to pay a physician's fees on the grounds that the physician was negligent and the physician sues for money owed and wins, the patient cannot then sue the physician for negligence. However, if the patient fails to respond to the suit (defaults) or does not allege negligence in his or her defense, then usually he or she may sue the physician for negligence. If a physician has been sued by a nonpaying patient for negligence and does not file a counterclaim for the fee while defending the suit, the patient cannot be sued later for unpaid bills.

Statute of Limitations Since statutes of limitations vary with states, health care practitioners must be familiar with specific laws for their state. Statutory time limits apply to a number of legal actions, including collections, damages for child sexual abuse, retaining of medical records,

Release of Tortfeasor

A driver of an automobile was injured in an accident. A physician subsequently treated the driver's broken arm. The injured party sued the physician for malpractice, alleging that the physician was negligent in that he had severed a nerve in her arm.

Before trial, the plaintiff had signed a release of tortfeasor agreement with the insurer of the other driver involved in the accident, releasing that driver from any further liability.

Both a trial court and a superior court had granted summary judgment in favor of the physician in a medical malpractice action. The plaintiff appealed those decisions, alleging that the release of tortfeasor agreement she had signed did not also release the physician who was allegedly negligent in treating her injury.

The court of appeals that heard the final appeal reversed lower court rulings granting summary judgment in favor of the physician, based on the court's agreement that the release of tortfeasor did not include the physician and that the plaintiff had not been allowed to present expert witness testimony in previous hearings. The court remanded the case to the trial court for rehearing.

Source: Depew v. Burkle, 786 N.E.2d 1144 (Ind. App. 2003).

---

wrongful death claims, medical malpractice, and many other causes of action. The **statute of limitations** for filing professional negligence suits varies with states but generally specifies one to six years, with two years being most common. In other words, patients may not file suit for negligence against physicians if the designated length of time has elapsed.

Establishing when the statute of limitations begins also varies with state law, but the most common dates for marking the beginning of the statutory period are as follows:

> **statute of limitations** That period of time established by state law during which a lawsuit may be filed.

- The day the alleged negligent act was committed.

- When the injury resulting from the alleged negligence was actually discovered or should have been discovered by a reasonably alert patient.

- The day the physician–patient relationship ended or the day of the last medical treatment in a series.

In some states, statutory periods may be modified for minors, for persons who are legally insane, or in certain circumstances, such as imprisonment or a situation in which foreign objects were left in the body during surgery.

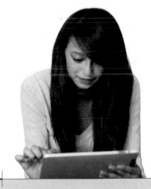

check your **progress**

5. What is the difference between an affirmative defense and a technical defense?

6. Identify the type of defense described in each of the following:

   One in which the defendant claims innocence.

   One in which the accused is allowed to present factual evidence that the physician's negligence did not cause the patient's condition.

   One in which the defendant claims that the patient contributed to his or her own injury.

   One in which informed consent is a vital factor.

   One that hinges on legal technicalities rather than factual evidence.

7. If a medical malpractice claim is dismissed due to a state's statute of limitations, does this imply that the defendant health care practitioner is exonerated? Explain your answer.

Action Dismissed Due to Statute of Limitations

A patient's family sued a physician in Texas for wrongful death for failure to diagnose the patient's cancer. A Texas state law passed in 1977, The Medical Liability and Insurance Improvement Act, established a two-year statute of limitations for medical malpractice claims; therefore, the Supreme Court of Texas barred the action because by the time the lawsuit reached the courts, the statute of limitations had run out.

The patient was first evaluated for anemia in 1986, but test results revealed a lesion in the stomach. A biopsy showed no sign of malignancy in the lesion. A second biopsy performed in 1987 was also negative for cancer, but on further examination two weeks later, cells from the lesion were found to be consistent with carcinoma.

Follow-up exams and another biopsy performed in 1988 revealed cancer cells in the patient's stomach lesion, which by then had ulcerated. Surgery was recommended, but was not performed because advanced cancer was found in the patient's lung and stomach. The patient died, and her family continued the lawsuit on her behalf.

The appellate court ruled that the statute of limitations period began at the time of the second biopsy in 1987. The claim was not brought until after 1989; therefore, the time limitation had run out.

Source: Bala v. Maxwell, 909 S.W.2d 889 (Texas Sup. Ct., Nov. 2, 1995).

Do you know where to find the statute of limitations for medical malpractice in your state?

Specific statutory time limits may be found in the state code, online, and in most public and university libraries.

The court case, "Action Dismissed Due to Statute of Limitations," illustrates the importance of statutes of limitations in determining whether or not a medical malpractice complaint can go to trial.

LO 6.3

Explain the purpose of quality improvement and risk management within a health care facility.

risk management The taking of steps to minimize danger, hazard, and liability.

quality improvement (QI) or quality assurance A program of measures taken by health care providers and practitioners to uphold the quality of patient care.

Risk Management

Since liability is a major factor in health care delivery, and since health care delivery systems and practitioners seek to minimize liability whenever possible, **risk management** has become a necessary practice component. Risk management is one approach to reducing the likelihood of a malpractice lawsuit. Risk management involves identifying problem practices or behaviors, then eliminating or controlling them. Risk management activities that may help avoid litigation include providing written job descriptions for health care practice employees and providing office procedures manuals and employee handbooks that can help avoid misunderstanding and mistakes that lead to liability risks. Other common health care facility activities that may affect the likelihood or course of litigation include medical record charting, patient scheduling, writing prescriptions, and communicating with patients.

How did EMT Daryl in the opening scenario practice risk management?

After Daryl's patient was delivered to the hospital, he documented exactly what was done to treat the man. Is this also a means of practicing risk management? Explain your answer.

Methods used to manage risk are part of **quality improvement (QI) or quality assurance:** a program of practices performed by health care providers and practitioners to uphold the quality of patient care and to reduce liability risk.

Most health care facilities and plans employ quality improvement and risk managers to oversee risk and quality issues relating to physicians and support staff. Quality improvement and risk managers may also assume responsibility for compliance with federal, state, and other health care regulatory agencies. A compliance plan is developed to help ensure that all governmental regulations are followed. Such a plan is especially beneficial for following coding and billing regulations for Medicare, Medicaid, and other government plans.

Most health care institutions and organizations also employ individuals who are responsible for credentialing. Credentialing may be done by risk management staff or by other departments within a health care organization. Credentialing is the process of verifying a health care provider's credentials. The process may be performed by an insurance company before a provider is admitted to the network, by medical offices prior to granting hospital privileges, or by other groups that routinely employ or contract with health care providers. Credentialing usually consists of the following:

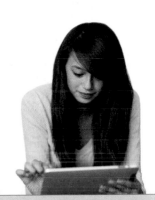

1. A provider fills out an application and attaches copies of his or her medical license, proof of malpractice insurance coverage, and other requested credentials.

2. The listed sources are asked to verify the information.

3. Medicare and Medicaid sanctions and malpractice history are checked via the National Practitioner Data Bank.

4. The findings are presented to a credentialing committee.

5. A peer review process completes the credentialing procedure.

check your **progress**

Circle the correct answer for each of the following questions.

8. Risk management has become a necessary health care practice component because

 a. Liability insurance is often unavailable

 b. Liability is a major factor in health care delivery

 c. Patients with bad outcomes always sue

9. Methods used to manage risk are part of

 a. The provisions in liability insurance policies

 b. Every health care provider's practice

 c. Quality improvement or quality assurance

10. Which of the following activities help health care providers avoid litigation?

 a. Vocal disclaimers before procedures are performed

 b. Medical record charting

 c. Issuing written denials in response to accusations of wrong-doing

11. Which of the following is *not* a duty of a medical practice's quality improvement and risk manager?

 a. Credentialing

 b. Checking compliance with health care regulatory agencies' requirements

 c. Scheduling patient appointments

12. Credentialing consists of

 a. Publishing health care provider job vacancies

 b. Filing health care employees' credentials with state agencies

 c. Verifying health care providers' credentials before hiring

Discuss five different types of medical liability insurance.

Professional Liability Insurance

Because costs for defending a medical malpractice lawsuit can be high, **liability insurance** may be purchased to cover the costs up to the limits of the policy. For example, if a medical professional liability insurance policy covers an insured physician up to $10 million, in the event that he or she loses a malpractice suit and must pay damages, the insurance company will not pay more than that amount.

The cost of liability insurance premiums for a physician is based on the physician's specialty and the dollar amount covered by the policy. Insurance for those physicians in the least risky insurance risk class (for example, family practitioners and specialists who do not perform surgery) is generally less costly than insurance for those in specialties considered riskier (for example, orthopedic surgeons and obstetricians). States vary regarding those medical specialties considered to carry the highest risk of liability and, therefore, are subject to the highest liability insurance premiums.

Some physicians drop liability insurance coverage when rates become too high. However, this can adversely affect a physician's practice, since most hospitals require proof of coverage up to a predetermined minimum amount to grant hospital privileges. In addition, managed care organizations require physicians to provide proof of liability insurance coverage as a prerequisite for entering into a contractual agreement and as a component of their credentialing process.

There are two main types of medical malpractice insurance:

1. **Claims-made insurance** covers the insured only for those claims made (not for any injury occurring) while the policy is in force. With this kind of insurance, the determining factor is when the claim is made, not when the injury occurs. For example, a policy in force during a previous year would cover only those claims made during that year.

2. **Occurrence insurance** (also known as claims-incurred insurance) covers the insured for any claims arising from an incident that occurred or is alleged to have occurred while the policy is in force, regardless of when the claim is made. For example, suppose an alleged incident of negligence by a physician occurred in September 2003, while the physician's occurrence insurance policy was in effect with XYZ Insurance Company. If a patient files a claim against the physician in January 2005, after the policy period has passed, the physician is covered under the terms of the occurrence insurance policy.

There are three types of insurance that health care practitioners can purchase to extend coverage of a canceled claims-made policy or for claims-made coverage when the insured switches to a different insurance carrier:

Tail coverage. When a claims-made policy is discontinued, tail coverage (sometimes called a reporting endorsement) is an option available to health care practitioners from their former carriers to continue coverage for those dates that claims-made coverage was in effect. Once a claims-made policy is canceled, coverage does not continue in the future for any claims that might be reported unless tail coverage or prior acts coverage is secured at the time the policy is canceled. If neither is purchased, any future claims that might arise from services performed during the policy period will no longer be covered.

Prior acts insurance coverage. This is a supplement to a claims-made policy that health care practitioners can purchase from a new carrier when they change carriers. Prior acts coverage, also known as "nose" coverage, covers incidents that occurred prior to the beginning of the new insurance relationship but have not yet been brought to the

liability insurance Contract coverage for potential damages incurred as a result of a negligent act.

claims-made insurance A type of liability insurance that covers the insured only for those claims made (not for any injury occurring) while the policy is in force.

occurrence insurance A type of liability insurance that covers the insured for any claims arising from an incident that occurred, or is alleged to have occurred, during the time the policy is in force, regardless of when the claim is made.

tail coverage An insurance coverage option available for health care practitioners: When a claims-made policy is discontinued, it extends coverage for malpractice claims alleged to have occurred during those dates that claims-made coverage was in effect.

prior acts insurance coverage A supplement to a claims-made insurance policy that can be purchased from a new carrier when health care practitioners change carriers.

insured's attention as a claim. Prior acts coverage is an alternative to a reporting period endorsement (also known as tail coverage), which is purchased from the original carrier when a change in carriers is made. Companies typically require the new insured to purchase either tail or nose coverage to protect against claims arising from prior acts.

Self-insurance coverage. As medical malpractice insurance premiums have continued to rise, self-insurance coverage has become an option for health care practitioners in some states. It works like this: An insurance company writes a policy with a limit of $X, and the insured parties contribute to a trust fund up to a limit of $X to be used in paying potential medical malpractice awards. The insurance company charges fees for managing the fund. One advantage to self-insurance coverage is that premiums are considerably lower than with traditional types of medical malpractice insurance. A disadvantage is that state laws regulating insurance do not always allow such plans, and even in states where such coverage is allowed, hospitals must agree to accept self-insurance plans for those physicians who apply for hospital privileges.

> **self-insurance coverage** An insurance coverage option whereby insured subscribers contribute to a trust fund to be used in paying potential damage awards.

Physicians and other health care practitioners should notify their insurance companies immediately if advised of the possibility of a malpractice lawsuit. Insurance companies almost always provide legal representation for covered physicians, and some insurance contracts require that the insurance company's attorneys represent the insured physician.

Once a lawsuit seems imminent, the health care practitioner and/or his or her employees should not mention the suit on the telephone or in correspondence unless the insurance company's legal counsel approves such a reference.

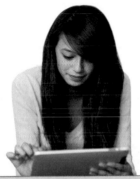

check your **progress**

13. If a health care practitioner covered by medical malpractice insurance receives notice of a lawsuit, he or she should first notify _____

14. Claims-made insurance pays for _____

15. Occurrence insurance pays for _____

16. Name two types of insurance that, in certain circumstances, extend coverage of claims made insurance. _____

17. Explain how physicians might insure themselves.

_____

[CHAPTER SUMMARY]

LO 6.1 What are the four Cs of medical malpractice prevention?

- Caring
- Communication
- Competence
- Charting

Why do patients sue?

- Unrealistic expectations.
- Poor rapport and poor communication.
- Greed.
- Lawyers and our litigious society.
- Poor quality of care—either in fact or in perception.
- Poor outcome.
- Failure to understand patients' and families' perspectives and devaluing their point of view.

What general categories of information should be documented for legal purposes?

- What treatment was performed and when.
- Referrals.
- Missed appointments.
- Dismissals.
- Treatment refusals.
- All other patient contact.

LO 6.2 What types of defense may be used in a medical malpractice lawsuit?

- Denial
- Affirmative
  - Contributory negligence
  - Comparative negligence
  - Assumption of risk
  - Emergency
- Technical
  - Release of tortfeasor
  - *Res judicata*
  - Statute of limitations

LO 6.3 What are the common risk management methods?

- Quality improvement (QI) or quality assurance.
- Credentialing.

LO 6.4 What types of professional liability insurance are available to medical providers?

- Claims-made
  - Tail coverage
  - Prior acts coverage
- Occurrence
- Self-coverage

ETHICS ISSUES Defenses to Liability Suits

Ethics ISSUE 1: According to the ethical guidelines for a number of professional organizations, incompetence, corruption, or dishonest conduct on the part of health care practitioners is unethical and never acceptable. In addition to posing a real or potential threat to patients, such conduct undermines the public's confidence in the health care professions, and could cause adverse events that in turn lead to lawsuits.

Discussion Questions

Determine whether each of the following behaviors is unethical, illegal, or both, and explain how each might lead to liability.

1. A physician intentionally enters a billing code on a patient's billing sheet for an examination that was not performed. The code entered means that the patient's insurance carrier will be billed for a more expensive exam than the one that was actually performed.

2. A hospital instructs its nurses to introduce themselves by name to each new patient in this manner: "I am Susan and I've been assigned to take care of you. I have an associate's degree in nursing [or substitute appropriate educational credentials]. I see your physician is Dr. Wellness, and I can assure you that he is an excellent doctor. Let me know if you need anything at all."

3. An anesthesiologist has never administered anesthesia to a child, but conceals this fact from a surgeon who likes her and requests her for an upcoming procedure on a six-year-old.

4. A nursing assistant slaps an elderly patient in a skilled nursing care facility for calling her a name.

5. A nurse begins a painful procedure on an elderly hospital patient and ignores the patient's requests for an explanation.

6. A phlebotomist mislabels a blood sample, but later denies any responsibility for the inappropriate medical treatments that result.

Ethics ISSUE 2: Principles of ethics and professional conduct for all health care professions emphasize that health care practitioners have a responsibility to promote and advance the patient's welfare.

After misreading an X-ray, a dentist mistakenly removes a healthy incisor from a patient's mouth, then fits the patient with a fixed bridge that will not stay in place and causes the patient great pain. The patient sees a second dentist who repairs the damage done by the first dentist and remarks about the "shoddy quality" of the first dentist's work. The patient sues the first dentist for medical malpractice, and the defendant is found not guilty. Several jurors who hear the case express the opinion that the patient bears some responsibility for his injuries simply for seeing the first dentist.

Discussion Questions

1. Was the second dentist acting ethically when she criticized the first dentist's work? Explain your answer.

_____

_____

2. Is the dentist who was found not guilty of medical malpractice thereby exonerated of any wrongdoing? Explain your answer.

_____

_____

3. Might the dentist found not guilty in the previous scenario be subject to sanctions from the professional organization to which he belongs? Explain your answer.

_____

_____

4. Do you agree that the patient in this case bears some responsibility for her injuries simply for seeing the dentist in question?

_____

_____

Ethics ISSUE 3: The American Medical Association's _Code of Medical Ethics_ states that physicians and other health care practitioners should not provide, prescribe, or bill for services they know are unnecessary. A recent poll commissioned by the Alpharetta, Georgia-based Jackson Healthcare consulting firm reported that 73 percent of doctors said they practice defensive medicine. Defensive medicine, a phenomenon born with the rise in malpractice lawsuits, includes ordering unnecessary tests and sometimes even unnecessary treatments. To be fair, it's not difficult to understand why a reasonable doctor would want to cover all his or her bases, so to speak, since the threat of a frivolous lawsuit is always looming. Whatever the reason, by the doctors' own estimate, unnecessary tests and treatments account for more than one-quarter of health care costs.

Not only is this practice expensive, it also can be dangerous. For instance, according to the U.S. Department of Health and Human Services, about 1 percent of people who have a coronary angiogram experience a stroke as a result of the test; the procedure consists of a catheter threaded through the arteries which can then be X-rayed to determine if any blockage is present. This is only one example of a serious procedure with a fairly serious risk—not something you'd want a doctor to order flippantly.

James Wilson sees his physician for intermittent chest pain. Mr. Wilson's symptoms do not include sweating, difficulty breathing, or any other indications of heart problems. After a complete examination that includes a stress test and blood work, the physician is reasonably sure Mr. Wilson does not have heart problems. To protect against liability, however, Mr. Wilson's physician orders a coronary angiogram.

Discussion Question

1. Is it ethical for a physician or any other health care practitioner to prescribe or administer a medical treatment or test just to protect against potential liability? Explain your answer.

_____

_____

Go to **www.mhhe.com/judson6e** to practice your case review skills. Then read on for more information.

[KEY TERMS]

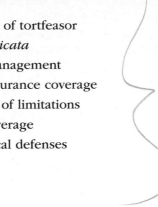

affirmative defenses
assumption of risk
claims-made insurance
comparative
  negligence
contributory
  negligence
denial

emergency
liability insurance
occurrence insurance
prior acts insurance
  coverage
quality improvement
  (QI) or quality
  assurance

release of tortfeasor
res judicata
risk management
self-insurance coverage
statute of limitations
tail coverage
technical defenses

[CHAPTER 6 REVIEW]

Applying Knowledge

LO 6.1

Name the four Cs of medical malpractice prevention, and after each term, list at least one way you can comply.

1. _____

2. _____

3. _____

4. _____

Name eight guidelines for physicians and other health care practitioners to follow that may help prevent malpractice lawsuits.

5. _____

6. _____

7. _____

8. _____

9. _____

10. _____

11. _____

12. _____

LO 6.2

13. Under _____ a claim may not be retried between the same two parties if it has been legally resolved.
    a. Common law
    b. *Res ipsa loquitur*
    c. *Res judicata*
    d. Arbitration

14. The _____ is the time limit for filing a lawsuit.
    a. Affirmative defense
    b. Assumption of risk
    c. Statute of limitations
    d. technical defense

15. Which of the following is *not* a form of affirmative defense to a professional liability suit?
    a. Contributory negligence
    b. Denial
    c. Assumption of risk
    d. Emergency

16. Under the _____ defense, a health care practitioner who comes to the aid of an accident victim at the scene would not be held liable.
    a. *Res judicata*
    b. *Res ipsa loquitur*
    c. Emergency
    d. Denial

17. When the defendant alleges that he or she did no wrong, that defense is called
    a. Negligence
    b. Contributory negligence
    c. Denial
    d. Assumption of risk

18. If the patient knew the inherent risk before treatment, the defendant may use _____ as a defense in a lawsuit.
    a. Negligence
    b. Contributory negligence
    c. Denial
    d. Assumption of risk

19. Which of the following is an affirmative defense?
    a. Release of tortfeasor
    b. Emergency
    c. *Res judicata*
    d. Statute of limitations

20. Which of the following is a technical defense?
    a. *Res judicata*
    b. Contributory negligence
    c. Comparative negligence
    d. Assumption of risk

21. When damages are apportioned according to the degree a plaintiff contributed to his or her injury, this is called
    a. Negligence
    b. Contributory negligence
    c. Denial
    d. Assumption of risk

22. The statute of limitations
    a. Is the same in each state
    b. Is a federal law
    c. Is determined by the courts
    d. Is different depending on the state

23. *Res judicata* is Latin for
    a. Buyer beware
    b. The judge is in charge
    c. The jury is in charge
    d. The thing has been decided

LO 6.3

24. Risk management is a process
    a. To assess liability insurance
    b. To manage difficult patients
    c. To minimize danger, hazard, and liability
    a. None of the above

LO 6.4

25. Medical malpractice insurance that covers the insured only for those claims made while the policy is in force is called
    a. Prior acts coverage
    b. Self-insurance coverage
    c. Claims-made coverage
    d. Occurrence insurance

26. Medical malpractice insurance that covers the insured for any claims arising from an incident that occurred, or is alleged to have occurred, during the time the policy was in force, regardless of when the claim is made, is called
    a. Prior acts coverage
    b. Self-insurance coverage
    c. Claims-made coverage
    d. Occurrence insurance

27. Which of the following is a supplemental insurance to medical liability insurance?
    a. Occurrence coverage
    b. Prior acts coverage
    c. Claims-made coverage
    d. Self-insurance coverage

[CASE STUDIES]

Use your critical thinking skills to answer the questions that follow each case study.

LO 6.1

A patient in her midtwenties saw an ophthalmologist for a routine eye exam. Due to her young age, a glaucoma test was not performed. She later was diagnosed with glaucoma and sued the ophthalmology group, alleging negligence in failing to perform a glaucoma test.

The defense argued that the standard of care was to not administer the test to patients younger than 40 because the instance of glaucoma at younger ages was rare.

Which of the following statements do you think best describes the applicable standard of care in this case? Explain your choice.

28. The defense should prevail because the reasonable, customary, and prudent course of action followed by practitioners in the same or similar circumstances would be the same.

_____

_____

29. The plaintiff should prevail because all patients should be protected against glaucoma, regardless of age.

_____

_____

You are a phlebotomist for a community laboratory, and you report for work on an extremely busy day. You travel daily from the lab where you work to the hospital to draw blood, and then back to the lab. You have finished drawing blood at the hospital and are on your way back to the lab when you get a cell phone call that the hospital needs a complete blood count (CBC) and electrolytes drawn STAT for a patient who has just come into the emergency room (ER).

30. Would you turn around and go back to the ER or drop off your current blood samples and then go back to the ER? Explain your answer.

_____

_____

31. What does question 31 have to do with preventing medical malpractice lawsuits?

_____

_____

LO 6.3

A nurse on the night shift in a busy hospital sees a physician's order to administer an intravenous medication to a patient who has just been admitted through the emergency room. She does not recognize the name of the drug, but notes a charge of $4,000 for the drug. Her curiosity aroused, the nurse checks the drug and discovers it should not be administered more frequently than every six weeks, and any patient receiving it should be carefully monitored at fifteen-minute intervals. The patient tells her he received the same medication just two weeks previously.

32. What should the nurse do?

_____

_____

33. In checking the drug is the nurse practicing risk management? Explain your answer.

_____

_____

Complete the activities and answer the questions that follow.

34. Do a Web search for "medical errors." List at least two ways to prevent medical errors from the online material you find. If you see statistics for the number of deaths from medical errors in 2009 or 2010, record that figure.

_____

_____

35. Search the Web site of the American Tort Reform Association (ATRA). Use the site to find out if your state has passed civil justice reform acts that pertain specifically to health care practitioners. If so, briefly describe the acts and how they might affect health care practitioners.

_____

_____

36. Do a Web search for "physician malpractice insurance" to find out how malpractice insurance premium rates vary among states. Which states seem to be in crisis regarding the cost of medical malpractice insurance? In states with lower rates, what is credited with keeping costs lower than they are in other states? What is the situation in the state where you plan to practice? Should all health care practitioners carry medical malpractice insurance? Explain your answer.

_____

_____

RESOURCES

Boumil, Marcia M., Clifford E. Elias, and Diane Bissonnette Moes. *Medical Liability in a Nut Shell*. St. Paul, MN: West/Thomson, 2003.

Joel, Lucille A. *Kelly's Dimensions of Professional Nursing*. New York: McGraw-Hill, 2011.

Kubasek, Nancy, et al. *Dynamic Business Law*. New York: McGraw-Hill, 2011.

Mallor, Jane P., et al. *Business Law and the Legal Environment*. New York: McGraw-Hill, 2002.

Melvin, Sean. *The Legal Environment of Business*. New York: McGraw-Hill, 2010.

Hastings, Richard. "Seven Reasons Physicians Are Sued for Medical Malpractice," March 24, 2009: **www.articlesbase.com/personal-injury-articles/seven-reasons-physicians-are-sued-for-medical-malpractice-832271.html#ixzz19FT844BA.**

Hickson, Gerald B., et al. "Factors That Prompted Families to File Medical Malpractice Claims Following Perinatal Injuries." *Journal of the American Medical Association* 267 (1992), p. 1359.

Litman, Ronald S. "Physician Communication Skills Decrease Malpractice Claims."

http://depts.washington.edu/asaccp/prof/asa73_12_20_21.shtml.

Lowry, John R. "Why People Sue Hospitals and Health Care Professionals." *Health Industry Online*, January 10, 2007: **www.strasburger.com/p4p/publications/why_people_sue_hospitals.**

Randolph, Adrienne G. *A Family's Search for Truth,* **www.psqh.com/novdec06/communication.html.**

Vincent, Charles, et al. "Why Do People Sue Doctors? A Study of Patients and Relatives Taking Legal Action." *The Lancet* 343 (1994), pp. 1609, 1611.

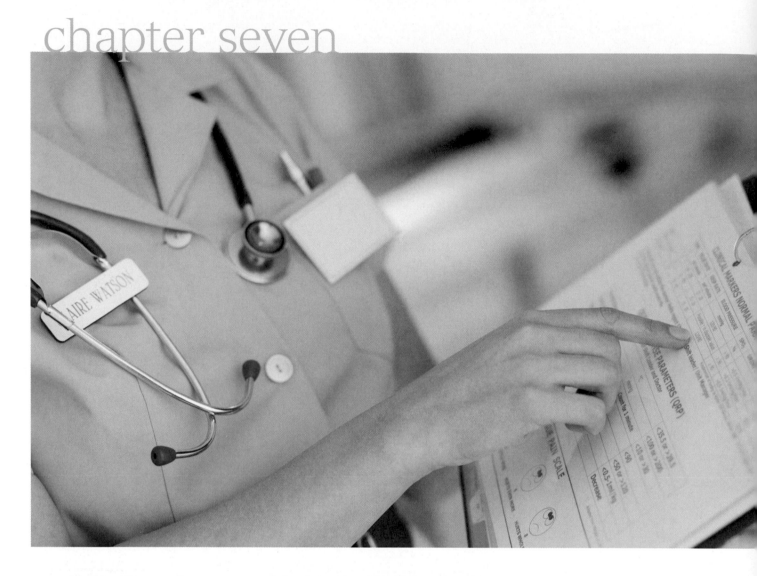

MEDICAL RECORDS AND INFORMED CONSENT

Learning Outcomes

After studying this chapter, you should be able to:

LO 7.1 Explain the purpose of medical records and the importance of correct documentation.

LO 7.2 Identify ownership of medical records and determine how long a medical record must be kept by the owners.

LO 7.3 Describe the purpose of obtaining a patient's consent for release of medical information, and explain the doctrine of informed consent.

LO 7.4 Describe the necessity for electronic medical records and the efforts being made to record all medical records electronically.

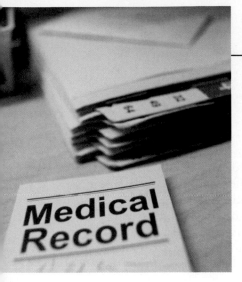

from the perspective of . . .

SALLY, MICHAEL, AND TERESA handle requests for release of patients' medical records for a midwestern hospital serving a five-state area. They emphasize that they can release records only with signed authorization from the patient or on subpoena, and that they may then release photocopies, but never original medical records. When someone visits the hospital to pick up copies of a patient's records, that person is asked to show identification.

Michael lets experience be his guide and checks out any request for release of records that "doesn't feel right." For example, if a husband brings an authorization form for release of medical records that he says his wife signed, her signature should be checked against the signature on hospital admission forms. It could be that a divorce is in progress in such a situation, and the husband or wife is seeking medical records to prove the spouse an unfit parent.

"Never release medical records because the person making the request has intimidated you," adds Teresa. "The most officious person I've dealt with was an FBI agent who told me, 'I want this record. If you don't give it to me, I'll get it myself.' I said, 'Go for it.' Later the agent called and apologized to me."

Since the employing hospital is located in a city with an air force base, Sally, Michael, and Teresa often receive requests for medical records for active duty military personnel. "We have now been told that the military can get the records they request on any active duty person," adds Sally. "We still ask for an authorization, but it is not required, since the active duty person signs away that right when he or she signs up for the military. This applies to active duty personnel on duty or on leave, but it does not include dependents of the person in the military."

Michael, Teresa, and Sally know that medical records contain information that can be used in ways not intended when the health care data were collected. They also know that the hospital that employs them can be legally liable for improper release of medical records. Therefore, they are extremely careful about always obtaining proper consent before releasing records.

From the perspective of individuals seeking medical records for their own purposes, not related to health care or the welfare of patients, Michael, Teresa, and Sally are unrelenting obstacles. From the perspective of the patients whose confidential medical records are conscientiously protected, Michael, Teresa, and Sally are performing their jobs well.

As a medical records or health information technician, how would you react to a person demanding her estranged husband's medical records and threatening to sue you if you did not comply?

Should family members be entitled to obtain loved ones medical records on request, no questions asked? Explain your answer.

Medical Records

A **medical record** is a collection of data recorded when a patient seeks medical treatment. Hospitals, surgical centers, clinics, physician offices, and other facilities providing health care services maintain patients' medical records. Medical records serve many purposes:

1. They are required by licensing authorities and provide a format for tracking, documenting, and maintaining a patient's communication data, both inside and outside a health care facility.

LO 7.1

Explain the purpose of medical records and the importance of correct documentation.

> **medical record** A collection of data recorded when a patient seeks medical treatment.

2. They provide documentation of a patient's continuing health care, from birth to death.

3. They provide a foundation for managing a patient's health care.

4. They serve as legal documents in lawsuits.

5. They provide clinical data for education, research, statistical tracking, and assessing the quality of health care.

Entries

As a legal document, a patient's medical record may be subpoenaed (via subpoena *duces tecum*) as evidence in court. When they are conscientiously compiled, medical records can prevail over a patient's recollection of events during a trial. When there is no entry in the record to the effect that something was done, there is a presumption that it was not done, and when there is an entry that something was done, the presumption is that it was done. Therefore, what is omitted from the record may be as important to the outcome of a lawsuit as what is included.

Records may be kept on paper, microfilm, or computer tapes or disks. For legal protection as well as continuity of care, the following information must be recorded in a patient's record:

- Contact and identifying information: the patient's full name, Social Security number, date of birth, and full address. If applicable, include e-mail address, home and work telephone numbers, marital status, and name and address of employer.

- Insurance information: name of policy member and relationship to patient, details such as certificate and group numbers, telephone numbers, copy of insurance card, Medicaid or Medicare numbers if applicable, and secondary insurance.

- Driver's license information, state, and number.

- Person responsible for payment and billing address.

- Emergency contact information.

- The patient's health history.

- The dates and times of the patient's arrival for appointments.

- A complete description of the patient's symptoms and reason for making an appointment.

- The examination performed by the physician.

- The physician's assessment, diagnosis, recommendations, treatment prescribed, progress notes, and instructions given to the patient, plus a notation of all new prescriptions the physician writes for the patient and of refills the physician authorizes.

- X-rays and all other test results.

- A notation for each time the patient telephoned the medical facility or was telephoned by the facility, listing date, reason for the call, and resolution.

- A notation of copies made of the medical record, including date copied and the person to whom the copy was sent.

- Documentation of informed consent, when necessary.

- Name of the guardian or legal representative to be contacted if the patient is unable to give informed consent.

- Other documentation, such as complete written descriptions; photographs; samples of body fluids, foreign objects, and clothing in cases involving criminal investigations; and so on. All items should be carefully labeled and preserved.

- Condition of the patient at the time of termination of treatment, when applicable, and reasons for termination, including documentation if the physician–patient contract was terminated before completion of treatment.

Five Cs (Figure 7-1) can be used to describe the necessary attributes of entries to patients' medical records. These entries must be

1. Concise.
2. Complete (and objective).
3. Clear (and legibly written).
4. Correct.
5. Chronologically ordered.

Medical records should never include inappropriate personal judgments or observations or attempts at humor.

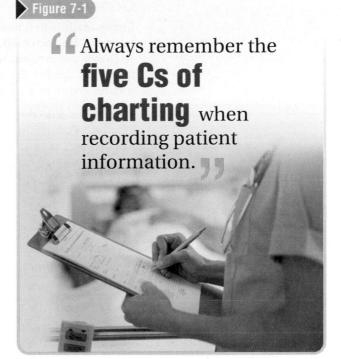

" Always remember the **five Cs of charting** when recording patient information. "

Photographs, Videotaping, and Other Methods of Patient Imaging

In today's health care environment, it has become increasingly common to record patients' images through the use of photography, videotaping, digital imaging, and other visual recordings. For example, surgeons may photograph, videotape, or otherwise record procedures used during an operation for purposes of education or review. Cosmetic surgeons and physicians who treat accident victims may want to document visually the patient's condition "before" and "after" the incident. Such images then become part of the patient's medical record, subject to the same requirement for written release as the rest of the record. (See the section in this chapter entitled "Routine Release of Information" on page 200.)

Photographing or otherwise recording a patient's image without proper consent may be interpreted in a court of law as invasion of privacy. Invasion of privacy charges are most often upheld in court if the patient's image was used for commercial purposes, but such claims have also been upheld under public disclosure of embarrassing private facts. For example, "before" and "after" photographs published by a cosmetic surgeon may cause embarrassment to the patient if he or she did not give consent for the photographs to be published.

If a health care facility routinely photographs patients to document care, a special consent form should be signed stating that

- The patient understands that photographs, videotapes, and digital or other images may be taken to document care.

- The patient understands that ownership rights to the images will be retained by the health care facility, but that he or she will be allowed to view them or to obtain copies.

- The images will be securely stored and kept for the time period prescribed by law or outlined in the health care facility's policy.

- Images of the patient will not be released and/or used outside the health care facility without written authorization from the patient or his or her legal representative.

If the images will be used for teaching or publicity, a separate consent form should be used.

Corrections

Errors made when making an entry in a medical record or errors discovered later can be corrected, but corrections must be made in a specific manner, so that if the medical records are ever used in a medical malpractice lawsuit, it will not appear that they were falsified. Follow these guidelines when correcting errors in a client's medical record:

- Draw a line through the error so that it is still legible. Do not black out the information or use correction fluid to cover it up.

- Write or type in the correct information above or below the original line or in the margin. If necessary, you may attach another sheet of paper or another document with the correction on it. In this case, note in the record "See attached document A" to indicate where the corrected information can be found.

- Note near the correction why it was made (for example, "error, wrong date," or "error, interrupted by a phone call"). You can place this note in the margin or, again, add an attachment. Do not make a change in the record without noting the reason for it.

- Enter the date and time, and initial the correction.

- If possible, ask another staff member or the physician to witness and initial the correction to the record when you make it.

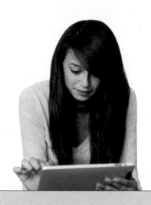

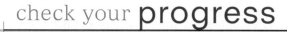

check your **progress**

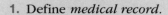

1. Define *medical record*.

2. List five purposes served by a patient's medical record.

3. As the person responsible for charting in a medical office, would you record a patient's statement that she often feels "woozy" and thinks she has "dropsy"? Why or why not?

4. If a reconstructive surgeon wants to publish "before" and "after" photographs of patients in a brochure left in the waiting room for distribution to prospective patients, what must she do?

5. If a patient makes critical remarks to you, a medical assistant, about your physician/employer, would you record the remarks in the patient's medical record? Why or why not?

6. You are charting after a patient's office visit and you are interrupted by a telephone call. The interruption causes you to incorrectly record results of the patient's blood tests. When you discover your mistake, can you correct it? If so, how?

LO 7.2

Identify ownership of medical records and determine how long a medical record must be kept by the owners.

Medical Records Ownership, Retention, and Storage

Ownership

Patients' medical records are considered the property of the owners of the facility where they were created. For example, a physician in private practice owns his or her records; records in a clinic are the property of the clinic. Hospital records are the property of the admitting hospital. The facility where the medical records were created owns the documents, but *the patient owns the information they contain*. On signing a release, patients may usually obtain access to or copies of their medical records, depending on state law. However, under the **doctrine of professional discretion,** courts have held that in some cases, patients treated for mental or emotional conditions may be harmed by seeing their own records. Under HIPAA, patients who ask to see and/or copy their medical records must be accommodated, with a few exceptions. HIPAA is discussed in detail in Chapter 8. If patients need clarification, records may be reviewed in the presence of a trusted health care professional, but this is not a requirement for allowing patients to see their records.

When a physician in private practice examines a patient for a job-related physical, scheduled and paid for by the patient's employer or prospective employer, those records are still the physician's property, but the employer is entitled to a copy of the record that is pertinent to the job-related exam. Medical records should never be kept in an employer's general personnel files. The patient must obtain permission from the employer to release information contained in the records.

Under HIPAA, patients are entitled to access any health care information a physician generates about them, with a few exceptions, which are discussed in Chapter 8.

doctrine of professional discretion A principle under which a physician can exercise judgment as to whether to show patients who are being treated for mental or emotional conditions their records. Disclosure depends on whether, in the physician's judgment, such patients would be harmed by viewing the records.

Retention and Storage

As a protection in the event of litigation, records should be kept until the applicable statute of limitations period has elapsed, which generally ranges from two to seven years. In some cases, this involves keeping the medical records for minor patients for a specified length of time after they reach

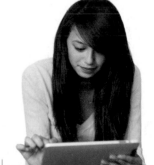

check your **progress**

7. How long should medical records be retained?

8. Who owns a patient's medical record?

9. Define *doctrine of professional discretion.*

10. Are you entitled to a copy of your own medical records on request? Explain your answer.

11. If medical records are lost prior to the filing of a medical malpractice lawsuit where the records are necessary, what might result?

legal age. Some states have enacted statutes for the retention of medical records. However, most physicians retain records indefinitely, since, in addition to their value as documentation in medical professional liability suits and for tax purposes, the patient's medical history may be vital in determining future treatment.

As illustrated in the court case, "Loss of Medical Records," medical malpractice is impossible to prove without medical records:

LO 7.3

Describe the purpose of obtaining a patient's consent for release of medical information, and explain the doctrine of informed consent.

Confidentiality and Informed Consent

Since medical office personnel have a duty to protect the privacy of the patient, medical records should not be released to a third party without written permission, signed by the patient or the patient's legal representative. Only the information requested should be released.

Requests for release of records may ask for records concerning a specific date or time span. Records may also be requested for a specific diagnosis, symptom, or body system, or for results of certain diagnostic tests. Medical records personnel should not send unsolicited records. They should carefully review the signed release form to ensure that the correct records are sent.

When medical records are requested for use in a lawsuit, a signed consent for the release of the records must be obtained from the patient, unless a court subpoenas the records. In this case, the patient should be notified in writing that the records have been subpoenaed and released.

Routine Release of Information

Medical information about a patient is often released for the following purposes:

Insurance Claims. The medical office supplies specific requested information, but does not usually send the patient's entire medical record. An authorization to release information, signed by the patient, is required before records may be released, but most health care providers incorporate the release into the patient registration form so that information can be provided in a timely manner.

Transfer to Another Physician. The physician may photocopy and send all records, or may send a summary. The patient must sign an authorization to release records.

Use in a Court of Law. When a subpoena *duces tecum* is issued for certain records (the subpoena commands a witness to appear in court and to bring certain medical records), the patient's written consent to release the records is waived.

The classic court case, "Not Guilty of Breach of Confidentiality," illustrates that physicians who produce patients' medical records for use in court, or those who testify in court as expert witnesses, are not liable for breach of confidentiality.

As illustrated in the chapter's opening scenario, individuals responsible for releasing medical information must follow procedure to protect against unauthorized release, even in the previous situations where medical records are routinely requested.

Not Guilty of Breach of Confidentiality

A physician cannot be sued for breach of confidentiality when required to produce a patient's medical records for use in court testimony.

A patient (Cruz) sued a physician (Agelides) for breach of fiduciary duty. (**Fiduciary duty** is a physician's duty to his or her patient, based on trust and confidence.) In a previous malpractice action brought by Cruz against another physician, Agelides had given a sworn pretrial affidavit and video deposition in favor of the defending physician. The court held that Agelides was immune from any civil liability action as a result of his testimony as a witness in the previous trial.

Source: Cruz v. Agelides, 574 So.2d 278 (Fla. App. 3 Dist., 1991).

In your opinion, what would be the result if any health care practitioner could be sued for breach of confidentiality when required to produce patients' medical records for use in court?

The following court case, "Breach of Confidentiality Declared," determined that damages were properly awarded to the plaintiff in a suit against a nurse who released confidential medical information without authorization.

While Michael, Sally, and Teresa, medical records employees, are explicitly aware of the dangers of releasing confidential medical information, all health care practitioners, like the nurse in the court case, "Breach of

> **fiduciary duty** A physician's obligation to his or her patient, based on trust and confidence.

Breach of Confidentiality Declared—Damages Upheld

A 20-year-old unmarried woman who lived with her parents decided to terminate her pregnancy at the Long Island Surgi-Center. Because her parents strongly disapproved of premarital sex and were implacably opposed to abortion, she did not tell them of her decision. When she arranged for the procedure, the woman provided her cell phone number, but told the clinic never to call her at home. Nevertheless, a day after the abortion one of the clinic's nurses telephoned the young woman at home and spoke with a person she knew to be the woman's mother. Because blood test results had been received at the center that morning, but had not been entered in the patient's medical record, the nurse called the patient's home to determine (1) information about the patient's blood type, and (2) if the patient was experiencing vaginal bleeding. The nurse did not explicitly tell the patient's mother that her daughter had undergone an abortion, but the mother deduced the truth from the nurse's questions. The patient's relationship with her parents was irreparably damaged, and she sued the clinic, charging breaches of confidentiality, privacy, and fiduciary duty, and seeking compensatory and punitive damages. The center conceded liability, and the matter proceeded to trial on the question of damages. The jury awarded the plaintiff $65,000 for past and future emotional distress and $300,000 in punitive damages. The Surgi-Center appealed the damages awarded, but the appeals court upheld the awards.

Source: Randi A.J. v. Long Is. Surgi-Ctr., 2007 NY Slip Op 06953; 46 A.D. 3d 74.

What actions might the nurse have taken to prevent the breach of confidentiality that occurred?

Confidentiality Declared," also need to be constantly aware of protecting confidentiality of patients' medical records.

Physicians receive subpoenas for patient medical records for a variety of reasons, including accidents involving patients, workers' compensation claims, and other non-medical-liability reasons. When this occurs, the medical office sends a photocopy of the patient's medical records to the attorney who issued the subpoena.

When a physician is sued for medical malpractice, however, responsibility to comply with a subpoena to produce specified medical records in court may fall to the medical office employee in charge of medical records. In that case, the person in charge of medical records should follow these guidelines:

- Check the subpoena to be sure the name and phone number of the issuing attorney and the court docket number of the case are listed.

- If a carbon copy of the subpoena is received, verify with the issuing attorney that it is the same as the original in every way.

- Verify that the patient named was a patient of the physician named.

- Verify the trial date and time as listed on the subpoena.

- Notify the physician that a subpoena was received, and then notify the physician's insurance company or attorney, if so directed.

- Check all subpoenaed records to be sure they are complete, but never alter them in any way.

- Document the number of pages in the record and itemize its contents. Make a photocopy of the original to be submitted, if permitted by state law and the court.

- Offer sworn testimony regarding the record, if so instructed by the court.

Confidentiality of Alcohol and Drug Abuse, Patient Records A federal statute that protects patients with histories of substance abuse regarding the release of information about treatment.

Some state laws specifically address the release of confidential medical information, especially as it pertains to treatment for mental or emotional health problems, HIV testing, and substance abuse. In addition, the federal statute **Confidentiality of Alcohol and Drug Abuse, Patient Records** protects patients with histories of substance abuse regarding the release of information about treatment. Under no circumstances should information of this type be released without specific, written permission from the patient to do so. The patient also has the right to rescind (cancel) consent to release information, in which case the information should not be released.

The following rules for authorizations for the release of medical records can serve as a general guide for medical assistants, health information technicians, and other health care practitioners:

- Authorizations should be in writing.

- Authorizations should include the patient's name, address, and date of birth.

- The patient should sign authorizations, unless he or she is not a legal, competent adult. In that case, parents or guardians should sign authorizations.

- Only the information specifically requested should be released.

- Requests for information coming into the medical office from insurance companies, physicians, or other sources should be witnessed and dated and include the complete name, address, and signature of the party requesting the information, as well as that of the party asked to release the information.

- Include a specific description of the information that is needed. List the purpose for which the data will be used and the date on which the consent expires.

Consent

By giving **consent,** the patient gives permission, either expressed (orally or in writing) or implied, for the physician to examine him or her, to perform tests that aid in diagnosis, and/or to treat for a medical condition. When the patient makes an appointment for an examination, that patient has given implied consent for the physician to perform the exam. Likewise, when he or she cooperates with various diagnostic testing procedures, implied consent for the tests has been given.

consent Permission from a person, either expressed or implied, for something to be done by another.

Informed Consent For surgery and for some other procedures, such as a test for HIV, implied consent is not enough. In these cases, it is important to ask the patient to sign a consent form, thereby documenting informed consent (see Figure 7-2).

The **doctrine of informed consent** is the legal basis for informed consent and is usually outlined in a state's medical practice acts. Informed consent implies that the patient understands

doctrine of informed consent The legal basis for informed consent, usually outlined in a state's medical practice acts.

- Proposed modes of treatment.
- Why the treatment is necessary.
- Risks involved in the proposed treatment.
- Available alternative modes of treatment.
- Risks of alternative modes of treatment.
- Risks involved if treatment is refused.

Informed consent involves the patient's right to receive all information relative to his or her condition and then to make a decision regarding treatment based on that knowledge. Documents establishing that the patient gave informed consent prove that the patient was not coerced into treatment.

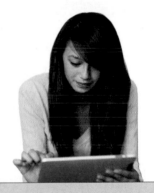

check your **progress**

12. Name three reasons a medical office might be requested to release a patient's medical records.

13. In which of the three situations named for question 12 might a patient's written consent to release records be waived?

14. What is needed before the medical office can send a patient's medical record to the insurer?

15. If an insurance company submits a request for medical records pertaining to an enrolled patient's outpatient foot surgery and you are responsible for sending the records, should you send the patient's entire file to be on the safe side? Why or why not?

16. As the person who reviews requests for patients' medical records, do you need to know the purpose for which the data will be used? Explain your answer.

Figure 7-2 A Sample Consent Form

INFORMED CONSENT for SURGERY and PROCEDURES

1. I hereby authorize staff physicians and resident staff at _____ to perform upon
                                                            (Name of Hospital or Facility)
_____ , such treatment, procedures and/or operations necessary to treat or diagnose the
        (Name of patient)
condition(s) which appear indicated.

2. The operation(s) or procedure(s) necessary to treat and/or diagnose my condition and the risks, benefits/alternatives and options associated with them have been explained to me by_____ , and I understand the operation(s) or
                                                        (Name of Physician or provider)
procedure(s) to be: _____

3. Different Provider: ☐ Not Applicable
I understand and approve that a different provider other than the physician named above may actually perform the procedure.

4. Operative Side: ☐ Not Applicable   ☐ Left   ☐ Right

5. Sedation & Local Anesthetics: I authorize the administration of sedation and the use of local anesthetics, drugs and medicines as may be deemed appropriate. If they will be used, the risks and benefits/alternatives of sedation have been explained to me by the procedural physician.

6. Blood and Blood Products: ☐ Not Applicable
I understand certain surgeries, procedures, or illnesses may result in loss of blood. I authorize the administration of blood and/or blood components during the procedure as well as during the course of my hospital stay. If blood will be used, the risks, benefits/alternatives have been explained to me by the physician.
Patient Initials: _____

7. No Blood Products: ☐ Not Applicable
I request that No blood derivative be administered to me. I hereby release the hospital, its personnel, the attending physician and its agents from any responsibility whatsoever for unfavorable reactions or any untoward results due to my refusal to permit the use of blood or its derivatives. The possible risks and consequences of such refusal on my part have been fully explained and I fully understand such risks and consequences may occur as a result of my refusal.

Signature of Patient/Responsible Person: _____   Relationship: _____

8. Unforeseen Conditions: It has been explained to me that during the course of the operation(s) or procedure(s) unforeseen conditions may be revealed that necessitate an extension of the original procedure(s) or different procedure(s) than those set forth above. I am aware that the practice of medicine is not an exact science and I acknowledge that no guarantees have been made to me concerning the result of the operation(s) or procedure(s).

9. Photography: I consent to the use of photography, closed circuit television recording and to use the photographs and other materials for study, educational and scientific purposes, in accordance with ordinary practices of the facility.

10. I consent to have my procedure/operation observed, for educational purposes, by individual(s) other than those assisting the physician during the procedure/operation.

Physician or Provider Signature	Patient's Signature (if competent)	Witness	Date	Time
Signature of Interpreter (if applicable)	Date	Time	Signature of Person Responsible Relationship	Date	Time
Witness (Telephone consent)	Date	Time	Second Physician or Provider Signature for Emergencies for incompetent patient and No family	Date	Time

Physician must initial faxed copy

Adults of sound mind are usually able to give informed consent. Those individuals who cannot give informed consent include the following:

Minors, Persons under the Age of Majority. Exceptions include

- Emancipated minors—those who are living away from home and responsible for their own support. A minor becomes "emancipated" through a court hearing where evidence is presented that the minor should be emancipated, and a judge makes a determination that the minor has met certain criteria. The minor is then declared "emancipated" and can consent to his or her health care treatment just as any adult of sound mind determines his or her health care treatment.

- Married minors.

- Mature minors—those who, through the doctrine of mature minors, have been granted the right to seek birth control or care during pregnancy, treatment for reportable communicable diseases, or treatment for drug- or alcohol-related problems without first obtaining parental consent.

Persons Who Are Mentally Incompetent. Individuals judged by the court to be insane, senile, mentally challenged, or under the influence of drugs or alcohol cannot give informed consent. In these cases, a competent person may be designated by the court to act as the patient's agent.

Persons Who Speak Limited or No English. When a patient does not speak or understand English, an interpreter may be necessary to inform the patient and obtain his or her consent for treatment.

The rights of emancipated minors, married minors, and mature minors to consent to their own health care are discussed further in Chapter 10.

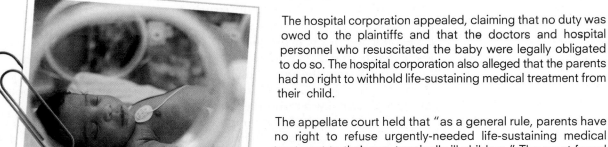

COURT CASE

Medical Malpractice/Consent and Informed Consent

A woman who was 23 weeks pregnant went into labor and was admitted to a Texas hospital. An obstetrician and a neonatologist informed both parents that if the "baby were born alive and survived, she would suffer severe impairments." Based on that information, the parents orally requested that no heroic measures be performed on the baby after birth. The request was entered in the medical record, and the neonatologist was dismissed. However, the obstetrician later concluded that if the baby were born alive and weighed over 500 grams, the medical staff would be obligated by law and hospital policy to administer life-sustaining procedures, even if the baby's parents did not consent to such procedures. The obstetrician later stated that this caveat was explained to the parents. A second neonatologist who assisted in the delivery determined that the child was "viable" and "instituted resuscitative measures." The child survived birth but, as predicted, suffered severe physical and mental impairments.

The parents filed suit against the corporation that owned the hospital, alleging, among other claims, that the physicians had treated their newborn without their consent. A jury trial held the hospital corporation liable for the baby's injuries, and the court awarded the parents $29,400,000 in past and future medical expenses, $13,500,000 in punitive damages, and $17,503,066 in "prejudgment interest."

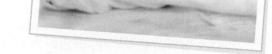

The hospital corporation appealed, claiming that no duty was owed to the plaintiffs and that the doctors and hospital personnel who resuscitated the baby were legally obligated to do so. The hospital corporation also alleged that the parents had no right to withhold life-sustaining medical treatment from their child.

The appellate court held that "as a general rule, parents have no right to refuse urgently-needed life-sustaining medical treatment to their non-terminally ill children." The court found that the physicians involved in resuscitating the newborn had acted reasonably and dismissed the vicarious liability action against the hospital corporation. Therefore, the parents received no award.

Source: HCA, Inc. v. Miller, 36 S.W.3d 187 (2000).

Other problems in obtaining informed consent may arise in situations such as when foster children need medical attention or a spouse seeks sterilization or an abortion. In each case, health care practitioners must determine who is legally able to give informed consent for treatment. When in doubt, seek legal advice.

Patient education is vital to the issue of informed consent. Stocking the medical office with brochures about various medical problems is not sufficient if the physician does not review the material with the patient. Patients who sue have successfully claimed lack of informed consent because they did not read the consent form they signed or did not read brochures handed to them. Health care personnel should be sure that patients understand all forms and all treatments/surgeries to be performed before signing.

The following U.S. Supreme Court decision illustrates the fact that before proceeding with treatment, health care practitioners must determine whether or not patients are competent to give informed consent.

COURT CASE

Patient Not Competent to Sign Forms

The U.S. Supreme Court overruled two lower federal courts, stating that a Florida mental patient had a cause of action. The patient claimed that he had been admitted to a state mental health treatment facility as a voluntary patient, based on forms he signed when he was heavily medicated, disoriented, and suffering from a psychotic disorder. His admission, he alleged, deprived him of his liberty, without due process of law, when he was incompetent to give informed consent.

The U.S. Supreme Court held that allegations that employees of the state hospital admitted him as a voluntary patient without taking steps to ascertain whether he was mentally competent to sign the admission forms stated a cause of action.

Source: Zinermon v. Burch, 110 S.Ct. 975 (U.S. Sup. Ct., Feb. 27, 1990).

Informed Consent and Abortion Law In *Planned Parenthood v. Casey,* U.S. 833 (1992), the U.S. Supreme Court upheld a 24-hour waiting period, an informed consent requirement, a parental consent provision for minors, and a record-keeping requirement for women seeking an abortion. At the same time, the Court struck down the spousal notice requirement of a Pennsylvania statute, in addition to other specific requirements. *Casey* and *Webster v. Reproductive Health Services* before it (1989) upheld *Roe v. Wade,* the 1973 Supreme Court decision that legalized abortion in the United States (see the following case, "Case Legalizes Abortion"), but allowed state regulation of abortion. A number of state legislatures took the cue and passed new abortion restrictions.

Among a long list of state-imposed abortion restrictions are laws that specify certain changes in informed consent. For example, some states require that a woman seeking an abortion be clearly informed of all alternatives to abortions and be told of all risks associated with such surgeries before she can give informed consent to the abortion. In addition, before a woman can consent to an abortion in many states, she must wait a certain length of time (usually 24 hours) before actually signing a consent form.

A more recent court case, "Case Allows State Regulation," upheld *Roe v. Wade,* and also allowed a state to regulate abortion.

In 1970 a single woman in Texas became pregnant. She had difficulty finding work because of her pregnancy and feared the stigma of an illegitimate birth. Under the fictitious name "Jane Roe," the woman sued Henry Wade, the district attorney in Dallas County, Texas, claiming that she had limited rights to an abortion and sought an injunction against the Texas statute prohibiting abortion except to save a woman's life.

It took three years for the case to reach the U.S. Supreme Court, which struck down the Texas statute. The ruling came too late for Jane Roe to have the abortion she originally sought, of course, but it affected the rights of all women who would seek abortions from that time on. The Court held that the constitutional right to privacy includes a woman's decision to terminate a pregnancy during the first trimester (three months), but that states could impose restrictions and regulate abortions after that.

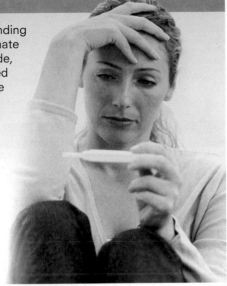

Source: Roe v. Wade, 410 U.S. 113, 144 "n.39" (1973).

Technically, abortion is legal in all 50 states, but state legislatures have added restrictions, as shown in Table 7-1.

Since abortion law is constantly changing, health care practitioners must stay informed about current abortion laws in their respective states.

HIV and Informed Consent State public health law varies for human immunodeficiency virus (HIV) testing, but, generally, health care practitioners must consider the following factors:

Can a minor (aged less than 18 in some states, 21 in others) consent to his or her own HIV test? Informed consent law for minors vary, but this determination may sometimes be made without regard to age, depending on the minor's situation:

The Pennsylvania legislature amended its abortion control law in 1988 and 1989. Among the new provisions, the law required informed consent and a 24-hour waiting period prior to the procedure. A minor seeking an abortion required the consent of one parent (the law allowed for a judicial bypass procedure). A married woman seeking an abortion had to indicate that she notified her husband of her intention to abort the fetus. These provisions were challenged by several abortion clinics and physicians. A federal appeals court upheld all the provisions except the husband notification requirement.

The question in this case was, can a state require women who want an abortion to obtain informed consent, wait 24 hours, and, if minors, obtain parental consent without violating their right to abortions as guaranteed by *Roe v. Wade?* In a bitter 5-to-4 decision, the Court again reaffirmed *Roe,* but it upheld most of the Pennsylvania provisions. For the first time, the justices imposed a new standard to determine the validity of laws restricting abortions. The new standard asks whether a state abortion regulation has the purpose or effect of imposing an "undue burden," which is defined as a "substantial obstacle in the path of a woman seeking an abortion before the fetus attains viability." Under this standard, the only provision to fail the undue-burden test was the husband notification requirement.

Source: Planned Parenthood v. Casey, 505 U.S. 833 (1992).

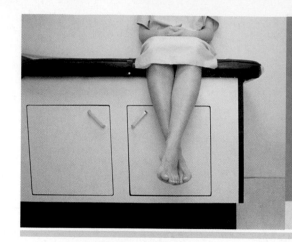

A SUMMARY OF STATE ABORTION LAWS, AS OF JUNE 2010

Table 7-1

34 states require parental notification or consent. 7 states—AK, CA, IL, MT, NV, NJ, and NM—have parental notification laws that are not enforced. 10 states—CT, HA, ME, MD, NH, NY, OR, VT, WA, and Washington, DC—have no parental notification or consent laws. (Parental notification laws require that a parent is notified before a minor daughter can receive an abortion. Parental consent laws require that the parent consent to a minor daughter's abortion.)

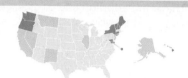

■ Parental Notification Law ■ No Parental Notification Laws

30 states ban partial-birth:* AL, AK, AZ, AR, FL, GA, ID, IL, IN, IA, KS, LA, MI, MS, MO, MT, NB, NJ, NM, ND, OH, OK, RI, SC, SD, TN, UT, VA, WV, and WI. Of these bans, 16 are actually enforced: AK, GA, IN, KS, LA, MS, MT, NM, ND, OH, OK, SC, SD, TN, UT, and VA.

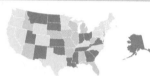

■ Partial-birth banned ■ Partial birth ban enforced

17 states require counseling for women seeking an abortion: AL, AR, GA, IN, KS, KY, LA, MI, MS, MO, OK, SC, SD, TX, UT, WV, and WI. (Counseling must include information on at least one of the following: the link between abortion and breast cancer, the ability of a fetus to feel pain, the mental health consequences of abortion, or the availability of ultrasound.) 5 states require that abortion counseling be done in person: IN, LA, MS, UT, and WI.

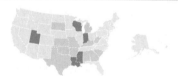

■ Required abortion counseling ■ Required in person abortion counseling

24 states require women to wait a specified amount of time (usually 24 hours) between receiving counseling and obtaining an abortion: AL, AK, GA, ID, IN, KS, KY, LA, MI, MN, MS, MO, NB, ND, OH, OK, PA, SC, SD, TX, UT, VA, WV, and WI.

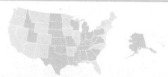

■ States requiring 24 hour waiting period

17 states use public funds to pay for abortions: AK, AZ, CA, CT, HA, IL, MD, MA, MN, MT, NJ, NM, NY, OR, VT, WA, and WV. 33 states prohibit using public funds to pay for abortions except in cases when federal funds are available: AL, AR, CO, DE, FL, GA, ID, IN, IA, KS, KY, LA, ME, MI, MS, MO, NB, NV, NH, NC, ND, OH, OK, PA, RI, SC, SD, TN TX, UT, VA, WI, and WY.

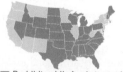

■ Public funds to pay for abortions ■ Prohibit public funds to pay for abortions

46 states allow some health care providers to refuse to provide abortion services if such services go against religious and/or ethics beliefs.

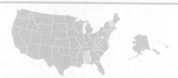

■ States that allow abortion refusal due to religious and/or ethnic beliefs

*Partial-birth abortion is a lay term. The medical term for the procedure is dilation and extraction (D&X). *Merriam-Webster's Medical Dictionary* defines partial-birth abortion as "an abortion in the second or third trimester of pregnancy in which the death of the fetus is induced after it has passed partway through the birth canal." Since abortion law is constantly changing, health care practitioners must stay informed about current abortion laws in their respective states.

- Infants and young children do not have the capacity to consent, because they do not yet have the ability to make informed decisions. The person legally designated to make health care decisions for the child has the right to decide whether the child should be tested for HIV.

- Married minors, emancipated minors, and minor parents may have the right to give consent for HIV testing, depending on state law.

Can an HIV-infected minor consent to his or her treatment? Generally, parental or guardian consent is required for a physician to treat a minor for HIV/AIDS, including treatment in school-based clinics. Married, emancipated, and mature minors can usually consent to their own care.

When Consent Is Unnecessary In emergency situations, when the patient is in immediate danger, the physician is not expected to obtain consent before proceeding with treatment.

All 50 states have passed **Good Samaritan acts.** These acts were intended to protect physicians and, in some states, other health care practitioners and laypersons from charges of negligence or abandonment if they stop to help the victim of an accident or other emergency (Figure 7-3), provided they

- Give such care in good faith.
- Act within the scope of their training and knowledge.
- Use due care under the circumstances.
- Do not bill for their services. (If a physician treats a patient as a "Good Samaritan" and later bills the patient for services, he or she may be held as having established a physician–patient relationship and may not have the immunity from civil damages that a Good Samaritan law would otherwise provide.)

While some states offer immunity to Good Samaritans, sometimes the act of rescuing an accident victim can result in a legal claim of negligent care if the injuries or illness were made worse by the volunteer's actions. Statutes typically don't exempt a Good Samaritan who acts in a wilful and wanton or reckless manner in providing emergency care, advice, or assistance. Furthermore, Good Samaritan laws usually don't apply to a person rendering emergency care, advice, or assistance during the course of regular employment, such as services rendered by a health care provider to a patient in a health care facility.

Good Samaritan in legal terms refers to someone who renders aid in an emergency to an injured person on a voluntary basis. Usually, if a volunteer comes to the aid of an injured or ill person who is a stranger, the person giving the aid owes the stranger a duty of being reasonably careful. A person is not obligated by law to do first aid in most states, unless it's part of a job description. However, some states will consider it an act of negligence if a person doesn't at least call for help. Generally, where an unconscious victim cannot respond, a Good Samaritan can help on the grounds of implied consent. However, if the victim is conscious and can respond, a person should first ask permission to help.

▶ **Figure 7-3**

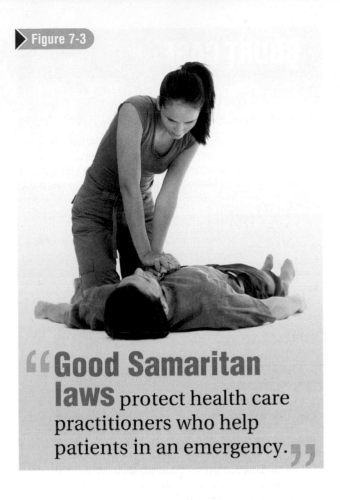

"Good Samaritan laws protect health care practitioners who help patients in an emergency. **"**

Good Samaritan acts State laws protecting physicians and sometimes other health care practitioners and laypersons from charges of negligence or abandonment if they stop to help the victim of an accident or other emergency.

Good Samaritans Can Be Liable for Damages to Person Injured during Rescue Attempt

Good friends Alexandra Van Horn and Lisa Torti spent the evening partying in a bar; then each woman left the bar in her own car. Van Horn drove away first, and crashed into a curb and streetlight standard at 45 mph. Torti, behind Van Horn in the second car, saw the accident and, afraid the wrecked car was about to "blow up," she removed Van Horn. As a result, Van Horn was paralyzed.

Van Horn sued Torti. Torti's defense was based on California's Good Samaritan law, Health & Safety Code section 1799.102, which provides: "No person who in good faith, and not for compensation, renders emergency care at the scene of an emergency shall be liable for any civil damages resulting from any act or omission. The scene of an emergency shall not include emergency departments and other places where medical care is usually offered."

Based on this statute, the trial court granted summary judgment for the defendant. The plaintiff appealed, and the case eventually reached the California Supreme Court, where justices interpreted the state's Good Samaritan law to apply strictly to *medical* care, because the statute appears in the Health & Safety Code, in the division entitled "Emergency Medical Services." (A statute providing broad immunity would likely appear in the Civil Code.) Torti did not render emergency medical care; she merely pulled Van Horn from her crashed car, and, therefore, she was found potentially liable. This ruling meant that Van Horn could take her case to a jury.

Common law principles applied were that the defendant's broad interpretation of Health & Safety Code 1799.102 would undermine established common law regarding liability for assisting others. There is no general duty to give assistance, but under the common law, a person who undertakes to help others has a duty to exercise due care. Nothing in the statute overcomes the judicial presumption that the legislature does not intend to overrule established common law principles when it enacts legislation. A broad interpretation, the court held, would also render superfluous other California "Good Samaritan" statutes, such as Govt.C. 50086 (immunity for a person trained in first aid who is summoned by authorities and renders emergency services) and Harb. & Nav.C. 656(b) (immunity for a person who assists at scene of vessel collision). (45 C.4th 333.)

Source: Trial Court: *Van Horn v. Watson* (2008) 45 C.4th 322, 86 C.R.3d 350, 197 P.3d 164. California Supreme Court: *Alexandra Van Horn, Plaintiff and Appellant, v. Anthony Glen Watson et al., Defendants and Respondents; Anthony Glen Watson, Cross-complainant and Appellant, v. Lisa Torti, Cross-defendant and Respondent,* Supreme Court of California, Dec. 18, 2008. Rehearing Denied Feb. 11, 2009.

As a result of the ruling, the California legislature changed the state's Good Samaritan law. Health and Safety Code section 1799.102 now reads in part: "No person who in good faith, and not for compensation, renders emergency medical or nonmedical care or assistance at the scene of an emergency shall be liable for civil damages resulting from any act or omission other than an act or omission constituting gross negligence or wilful or wanton misconduct."

In your opinion, why have all states enacted Good Samaritan laws?

If a person helps a victim in an emergency and is later sued, whether or not the defendant can use a state Good Samaritan law for his or her defense may depend on the court's definition of the state's law, as shown in the case, "Good Samaritans Can Be Liable for Damages."

LO 7.4

Describe the necessity for electronic medical records and the efforts being made to record all medical records electronically.

Health Information Technology (HIT)

When Hurricane Katrina, a Category 5 storm, hit the Louisiana and Mississippi coasts on August 29, 2005, the widespread destruction that resulted included the loss of countless numbers of paper medical records. As a result, many of the survivors gathered in the Superdome couldn't remember the names of lost prescriptions, or when they had last been immunized against tetanus and other diseases—information that was vital to maintaining their health. In addition, Katrina victims who reported to physicians had virtually no medical records health care providers could use as a basis for treatment. Furthermore, reconstruction would take valuable time.

It was obvious after this record-breaking storm that health information technology, and especially the use of electronic medical records, could prevent such huge medical record losses in the future.

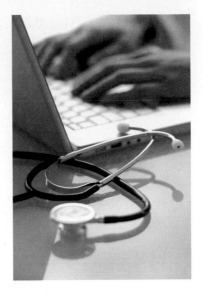

According to the U.S. Department of Health and Human Services, **health information technology (HIT)** is "the application of information processing involving both computer hardware and software that deals with the storage, retrieval, sharing, and use of health care information, data, and knowledge for communication and decision-making." The broad category *health information technology* also includes telemedicine and use of the Internet for health information purposes. A central component of HIT is the patient's medical file, and as electronic medical records become more widely adopted, confidentiality and privacy concerns must be addressed.

As of 2004, President George W. Bush had set a 10-year goal for the broad adoption of electronic health records in the United States. President Barack Obama, who took office January 1, 2009, continued to urge health care providers to convert records to electronic form. In fact, under the Patient Protection and Affordable Care Act signed into law in 2010, physicians could receive up to $44,000 from the government to help with the cost of converting to electronic health records.

health information technology (HIT) The application of information processing, involving both computer hardware and software, that deals with the storage, retrieval, sharing, and use of health care information, data, and knowledge for communication and decision making.

Government-initiated steps toward broad adoption of electronic health information include the following:

1. **The Health Insurance Portability and Accountability Act (HIPAA).** Passed in 1996 and implemented in stages through 2005, HIPAA addresses privacy of health information and mandates certain procedures and standards for the electronic transmission and storage of health care information. (See HIPAA details in Chapter 8.)

2. **Executive Orders.** In April 2004, President George W. Bush signed an executive order establishing the position of National Coordinator for Health Information Technology. The coordinator was charged with the development, maintenance, and oversight of a plan for nationwide adoption of health information technology.

   In August 2006, a second executive order stated that all federal agencies would utilize, where available, health information technology

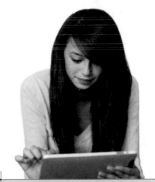

check your **progress**

17. Who may give informed consent?

18. Who may not give informed consent?

19. Must consent to perform routine medical care, such as a physical examination, always be in writing? Explain your answer.

20. In which health care situations is implied consent not sufficient?

21. What consequences generally ensue if a legally competent adult is treated without consent and an adverse event occurs?

systems and products meeting certain "recognized" standards. These HIT systems and products "shall be used for implementing, acquiring, or upgrading health information technology systems used for the direct exchange of health information between agencies and with nonfederal entities." The order further stipulated that federal agencies shall require in contracts or agreements with health care providers, health plans, or health insurance issuers that, where available, health information technology systems and products meeting recognized standards shall be used.

3. **Adoption of the Health Information Standards Developed by Health and Human Services (HHS).** As part of this effort, HHS has negotiated and licensed a comprehensive medical vocabulary and made it available to everyone in the United States at no cost. The results of these projects include standards for the following types of information:

- Transmitting X-Rays over the Internet: Today, a patient's chest X-ray can be sent electronically from a hospital or laboratory and read by the patient's doctor in his or her office.

- Electronic Laboratory Results: Laboratory results can be sent electronically to the physician for immediate analysis, diagnosis, and treatment, and could be automatically entered into the patient's electronic health record if one existed. For example, a doctor could retrieve this information for a hospitalized patient from his or her office, ensuring a prompt response and eliminating errors and duplicative testing due to lost laboratory reports.

- Electronic Prescriptions: Patients will save time because prescriptions can be sent electronically to their pharmacists. By eliminating illegible handwritten prescriptions, and because the technology automatically checks for possible allergies and harmful interactions with other drugs, standardized electronic prescriptions help avoid serious medical errors. The technology also can generate automatic approval from a health insurer.

4. **Use of the Federal Government to Foster the Adoption of Health Information Technology.** As one of the largest buyers of health care—in Medicare, Medicaid, the Community Health Centers program, the Federal Health Benefits program, veterans' medical care, and programs in the Department of Defense—the federal government can create incentives and opportunities for health care providers to use electronic records.

The federal government maintains that the broad use of health information technology will improve individual patient care by

- Improving health care quality.
- Preventing medical errors.
- Reducing health care costs.
- Increasing administrative efficiency.
- Decreasing paperwork.
- Expanding access to affordable care.

The previous benefits can be seen in the following examples:

- When arriving at a physician office, new patients do not have to enter their personal information, allergies, medications, or medical history, since these facts are already available.

- A parent, who previously may have had to carry a large folder containing the child's medical records and X-rays by hand when seeing a new physician, can now keep the most important medical history on a keychain, or simply authorize the new physician to retrieve the information electronically from previous health care providers.

- Arriving at an emergency room, an elderly patient with a chronic illness and memory difficulties can authorize his or her physicians to access her medical information from a recent hospitalization at another hospital—thus avoiding a potentially fatal drug interaction between the planned treatment and the patient's current medications.

Public health benefits will include

- Early detection of infectious outbreaks around the country. For example, three patients experience unusual sudden-onset fever and cough that would not individually be reported. They show up at separate emergency rooms, and through access to electronic health information, the trend is instantly reported to public health officials, who alert authorities of a possible disease outbreak or bioterror attack.

- Improved tracking of chronic disease management.

- Evaluation of health care based on comparisons of price and quality.

While the goal of widespread adoption of electronic health records by 2014 seems beneficial, many physicians and hospitals have not been eager to digitalize written records because the process is expensive and often fraught with information technology headaches, such as susceptibility to hackers who would steal private information, software that doesn't always perform as expected, and other threats to confidentiality when medical records are maintained and transported electronically.

According to Kathleen Sebelius, secretary of the U.S. Department of Health and Human Services, as quoted in the July 13, 2010, issue of the *New York Times,* just 20 percent of doctors and 10 percent of hospitals use even the most basic electronic records. Under federal legislation passed in 2009, the Department of Health and Human Services set aside $27 billion to help health care providers convert patients' records to **electronic health records (EHRs)**. Doctors can receive up to $44,000 under Medicare and $63,750 under Medicaid, and hospitals can receive millions, depending on

electronic health record (EHR) Contains the same information as any medical record, but in electronic form.

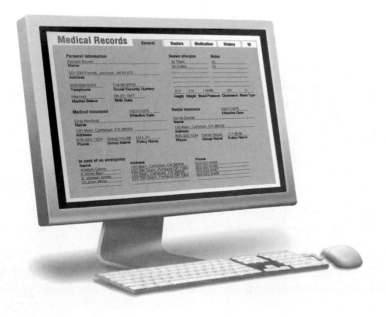

the size of the facility, to convert health records to electronic form. Health care providers who treat Medicare patients must comply by 2015 or face lower fee reimbursements from the federal government.

Technological Threats to Confidentiality

Increasingly, as the federal government mandates and encourages health information technology, modern health care facilities rely on technology for creating, maintaining, and transporting patients' medical information. The implementation of HIPAA imposes penalties for breaches of confidentiality regarding medical records that identify patients by name. The following guidelines can help ensure that confidentiality is not breached when employees use photocopiers, fax machines, computers, and printers to reproduce and send medical records.

Photocopiers

- Do not leave confidential papers anywhere on the copier where others can read the information.
- Do not discard copies in a shared trash container; shred them.
- If a paper jam occurs, be sure to remove from the machine the copy or partial copy that caused the jam.

Fax Machines

- Always verify the telephone number of the receiving location before faxing confidential material.
- Never fax confidential material to an unauthorized person.
- Do not fax confidential material if others in the room can observe the material.
- Do not leave confidential material unattended on a fax machine.
- Do not discard fax copies in a shared trash container; shred them.
- Use a fax cover sheet that states, "Confidential: To addressee only. Please return if received in error."

Computers

- Locate the monitor in an area where others cannot see the screen.
- Do not leave a monitor unattended while confidential material is displayed on the screen.

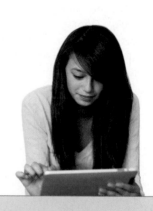

check your **progress**

- Because it is difficult to ensure the privacy of e-mail messages, sending confidential patient information via e-mail is not recommended.
- When computers are sold or otherwise recycled, it's vital that hard drives be erased or removed and destroyed.

Printers

- Do not print confidential material on a printer shared by other departments or in an area where others can read the material.
- Do not leave a printer unattended while printing confidential material.
- Before leaving the printing area, check to be sure all computer disks containing confidential material and all printed material have been collected.
- Be certain that the print job is sent to the right printer location.
- Do not discard printouts in a shared trash container; shred them.

Since medical records are legal documents, and their confidentiality is protected by law, health care practitioners must take every precaution to properly enter information into medical records and to keep that information confidential.

[CHAPTER SUMMARY]

LO 7.1 What purposes do medical records serve?

- They are required by licensing authorities and provide a format for tracking, documenting, and maintaining a patient's communication data, both inside and outside a health care facility.
- They provide documentation of a patient's continuing health care, from birth to death.
- They provide a foundation for managing a patient's health care.
- They serve as legal documents in lawsuits.
- They provide clinical data for education, research, statistical tracking, and assessing the quality of health care.

What information is entered into a patient's medical record?

- Contact and identifying information.
- Insurance information.
- Driver's license information.
- Person responsible for payment and billing.
- Emergency contact information.
- Patient's health history.
- Dates and times of appointments.
- Descriptions of patient's symptoms and reasons for appointments.
- Examinations performed.
- Physician's assessment, diagnosis, recommendations, treatment, progress notes, prescriptions, and instructions to patient.
- X-rays and all test results.

- Notations for telephone calls.
- Notations of copies made.
- Documentation of informed consent.
- Names of guardians or legal representatives if patient unable to give informed consent.
- All other documentation.
- Condition of patient at time of termination of treatment.

What are the five Cs of entries in medical records?

- Concise
- Complete
- Clear
- Correct
- Chronologically ordered

What is the accepted manner for correcting errors in a medical record?

- Draw a line through the error.
- Write correct information above or below original line.
- Note why correction was made.
- Enter the date, time, and initial the correction.
- Ask a coworker to witness and intial the correction when it is made.

LO 7.2 Who owns a person's medical record?

- The owners of the facility where the records were created.

How long should medical records be kept?

- Until the applicable statute of limitations period has elapsed.

LO 7.3 For what purposes is medical information routinely released?

- Insurance claims.
- Transfer of the patient to another physician.
- Use in a court of law.

What information does the patient need to give informed consent?

- Proposed modes of treatment.
- Why the treatment is necessary.
- Risks involved.
- Available alternatives.
- Risks of alternatives.
- Risks involved if treatment is refused.

Who cannot give informed consent?

- Minors.
- Persons who are mentally incompetent.
- Persons who speak limited or no English.

When do Good Samaritan laws protect health care practitioners who stop to help in emergencies?

- When care is given in good faith.
- When caregivers act within the scope of their training and knowledge.
- When caregivers use due care under the circumstances.
- When caregivers do not bill for their services.

LO 7.4 What benefits does the federal government ascribe to the adoption of health information technology, including the conversion to electronic health records?

- Improving health care quality.
- Preventing medical errors.
- Reducing health care costs.
- Increasing administrative efficiency.
- Decreasing paperwork.
- Expanding access to affordable care.

What machines require special care in preventing technological threats to confidentiality?

- Photocopiers
- Fax machines
- Computers
- Printers

ETHICS ISSUES Medical Records and Informed Consent

A basic tenet of medical law and ethics is that patients have the right of self-determination. That right, however, can be effectively exercised only if patients have enough information to make an intelligent, informed choice about medical treatment. Health care practitioners do not have the right to withhold information because full disclosure might prompt the patient to forgo needed therapy.

Dr. Carmen Paradis, a bioethicist with the Cleveland Clinic, says the following to health care practitioners regarding informed consent:

> Make information relevant to how the patient thinks. For example, "3 percent" may mean nothing to a patient, where "3 out of 100" will. You may also want to say, "97 out of 100 will not have this problem."

Benefits must be weighed against risks for the patient. How risky is the treatment under consideration? Is the benefit marginal? In addition, make the information available over time, so the patient is not overwhelmed with information all at once. And in addition to verbal explanations use alternative methods of giving information, such as videos, CDs, written material, and so on.

Medical providers at the Cleveland Clinic are fortunate, in that the clinic has an international center practitioners can call on for translations of medical documents into languages other than English, and for translators who can relate to a patient's native culture and language.

Ethics ISSUE 1: A nurse working in a physician office is helping the physician explain a medical diagnosis and proposed treatment plan to a middle-aged woman who is a recent immigrant from Thailand. The woman speaks no English, and her daughter is attempting to translate the conversation. The woman has metastasized lung cancer, and her prognosis is not good. The nurse notices a pronounced hesitation in the daughter's translation of this news to her mother, and she suspects the daughter has not relayed the information correctly, because the patient seems undisturbed by the news.

Discussion Questions

1. As the nurse helping the physician in this scenario, what would you do?

_____

_____

2. Assume that the nurse and the physician must obtain informed consent from the patient in the scenario. Should they rely solely on the daughter's ability to translate? Explain your answer.

_____

_____

Ethics ISSUE 2: You are an LPN in a reproductive services clinic, and a pregnant patient is suffering a medical condition wherein the pregnancy threatens her life. Her physician suggests that she undergo an abortion.

Discussion Questions

1. Will your personal values allow you to assist with the procedure? Explain your answer.

_____

_____

2. If your answer to question 3 is no, what are your alternatives?

_____

_____

Ethics ISSUE 3: You have observed an LPN with whom you work in a hospital attempting to erase an entry she has made in a patient's medical record. She asks you not to tell that you saw her attempting to erase the entry.

Discussion Question

1. What will you do next?

_____

_____

Ethics ISSUE 4: You have faxed a patient's medical record to another physician office and discover you have used the wrong fax number.

Discussion Question

1. What will you do next?

_____

_____

Go to **www.mhhe.com/judson6e** to practice your case review skills. Then read on for more information.

KEY TERMS

Confidentiality of Alcohol and Drug Abuse, Patient Records

consent

doctrine of informed consent

doctrine of professional discretion

electronic health record (EHR)

fiduciary duty

Good Samaritan acts

health information technology (HIT)

medical record

CHAPTER 7 REVIEW

Applying Knowledge

LO 7.1

Answer the following questions in the spaces provided.

1. Assume you are in charge of recording medical information in a patient's record after the patient has seen his or her physician. What seven items will you be sure to record?

_____

_____

2. What are the five Cs for correctly entering information into a medical record?

_____

_____

Circle the correct answer for each of the following questions.

3. After an entry in the medical record has been written or keyed and an error is discovered, what procedure should be followed to correct the error?
   a. Use a pencil eraser to remove the entry on a written record; then write in the correction.
   b. Use the delete or backspace key if the entry was keyed in; then key in the correction.
   c. Draw a line through the error; then call the patient's physician.
   d. None of the above.

4. Which of the following comments should *not* be included in a patient's medical record?
   a. "Patient complained of pain in her right index finger."
   b. "Blood drawn for CBC."
   c. "Patient requests no more Jell-O."
   d. "Patient is big as a blimp."

LO 7.2

5. Dr. Wellness works as an employee of Anytown Medical Clinic. Who owns the records of his patients?
   a. Dr. Wellness
   b. Anytown Medical Clinic
   c. Each of Dr. Wellness's patients
   d. The state in which Dr. Wellness practices

6. Dr. Wellness also sees patients at Anytown General Hospital, where he maintains records of hospital stays, procedures, and emergency room visits. To whom do these records belong?
   a. Dr. Wellness
   b. Each of Dr. Wellness's patients
   c. Anytown General Hospital
   d. The American Hospital Association

7. Jan B. is a patient of Dr. Wellness, who practices alone. She is moving, and wants to transfer her medical records from Dr. Wellness to her new physician, Dr. Good, who works for the Good Samaritan Clinic. Does Jan have the right to obtain copies of her medical records?
   a. Yes, but she must sign a consent form.
   b. No.
   c. Only with a subpoena.
   d. None of the above.

8. In the situation in question 7, who owns Jan's medical records before she moves?
   a. Jan
   b. Dr. Wellness
   c. The state in which Dr. Wellness is licensed
   d. None of the above

9. Who owns the medical records after Jan moves and begins to see Dr. Good?
   a. Jan
   b. Dr. Wellness
   c. Dr. Good
   d. The Good Samaritan Clinic

10. Which of the following is *not* necessary for Jan's medical records to be transferred to her new physician?
    a. Jan must sign a form, requesting the transfer of her medical records and giving her consent.
    b. Dr. Wellness must be informed that Jan is moving, and that her records will be transferred.
    c. Dr. Wellness's office personnel must follow up after the records have been transferred, to be sure Dr. Good received them.
    d. Jan's attorney must be present when she signs the request to transfer her records.

LO 7.3

11. In a court of law, which one of the following types of testimony will prevail?
    a. A patient's recollection of events
    b. A nurse's oral recollection of events
    c. A physician's testimony
    d. The written documentation in a medical record

12. Medical records are often subpoenaed in court because a patient's medical record is what kind of document?
    a. Confidential document
    b. Professional document
    c. Error-free document
    d. Legal document

13. Which of the following statements is *not* true of statute of limitations laws?
    a. They vary with states.
    b. They determine the period of time during which a lawsuit may be filed.
    c. The most common time periods specified in such laws are two to seven years.
    d. All specify that the time period for filing a medical malpractice lawsuit is two years.

14. Which of the following is *not* true of requests for medical records?
    a. They should not be released to a third party without written permission.
    b. A patient's legal representative can give written consent to release records.
    c. Requests for release of records may ask for specific records.
    d. A patient's complete medical record should always be released on request.

15. The copier malfunctions while you are photocopying a patient's medical records and prints too many copies of several pages. What will you do with the extra copies?
    a. File them with the original copy of the patient's medical records.
    b. Staple them to the photocopies, because you cannot destroy them.
    c. Shred them in a paper shredder.
    d. None of the above.

16. Assume you are in charge of releasing medical records to a third party. Which of the following does *not* require the patient's written consent?
    a. Release of the records to the patient's insurance company
    b. Release of the records for use in a lawsuit, in response to a court's subpoena
    c. Release of the records for research purposes
    d. All of the above require the patient's written consent

17. Which of the following is *not* a threat to the confidentiality of a patient's medical record?
    a. Written records are left open on a coder's desk when she takes her coffee break.
    b. A medical transcriptionist allows a friend from another office to read over his shoulder while he transcribes a physician's dictation.
    c. A medical office employee inadvertently leaves pages from a patient's medical record in the fax machine tray.
    d. A physician shows a patient's medical record to a consulting specialist.

18. Which of the following individuals may not be able to give informed consent for medical treatment?
    a. A married woman who falls in her home
    b. A child injured on a school playground
    c. A pregnant teenager
    d. A person who speaks a foreign language

LO 7.4

19. Health information technology (HIT) includes
    a. Telemedicine
    b. Use of the Internet
    c. Digital versions of patients' medical files
    d. All of the above

20. According to the federal government, which of the following is *not* a benefit of HIT with the wide adoption of technology?
    a. Preventing medical errors
    b. Reducing health care costs
    c. Improving health care quality
    d. Reducing discrimination in health care workplaces

Match each definition with the correct term by writing the letter in the space provided.

_____ 21. Addresses the electronic storage and transmission of health information.

_____ 22. Protects patients from being coerced into treatment.

_____ 23. Protects health care providers from lawsuits when providing care at an accident or emergency.

_____ 24. Provides for a continuum of medical care for patients.

_____ 25. Allows physicians to decide whether or not to show medical records to those patients treated for mental or emotional disorders.

_____ 26. A federal statute that protects the confidentiality of medical records of patients with histories of substance abuse.

a. Good Samaritan act

b. HIPAA

c. Uniform Anatomical Gift Act

d. Doctrine of informed consent

e. Confidentiality of Alcohol and Drug Abuse, Patient Records

f. Doctrine of professional discretion

g. Medical record

CASE STUDIES

Use your critical thinking skills to answer the questions that follow each case study.

LO 7.3

A 10-year-old girl suffered from a rare malignancy in her brain and around her spinal cord. She had surgery, and most of the tumor mass was removed, but residual tumor remained in the brain and around the spinal cord. The girl's doctors informed her parents that chemotherapy and radiation were possible treatment options but could cause serious problems such as sepsis, a permanent loss of IQ and stature, and even death. The parents wished to proceed with the therapy.

While their child was undergoing aggressive chemotherapy and radiation, the parents did independent research and read of several drugs being administered for cancer in other states that were unapproved by the Federal Drug Administration (FDA) and were illegal in their home state but were touted by physicians using them as "miracle cures." The couple sued their child's physician for failure to disclose alternative treatments, thus depriving them of informed consent.

A court awarded summary judgment to the physician.

27. In your opinion, does the court's decision seem warranted? Why or why not?

\
\

28. Did the physician involved follow the law? Did he or she act ethically? Explain your answer.

\
\

29. Under the doctrine of informed consent, should a physician be responsible for informing patients of all treatment options, even if some of the treatments are illegal or not yet proven effective? Explain your answer.

\
\

When Ruth applied for health insurance, she listed a colonoscopy examination as part of her medical history. The insurance company asked for more information. Ruth requested, in writing, that the clinic where she had been examined send only the colonoscopy records to her insurance company. In addition to the requested information on her colonoscopy, the clinic sent all of Ruth's medical records for the past five years, which included the diagnoses of fibrocystic breast disease and obesity. As a result, the insurance company issued Ruth a policy, but attached riders stipulating that it would not pay for any illnesses arising from the fibrocystic breast disease or obesity.

Ruth complained to the clinic administrator, explaining that she had requested that only those records concerning her colonoscopy be forwarded to the insurance company. The administrator apologized and assured Ruth that the clinic's policy concerning release of medical records would be reviewed. He also told Ruth that should she ever incur medical expenses for those conditions excepted in her insurance policy, she should contact him.

30. Did the clinic err in sending all of Ruth's medical records to the insurance company? Why or why not?

_____

_____

31. In your opinion, did Ruth have a legal cause for action against the clinic? Explain.

_____

_____

32. What would you do, in the clinic administrator's place, to rectify the situation and make sure that similar problems did not arise in the future?

_____

_____

A patient asked her dermatologist for the name of an internist. She visited the recommended internist several times and then learned that, without informing her, he had sent the dermatologist two detailed reports on her condition and family medical history. Since her gastrointestinal condition had nothing to do with her dermatological complaint, she believed the internist had sent the records to show his appreciation for the referral. She told the internist that she felt her privacy had been violated.

33. Do you agree with the patient? Why or why not?

_____

_____

INTERNET ACTIVITIES LO 7.2 and LO 7.4

Complete the activities and answer the questions that follow.

34. Determine how long medical records must be kept in your state. Begin your search with the question: "How long are medical records kept in [*fill in your state*]"?

_____

_____

35. Search online for "health information technology occupations." What occupations are listed under HIT? List three advantages to pursuing an education in HIT. If your primary interest is in patient care, would a career in HIT interest you? Explain your answer.

_____

_____

35. Visit the Web site for the American Medical Informatics Association (AMIA) at **www.amia.org/inside/code/.** Locate the association's Code of Ethics and briefly describe the AMIA's stance on maintaining confidentiality of electronic records.

_____

_____

[RESOURCES]

California's Good Samaritan Law:

www.portersimon.com/writ/writ-02-2011.pdf.

Telephone interview November 5, 2007, with Dr. Carmen Paradis, Dept. of Bioethics, Cleveland Clinic.

Content of medical records:

www.sh.lsuhsc.edu/policies/policy_manuals_via_ms_word/ hospital_policy/h_6.5.0.pdf.

Informed consent:

www.ama-assn.org/ama/pub/physician-resources/legal-topics/ patient-physician-relationship-topics/informed-consent.shtml.

Sebelius quote:

Pear, Robert. "Standards Issued for Electronic Health Records." _The New York Times,_ July 13, 2010, **www.nytimes.com/2010/07/14/health/ policy/14health.html.**

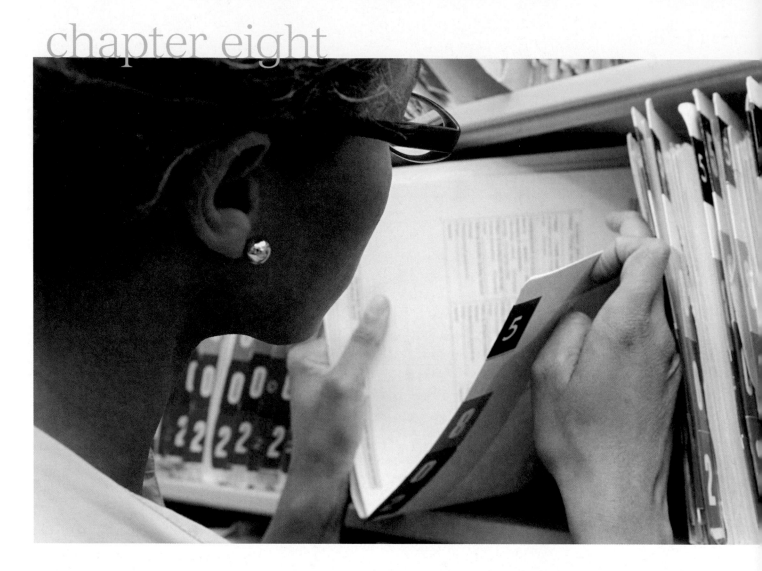

PRIVACY LAW AND HIPAA

Learning Outcomes

After studying this chapter, you should be able to:

LO 8.1 Discuss U.S. constitutional amendments and privacy laws that pertain to health care.

LO 8.2. Explain how the language provisions and standards of the Health Insurance Portability and Accountability Act (HIPAA) mandates apply to your profession.

LO 8.3 Discuss the special requirements for disclosing protected health information.

LO 8.4 Discuss the patient rights defined by HIPAA.

LO 8.5 Recognize and dispel some of the more prevalent myths concerning HIPAA.

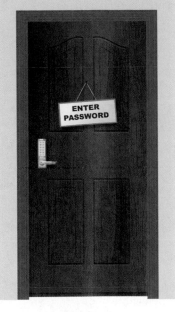

from the perspective of . . .

ANN HAS BEEN A NURSE IN A TEXAS HOSPITAL FOR 20 YEARS. "When I started," she says, "we posted the names of patients on the doors to their rooms." Now, as the result of laws passed to protect the privacy of patients and the confidentiality of medical records, Ann and her coworkers must not even admit to unauthorized callers or visitors that a person is a patient in the hospital.

"When patients authorize a certain family member or friend to visit them in the hospital, we ask them to come up with a password that only the two of them know," Ann explains. "Then when that person calls to ask how the patient is doing, or shows up on the floor to visit, we ask them for the password. If they have the correct password, we can talk to them on the telephone or admit them to the patient's room."

"Sometimes patients' family members call from distant states," Ann continues, "and if they don't have a password, we can't tell them a thing—not even that their loved one is a patient. We catch lots of flak from callers because of this, but it's the law, and we have to follow it."

Ann admits that once in a while, if she knows a caller has been in to visit a patient, she will say, "your dad/mom is resting comfortably." "But I know I'm walking a fine line when I do that, and I don't do it often."

"We have to be so careful about releasing any information," Ann adds, "that when my father's dear friend was admitted to my floor in the hospital where I work, I couldn't tell him that his friend had been admitted."

Ann emphasizes, however, that for certain patients, confidentiality laws are shields that they appreciate. "For example, the patient who has tried to commit suicide and failed, who doesn't want anyone to know he is in the hospital. Or the battered spouse, who doesn't want her abusive husband to find her."

From Ann's perspective, because she genuinely cares about her patients, she would like to be permitted to talk more freely with family members or friends who also care about her patients. But she is duty bound to follow the law, and she knows the benefits to patients for laws that guard their health information.

From the perspective of friends and family members who call for information about a patient, the law is harsh and hard to understand. They are often angry, and ask why they are not allowed to learn the status of a friend or loved one.

From the perspective of some patients, the law sometimes feels overprotective and unnecessarily intrusive, but for others it's a safety net they can depend on.

In your opinion, why have laws protecting patients' privacy become necessary?

If in a position to change health care confidentiality law, what changes, if any, would you make and why?

Privacy and the United States Constitution

LO 8.1

Discuss U.S. constitutional amendments and privacy laws that pertain to health care.

Contrary to popular belief, the term **privacy** (freedom from unauthorized intrusion) does not appear in the U.S. Constitution or the Bill of Rights. However, the U.S. Supreme Court, the court responsible for determining constitutional issues, has ruled in favor of privacy interests (and occasionally against them), deriving the right to privacy from the First, Third, Fourth, Fifth, Ninth, and Fourteenth Amendments to the Constitution. The U.S. Supreme Court first declared that a constitutional right to privacy was implied in the following case, *Griswold v. Connecticut*.

LANDMARK COURT CASE

The Constitution Protects the Right to Privacy

In November 1961, the executive director and the medical director of a Planned Parenthood clinic in Connecticut were charged with violating a state statute prohibiting the dispensing of contraceptive devices to a married couple. The defendants were convicted and fined $100 each. The U.S. Supreme Court heard the case in March 1965 and issued a written opinion on June 7, 1965. William O. Douglas, writing the majority opinion for the Court, held that the Connecticut statute was an unconstitutional violation of the right of privacy. Douglas noted that many rights are not expressly mentioned in the Constitution, but the Court has nevertheless found that persons possess such a right. In reviewing the many rights that Americans possess, Douglas noted the existence of "penumbras" or "zone(s) of privacy created by several fundamental constitutional guarantees."

As a result of the Supreme Court's decision in *Griswold v. Connecticut*, patients possess certain rights that affect the delivery of medical services and health care. For example, persons have the right to refuse medical treatment, and courts now recognize a person's right to die.

Source: Griswold v. Connecticut, 381 US 479, 85 S. Ct. 1978, 14 L. Ed.2d 510 (1965).

In your opinion, why is the case a "landmark" case?

The following amendments to the U.S. Constitution have particular implications in science, medicine, and the delivery of health care:

First Amendment: "Congress shall make no law respecting an establishment of religion, or prohibiting the free exercise thereof; or abridging the freedom of speech, or of the press; or the right of the people peaceably to assemble, and to petition the Government for a redress of grievances."

The First Amendment guarantees that information relevant to science and medicine can freely flow throughout the international marketplace of ideas. Furthermore, as a result of the Establishment and Freedom of Religion clauses, the government *cannot* fund or show preference for any religion (or discriminate against any religion), and religious tests are prohibited for anyone seeking a public office. Similarly, persons testifying in court or serving on juries cannot be required to take a religious oath or swear to a belief in any god.

Third Amendment: "No Soldier shall, in time of peace be quartered in any house, without the consent of the Owner, nor in time of war, but in a manner to be prescribed by law." This amendment has certain implications for privacy, but the U.S. Supreme Court has never had to decide a Third Amendment case.

Fourth Amendment: "The right of the people to be secure in their persons, houses, papers, and effects, against unreasonable searches and seizures, shall not be violated, and no Warrants shall issue, but on probable cause, supported by Oath or affirmation, and particularly describing the place to be searched, and the persons or things to be seized."

The Fourth Amendment protects persons from unreasonable searches. As a result, patient records are private, and the government must in most cases have a search warrant to obtain such records. Rules of evidence also govern the use of information obtained as a result of the doctor–patient relationship. Because of state licensing laws for medical offices, however, such offices are subject to administrative oversight by licensing agencies.

COURT CASE

Fourth Amendment Rights in Question

The Student Activities Drug Testing Policy adopted by the Tecumseh, Oklahoma, School District requires all middle and high school students to consent to urinalysis testing for drugs to participate in any extracurricular activity. Two Tecumseh High School students and their parents brought suit, alleging that the policy violates the Fourth Amendment, which states in part: "The right of the people to be secure in their persons, houses, papers, and effects, against unreasonable searches and seizures, shall not be violated." The district court granted the school district summary judgment. In reversing, the court of appeals held that the policy violated the Fourth Amendment. The appellate court concluded that before imposing a suspicionless drug-testing program a school must demonstrate some identifiable drug abuse problem among a sufficient number of those tested, such that testing that group will actually redress its drug problem, which the school district had failed to demonstrate.

The question before the court was: Is the Student Activities Drug Testing Policy, which requires all students who participate in competitive extracurricular activities to submit to drug testing, consistent with the Fourth Amendment?

The U.S. Supreme Court concluded that the answer to the question was yes. In a 5–4 opinion delivered by Justice Clarence Thomas, the Court held that, because the policy reasonably serves the school district's important interest in detecting and preventing drug use among its students, it is constitutional. The Court reasoned that the board of education's general regulation of extracurricular activities diminished the expectation of privacy among students and that the board's method of obtaining urine samples and maintaining test results was minimally intrusive on the students' limited privacy interest. "Within the limits of the Fourth Amendment, local school boards must assess the desirability of drug testing schoolchildren. In upholding the constitutionality of the Policy, we express no opinion as to its wisdom. Rather, we hold only that Tecumseh's Policy is a reasonable means of furthering the School District's important interest in preventing and deterring drug use among its schoolchildren," wrote Justice Thomas.

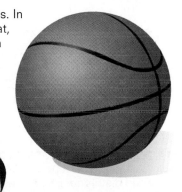

Source: Board of Education v. Earls, 536 U.S. 822 (2002).

In your opinion, what extenuating circumstances caused the Supreme Court justices to rule in favor of the school district?

Fifth Amendment: "No person shall be held to answer for a capital, or otherwise infamous crime, unless on a presentment or indictment of a Grand Jury, except in cases arising in the land or naval forces, or in the Militia, when in actual service in time of War or public danger;

nor shall any person be subject for the same offence to be twice put in jeopardy of life or limb; nor shall be compelled in any criminal case to be a witness against himself, nor be deprived of life, liberty, or property, without due process of law; nor shall private property be taken for public use, without just compensation."

The Miranda warning ("You have the right to remain silent. . . ."), so often heard recited on television crime shows, was derived from this amendment. The Fifth Amendment applies solely to criminal arrests and prosecutions. Since medical malpractice cases are argued in civil court, however, health care practitioners may be required to answer questions or submit documents to attorneys during the course of such a case.

Ninth Amendment: "The enumeration in the Constitution, of certain rights, shall not be construed to deny or disparage others retained by the people." That is, if a certain right is not explicitly mentioned in the Constitution that does not mean it doesn't exist. This amendment has not been used to uphold a specific right. Some constitutional scholars believe, however, that rights such as the right to health care or housing are implicit in the Ninth Amendment.

Fourteenth Amendment, Section 1: "All persons born or naturalized in the United States, and subject to the jurisdiction thereof, are citizens of the United States and of the State wherein they reside. No State shall make or enforce any law which shall abridge the privileges or immunities of citizens of the United States; nor shall any State deprive any person of life, liberty, or property, without due process of law; nor deny to any person within its jurisdiction the equal protection of the laws."

All states must provide rights for citizens that are at least equal to those in the U.S. Constitution, and under the philosophy called federalism states may grant citizens additional rights not specifically granted in the U.S. Constitution.

COURT CASE

Fourteenth Amendment at Issue

William Baird spoke at Boston University on the subject of birth control and overpopulation. At the end of his talk, Baird gave away Emko Vaginal Foam to a woman who approached him. Massachusetts charged Baird with a felony, distributing contraceptives to unmarried men or women. Under state law, only married couples could obtain contraceptives; only registered doctors or pharmacists could provide them. Baird was not an authorized distributor of contraceptives.

At issue was: Did the Massachusetts law violate the right to privacy acknowledged in *Griswold v. Connecticut,* and did it violate protection from state intrusion granted by the Fourteenth Amendment?

The case reached the U.S. Supreme Court, where justices struck down the Massachusetts law, but not on privacy grounds. The Court held that the law's distinction between single and married individuals failed to satisfy the "rational basis test" of the Fourteenth Amendment's Equal Protection clause. Married couples were entitled to contraception under the Court's *Griswold* decision. Withholding that right to single individuals without a rational basis proved the fatal flaw. Thus, the Court did not have to rely on *Griswold* to invalidate the Massachusetts statute. "If the right of privacy means anything," wrote Justice William J. Brennan, Jr., for the majority, "it is the right of the individual, married or single, to be free from unwarranted governmental intrusion into matters so fundamentally affecting a person as the decision to whether to bear or beget a child."

Source: Eisenstadt v. Baird, 405 U.S. 438 (1972).

Federal Privacy Laws

Concern about privacy has led to the enactment of federal and state laws governing the collection, storage, transmission, and disclosure of personal data. Privacy laws are generally based on the following considerations:

1. Information collected and stored about individuals should be limited to what is necessary to carry out the functions of the business or government agency collecting the information.

2. Once it is collected, access to personal information should be limited to those employees who must use the information in performing their jobs.

3. Personal information cannot be released outside the organization collecting it unless authorization is obtained from the subject.

4. When information is collected about a person, that person should know that the information is being collected and should have the opportunity to check the information for accuracy.

Table 8-1 is a summary of the major U.S. government laws concerning privacy.

As you can see from Table 8-1, most federal privacy laws have dealt with financial and credit information or the theft or illegal disclosure of electronic information. All states have laws governing the confidentiality of medical records, but laws vary greatly from state to state. HIPAA of 1996 was the first *federal* legislation to deal thoroughly and explicitly with the privacy of medical records. To ensure compliance, HIPAA provides for civil and criminal sanctions for violators of the law.

The American Recovery and Reinvestment Act (ARRA), passed in 2009, contained many key changes to HIPAA, as part of Title XIII, called the Health Information Technology for Economic and Clinical Health (HITECH) Act. The ARRA changes were grouped into four broad categories:

- Changes to HIPAA privacy and security regulations.
- Changes in HIPAA enforcement.
- Changes that address health information held by either covered entities or business associates not expressly covered by HIPAA.
- Changes relevant to HIPAA administration, and studies, reports, and educational initiatives related to health care.

These changes are detailed in the following sections.

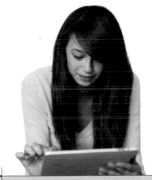

check your **progress**

1. Does the Constitution provide specifically for the protection of privacy? Explain your answer.

2. Name four common considerations for protecting privacy when federal and/or state legislation is written.

3. What was the first federal law to deal thoroughly and explicitly with the privacy of medical records?

4. Which constitutional amendment is most important in protecting Americans' privacy rights?

5. Which HIPAA standards were most affected by the changes legislated in ARRA?

6. Name one way in which your job as a health care practitioner is impacted by HIPAA privacy regulations. (For example, Ann, the hospital nurse in the chapter's opening scenario, is impacted by many HIPAA requirements, but especially by the prohibition against releasing patient information to unauthorized telephone callers or hospital visitors.)

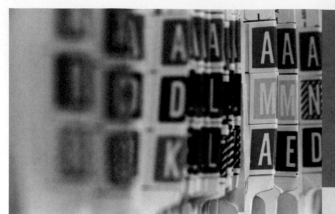

MAJOR FEDERAL PRIVACY LAWS

Table 8-1

Date Enacted	Law	Purpose
1970	Fair Credit Reporting Act	Prohibits credit reporting agencies from releasing credit information to unauthorized people, and allows consumers to review their own credit records
1974	Family and Privacy Act Educational Rights	Gives students and parents access to school records and limits disclosure of records to unauthorized parties
1974	Privacy Act	Forbids federal agencies from allowing information to be used for a reason other than that for which it was collected
1978	Right to Financial Privacy Act	Strictly outlines procedures federal agencies must follow when looking at customer records in banks
1984	Computer Fraud and Abuse Act	Forbids unauthorized access of federal government computers
1984	Cable Communications Policy Act	Regulates disclosure of cable television subscriber records
1986	Electronic Communications Privacy Act (ECPA)	Provides privacy protection for new forms of electronic communications, such as voice mail, e-mail, and cellular telephone
1988	Video Privacy Protection Act	Forbids retailers from releasing or selling video rental records without customer consent or a court order
1991	Telephone Consumer Protection Act	Restricts activities of telemarketers
1992	Cable Act	Extends the privacy provisions of the Cable Communications Policy Act of 1984 to include cellular and other wireless services
1994	Computer Abuse Amendments Act	Amends the 1984 act to forbid transmission of harmful computer code such as viruses
1996	National Information Infrastructure Protection Act	Penalizes theft of information across state lines, threats against networks, and computer system trespassing
1996	Health Insurance Portability and Accountability Act (HIPAA)	Guarantees that workers who change jobs can obtain health insurance. Increases efficiency and effectiveness of the U.S. health care system by electronic exchange of administrative and financial data. Improves security and privacy of patient-identifying information. Decreases U.S. health care system transaction costs

Date Enacted	Law	Purpose
1997	No Electronic Theft (NET) Act	Closed a loophole in the law that let people give away copyrighted material (such as software) on the Internet without legal repercussions
1998	Digital Millennium Copyright Act (DMCA)	Makes it illegal to bypass antipiracy measures in commercial software, and outlaws the sale of devices that copy software illegally
1999	Gramm-Leach-Bliley Act	Requires all financial institutions and insurance companies to clearly disclose their privacy policies regarding the sharing of nonpublic personal information with affiliates and third parties
2001	Provide Appropriate Tools Required to Intercept and Obstruct Terrorism (PATRIOT) Act	Gives law enforcement broad leeway in monitoring people's activities, including Internet use, e-mail, and library habits
First enacted in early 1970s, revised in 2002	Code of Federal Regulations (CFR), 42 (Public Health), Part 2	Provides for the confidentiality of medical records of patients treated for drug and alcohol dependency
2003	Do Not Call Implementation Act	Allows individuals to opt out of receiving calls from telemarketers by placing phone numbers on a national registry
2009	American Recovery and Reinvestment Act (ARRA), commonly called the Stimulus Bill	Title XIII, the Health Information Technology for Economic and Clinical Health (HITECH) Act, makes substantive changes to HIPAA, including privacy and security regulations, changes in HIPAA enforcement, provisions about health information held by entities not covered by HIPAA, and other miscellaneous changes
2010	Patient Protection and Affordable Care Act (PPACA)	Deals mostly with the availability of health insurance coverage for all Americans, but also reinforces privacy regarding protected health information
2010	Health Care and Education Reconciliation Act (HCERA)	A federal law that adds to regulations imposed on the insurance industry by PPACA

Health Insurance Portability and Accountability Act (HIPAA) History, Language, and Standards

HIPAA History

Circumstances that led to the 1996 passage of federal **Health Insurance Portability and Accountability Act (HIPAA)** legislation include the following:

- Health care has become a complicated business. Health care employees are faced with a quagmire of complex billing codes, a multitude of software programs in use for storing medical records and for processing billing and payment, and more time spent on administrative chores (and less on patient issues).

- Managed care adds yet another level to the many administrative duties necessary to administer patient care; personnel include case reviewers,

LO 8.2

Explain how the language provisions and standards of the Health Insurance Portability and Accountability Act (HIPAA) mandates apply to your profession.

claims and coding experts, billing personnel, committees to review every facet of service, employees trained to handle patient complaints, and so on. Before HIPAA was passed, nurses had assumed many of the duties associated with health care services reporting and administration, and both physicians and nurses had less time to spend on patient care.

- Patients gather information from television ads and the Internet, often expecting their physicians to prescribe medications and treatments not appropriate for their medical problems. A side effect has been that medical malpractice and risk management issues threaten to put some physicians and health care facilities out of business, due to the high cost of medical malpractice insurance and the rising costs of staying in the health care business.

- Health care consumers were and are increasingly dismayed over the rising cost of medical care and health insurance, to the point that millions of Americans do not seek necessary medical care for treatment their insurance plans will not cover, are underinsured, or do not have health insurance.

In the mid-1990s when groups of health care professionals, consumers, and others confronted members of the U.S. Congress about solving these serious health care problems, Congress responded with passage of the Health Insurance Portability and Accountability Act of 1996, to be administered by the *U.S. Department of Health and Human Services (HHS).* HHS has assigned enforcement activities for the Privacy and Security Rules to the *U.S. Office for Civil Rights (OCR).* A second agency within HHS, the *Centers for Medicare and Medicaid Services (CMS),* has enforcement authority for other HIPAA Administrative Simplification Standards, including transactions, code sets, and identifiers.

HIPAA Language

Covered Entities In HIPAA language, health plans, health care clearing-houses, and all health care providers that transmit HIPAA standard transactions electronically are called **covered entities.** Covered entities include:

- Hospitals, including academic medical centers.
- Nursing homes.
- Hospices.
- Pharmacies.
- Physician practices.
- Dental practices.
- Chiropractors.
- Podiatrists.
- Osteopaths.
- Physical therapists.
- Alternative medicine practitioners (acupuncturists, massage therapists).
- Laboratories.
- Health plans (payers).
- Health care clearinghouses.

Covered entities are people, businesses, or agencies that must comply with the HIPAA Standards and Privacy Rule. If a health care practice exchanges even one of the standard transactions via electronic means with any payer, that practice is a covered entity, no matter how small the practice.

For more complete information for determining covered entities, visit the home page for the Centers for Medicare and Medicaid Services at **www.cms.hhs.gov/**.

Covered Transactions Electronic exchanges of information between two covered-entity business partners using HIPAA-mandated transaction standards (explained below) are called **covered transactions.** HIPAA standard transactions include, but are not limited to, the following:

- A physician submitting an electronic claim to a health plan.

- A physician sending a referral or authorization electronically to another physician, lab, or hospital.

- A physician sending patient-identifying information to a billing service or to another physician.

- Any health care provider that employs another entity, such as a clearinghouse or billing agency, to send claims to payers or health plans.

Note that a patient sending an e-mail message to a physician that contains patient-identifying information would not be a HIPAA standards-covered transaction because patients are not covered entities.

Any physician, health care practitioner, or health care facility, regardless of size, that files even one electronic claim is a covered entity and must use HIPAA electronic transaction and code set standards.

Other Important HIPAA Terms A **designated record set** includes records maintained by or for a covered entity, including medical and billing records about individuals; a health plan's enrollment, payment, claims adjudication, case or medical management record systems; and records used by or for the covered entity to make decisions about an individual.

Notice of Privacy Practices (NPP) is a written document detailing a health care provider's privacy practices. Under HIPAA's Privacy Rule, every patient visiting his or her health care provider after April 14, 2003, must have received an NPP. The patient is asked to sign the form, and it is filed with the patient's medical records.

Protected health information (PHI) refers to information that contains one or more patient identifiers and can, therefore, be used to identify an individual. The Privacy Rule says that PHI must be protected whether it is written, spoken, or in electronic form. It is possible to **"de-identify"** health information, by removing the patient identifiers from it. Once patient identifiers are removed, the information is not considered PHI. Information that includes one or more of the following makes a patient's medical record identifiable (see Figure 8-1):

- Name.
- Zip code.
- Date of birth.
- Dates of treatment.
- Telephone numbers.
- Fax numbers.
- E-mail addresses.
- Social Security number.
- Medical record numbers.

covered transactions
Electronic exchanges of information between two covered-entity business partners using HIPAA-mandated transaction standards.

designated record set
Records maintained by or for a HIPAA-covered entity.

Notice of Privacy Practices (NPP) A written document detailing a health care provider's privacy practices.

protected health information (PHI) Information that contains one or more patient identifiers.

de-identify To remove from health care transactions all information that identifies patients.

Figure 8-1 Sample of a Medical Record

Medical Records

| General | Doctors | Medication | History | ID |

Personal Information

Ronald Brown
Name

521 SW Frewel, Jackson, WI 81475
Address

658-898-5484   744-60-8743
Telephone   Social Security Number

Married   06-22-1947
Marital Status   Birth Date

Known allergies
a) Trees
b) Grass

Notes
a)
b)

6'2"	212	118/98	120	O
Height	Weight	Blood Pressure	Cholesterol	Blood Type

Medical Insurance

03/31/1976
Effective Date

Etna Medical
Name

120 Main, Carlsbad, CA 98008
Address

876-322-1234   Group H4J66   HJ-L-31
Phone   Group Name   Policy Name

Dental Insurance

03/31/1976
Effective Date

Denta Dental
Name

120 Main, Carlsbad, CA 98008
Address

800-322-1234   Denta Group   111-654b
Phone   Group Name   Policy Name

In case of an emergency

Name	Address	Phone
Adalph Gayor	120 Main, Carlsbad, CA 98008	503-522-6484
K.Write Ben	533 SW Grant, Portland OR 7564	503-522-6485
S. William Smith	120 Main, Carlsbad, CA 98008	503-522-6487
Dr.John Write	533 SW Grant, Portland OR 7564	503-522-6489

---

state preemption If a state's privacy laws are stricter than HIPAA privacy standards, the state laws take precedence.

treatment, payment, and health care operations (TPO) A HIPAA term for qualified providers, disclosure of PHI to obtain reimbursement, and activities and transactions among entities. *Treatment* means that a health care provider can provide care; *payment* means that a provider can disclose PHI to be reimbursed; *health care operations* refers to HIPAA-approved activities and transactions.

- Health plan beneficiary numbers.
- Birth certificate and driver's license.
- Vehicle identification number and license plate number.
- Web site address.
- Fingerprints and voiceprints.
- Photos.

State preemption means that if a state's privacy laws are stricter than HIPAA privacy standards and/or guarantee more patients' rights, the state laws will take precedence.

Treatment, payment, and health care operations (TPO) is another important term. Within HIPAA, *treatment* means that a health care provider can provide care. *Payment* means that a provider can disclose PHI to obtain reimbursement for health care. *Health care operations* refers to a number of activities and transactions within and among entities, including conducting quality assessments, reviewing the competence or qualifications of health care practitioners, and managing the business.

Business associates conduct certain activities on behalf of covered entities. Contracts must specify that the business associate will safeguard protected health information according to HIPAA requirements.

Business associates of covered entities include, but are not limited to, services engaged in

Accounting

Accreditation

Benefit management

Billing

Claims processing

Consulting

Data aggregation

Data analysis

Dictation and transcription

Legal consultation

Practice management

Processing or administration

Quality assurance

Repricing

Utilization review

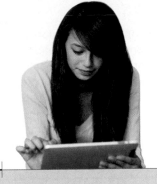

check your **progress**

7. Distinguish between *covered entities* and *covered transactions.*

8. Give two examples of covered entities.

9. Give two examples of covered transactions.

10. What is protected health information?

11. Define *state preemption.*

HIPAA Standards

HIPAA contains four sets of standards, with rules that health care facilities must have implemented within certain time frames. Under HIPAA, a **standard** is a general requirement; a **rule** is a document that includes the standards.

Standard 1. Transactions and Code Sets A **transaction** refers to the transmission of information between two parties to carry out financial or administrative activities. A **code set** is "any set of codes used to encode data elements, such as tables of terms, medical concepts, medical diagnostic codes, or medical procedure codes. A code set includes the codes and the descriptors of the codes." HIPAA provisions say that codes must now be uniform throughout the country, to make filling out insurance claim forms and billing for services much easier than before.

Before HIPAA, medical facilities filing and collecting on claims used different formats; this often held up payment while codes were explained and further information was submitted. (By the mid-1990s, there were over 400 different software formats for coding and billing in medical facilities.) HIPAA now mandates that all health care providers must ensure that they can send and receive information using standard data formats and data content. Health care providers, not software vendors, are responsible for compliance.

Code Sets Under HIPAA, all local code sets are eliminated. Code sets now fall into four categories:

1. Coding systems for diseases, impairments, or other health problems.

2. Causes of injuries, diseases, impairments, or other health problems.

3. Actions taken to prevent, diagnose, treat, or manage diseases, injuries, and impairments.

4. Substances, equipment, supplies, or other items used to perform these actions.

standard A general requirement under HIPAA.

rule A document that includes the HIPAA standards or requirements.

transaction Transmission of information between two parties for financial or administrative activities.

code set Under HIPAA, terms that provide for uniformity and simplification of health care billing and record keeping.

Health care practitioners required to use HIPAA code sets will need to consult HIPAA compliance officers in their facilities or areas for reference to HIPAA publications on coding.

Transaction Requirements Complying with HIPAA Transaction Standards means that covered entities must use the HIPAA-defined standards when using *electronic data interchange* (EDI) for electronic transmissions. **Electronic transmission** refers to the sending of information from one network-connected computer to another. **Electronic data interchange (EDI)** is the use of uniform electronic network protocols (formats) to transfer business information between organizations. Banking, financial, and retail businesses first began using electronic data interchange to transmit information in the mid-1960s, and it has been the transmission method of choice for businesses since the mid-1990s.

Under HIPAA, if a health care provider conducts one of the following general types of covered transactions electronically, that provider must use the HIPAA standards:

1. Claims or encounter information.
2. Eligibility requests.
3. Referrals and authorizations.
4. Claim status inquiries.

Health plans and clearinghouses must be able to receive the previously listed transactions and must also be able to conduct four additional transactions electronically:

1. Premium payment.
2. Claim payment and remittance advice.
3. Enrollment and disenrollment.
4. Coordination of benefits.

Since converting electronic transmissions to HIPAA standards is highly technical, health care practitioners and facilities need to rely on information technology (IT) staff or outside IT experts to be sure they are in compliance.

Standard 2. Privacy Rule As the electronic age progresses, individuals have become increasingly concerned about the privacy of their medical records. However, patient fears are not the underlying reason for the HIPAA Privacy Rule. Because Congress recognized that electronic transmission of health information is the rule in today's computerized society, legislators paid particular attention to ensuring that confidentiality of medical records would not be violated through electronic transmission or storage.

In the court case, "U.S. Attorney General Denied Medical Records," the U.S. attorney general claimed priorities under HIPAA for the health information requested, but the government did not prevail.

Health care providers and plans can use and disclose patient information (PHI), HIPAA legislators said, but they must identify a **permission**—a reason for each use and disclosure.

To *use* PHI means that you use patients' protected health information within the facility where you work in the normal course of conducting health care business. To *disclose* PHI means that patients' protected health information is sent outside of the office for legitimate business or health care reasons.

Permissions Using and disclosing PHI must fall within the following 11 HIPAA-defined permissions:

1. Required disclosures

    HIPAA *requires* just two types of PHI disclosures. The first is that you disclose PHI to representatives from HHS that want to see your books, records, accounts, and other documents. You must permit HHS

---

electronic transmission
The sending of information from one network-connected computer to another.

electronic data interchange (EDI) The use of uniform electronic network protocols to transfer business information between organizations via computer networks.

permission A reason under HIPAA for disclosing patient information.

In 2000, the U.S. Supreme Court found the Nebraska version of a partial-birth abortion ban unconstitutional, on grounds that this type of abortion may, in certain circumstances, be the safest means by which a medically necessary abortion can be performed, and the Nebraska law lacked such a safety clause. (The law defines partial-birth abortion as a method of abortion in which a second- or third-trimester fetus partially exits the womb and is then destroyed.)

When the U.S. Supreme Court has ruled, the matter is usually settled, but in response to the Court's Nebraska decision, Congress passed the federal Partial Birth Abortion Ban Act in 2003. Congress claimed it had made new factual findings that "partial-birth abortion is never necessary to preserve the health of a woman."

Immediately after President George W. Bush signed the act, a group of abortion providers challenged it in court. A federal district judge in New York City granted the group an injunction to stop enforcement of the law. In March 2004, however, the matter was ordered to trial to see if the Supreme Court's view of the facts still prevailed.

To defend the federal partial-birth abortion ban in court, U.S. Attorney General John Ashcroft sought the medical records of 45 patients at a Chicago hospital. He needed the records to dispute expert testimony for the plaintiffs' case, and he claimed that because he sought the records without patient-identifying information, he was not violating privacy laws.

However, on March 26, 2004, the U.S. District Court for the Northern District of Illinois disagreed. The court held that the Justice Department is not entitled to request patients' medical records, even with names and other identifying information removed.

In his opinion for the court, Judge Richard Posner explained that anonymity and privacy are not identical. Therefore, while the Justice Department would view the women's records without identifying information, the court still deemed their production a privacy violation.

Ashcroft's petition to obtain medical records was denied. In 2007, the Supreme Court issued a decision upholding the nationwide ban on partial-birth abortion enacted by Congress in 2003.

Source: Northwestern Memorial Hospital v. Ashcroft (Appeal from the United States District Court, for the Northern District of Illinois, Eastern Division, No. 04 C 55, Argued March 23, 2004, Decided March 26, 2004).

---

representatives to see the documents they request, but you should ask HHS representatives to show identification, and you should record the reason for the requested disclosure to HHS. The second type of PHI disclosure that HIPAA *requires* is to individual patients on request. (See number 2, "Disclosures to patients.")

Written authorization to disclose PHI to HHS representatives is not required.

2. Disclosures to patients

The second disclosure HIPAA *requires* is that PHI be disclosed to any patient who asks to see his or her own medical records (Figure 8-2) (unless the health care provider believes that access will do harm to the patient). This includes talking to the patient about his or her diagnosis, treatment, and medical condition, as well as allowing the patient to review his or her entire medical record. Some records, however, such as psychotherapy notes, may be withheld.

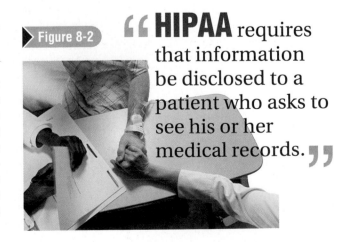

> Figure 8-2

"**HIPAA** requires that information be disclosed to a patient who asks to see his or her medical records."

3. Use or disclosure for treatment, payment, or health care operations (TPO)

Health care practitioners need to use PHI within the medical office, hospital, or other health care facility for coordinating care, consulting with another practitioner about the patient's condition, prescribing medications, ordering lab tests, scheduling surgery, or for other reasons necessary to conduct health care treatment or business, such as insurance claims and billing.

PHI disclosures for these purposes do not require written authorization.

4. Others' treatment, payment, operations

If other covered entities contact you or your employer for access to PHI, such as insurance plans, attorneys, medical survey representatives, and pharmaceutical companies, you must have the patient's written authorization to release PHI.

5. Personal representatives (friends, family)

Use professional judgment to determine if a family member, friend, or personal representative is participating in the care of a patient. For example, you saw the patient invite another person into the exam room, or you heard the patient ask that individual to pick up his or her prescription. You may share information with these individuals, in proportion to their involvement in the care of the patient. You should verify with the patient, if possible, before sharing information. If the patient objects, honor his or her wishes.

If a person claims to have the legal right to make medical decisions for a patient, including the right to review medical records, ask to see the legal document, and verify the representative's identity. A signature authorizing disclosure is recommended. If the patient is able, you can also verify with the patient.

6. Disaster relief organizations

Unless the patient objects, health care providers may disclose PHI to persons performing disaster relief notification activities. If the situation involves TPO, no authorization is needed.

7. Incidental disclosures

Guidelines for clarifying when incidental disclosures of PHI are permitted without authorization from patients include

- Nursing care center staff members can speak about patients' care if they take reasonable precautions to prevent unauthorized individuals, such as visitors in the area, from overhearing.

- Nurses and other health care practitioners can talk to patients on the phone or discuss patients' medical treatment with other providers on the phone if they are reasonably sure that others cannot overhear.

- Health care practitioners can discuss lab results with patients and other health care practitioners in a joint treatment area if they take reasonable precautions to ensure that others cannot overhear.

- Health care practitioners can leave messages on answering machines or with family members, but information should be limited to the amount necessary for the purpose of the call. (For detailed messages, it may be prudent to simply ask the patient to return a call.)

- You can ask patients to sign in, call patients by name in waiting rooms, or use a public address system to ask patients to come to a certain area. A patient sign-in sheet, however, must not ask for the reason for the visit.

- You can use an X-ray light board at a nursing station if it is not visible to unauthorized individuals in the area.

- You can place patient charts outside exam rooms if you use reasonable precautions to protect patient identity: face the chart toward the wall or place the chart inside a cover while it is in place.

8. Public purpose

Health care practitioners and facilities may be asked to disclose PHI "for the public good." If a state law does not prohibit releasing specific PHI, HIPAA allows this type of disclosure without patient authorization. Such disclosures include

- When disclosure is required by law. You should limit the PHI disclosed to the requirements of the law. Verify identification of representatives asking for PHI.

- Public health authority. Public health representatives are authorized by law to collect information to prevent or control disease, injury, birth, death, and for other public health investigations.

- Child abuse or neglect. You may release this information to public health authorities that are authorized to receive reports of child abuse or neglect.

- Victims of abuse, neglect, or domestic violence. If a health care practitioner has reason to believe a patient is a victim of abuse, neglect, or domestic violence, he or she may disclose PHI if

  - The disclosure is required by law.
  - The individual agrees to disclosure.
  - The disclosure is necessary to prevent serious harm, or the individual is physically or mentally unable to consent to disclosure. If PHI is disclosed in this situation, health care practitioners must notify the patient that they made the disclosure.

- Food and Drug Administration (FDA). Health care practitioners may disclose PHI to the FDA for safety, quality, or effectiveness such as reporting adverse events, product defects, product recalls, or monitoring patient response to a drug.

- Communicable diseases. If authorized by law to notify persons who may have been exposed to a communicable disease or are at risk of spreading a disease, health care practitioners may disclose PHI.

- Employee workplace medical surveillance. Health care practitioners may disclose PHI to a patient's employer under certain conditions. Consult the privacy officer for those conditions.

- Health oversight activities. These activities include audits, investigations, inspections, licensure, and disciplinary actions. You cannot disclose PHI about the person who is the subject of an investigation.

- Judicial and administrative proceedings. HIPAA adds special criteria that must be included in most subpoenas. Court orders generally have no additional criteria added by HIPAA. Consult your privacy official or your legal department if you receive a subpoena or court order to release PHI.

- Law enforcement. There are eight circumstances that apply concerning the disclosure of PHI to law enforcement officials:

  - Required by law, such as gunshot wounds, child abuse or neglect, or domestic violence.
  - Warrant or process.

- Government agency request.
- Identifying a suspect or material witness.
- Victims of a crime.
- Suspicious death.
- Crime on the premises.
- Medical emergency.

Consult your privacy official or legal department if law enforcement representatives ask for PHI.

- Coroners and funeral directors. You may disclose PHI to a coroner or medical examiner to identify a deceased person and to funeral directors to help them carry out their duties.
- Organ, eye, or tissue donation. You can disclose PHI to appropriate agencies to facilitate organ and tissue donations.
- Research. Consult your privacy officer for special conditions that apply.
- Avert a serious and imminent threat to health or safety. You can disclose PHI if you believe a serious and imminent threat to health or safety exists.
- Special government functions. Special circumstances apply to individuals in the military, veterans, and prison inmates. Consult your privacy officer to determine the appropriate response.
- Workers' compensation. You can disclose PHI to comply with state workers' compensation laws.

9. Authorization

A valid patient authorization allows you to disclose PHI. Use or disclose PHI as limited by the authorization. When in doubt, check with the privacy officer, and always document use or disclosure and those instances when access to PHI is denied.

10. De-identification

You can disclose certain types of patient information when identifying information has been removed, because once the identifiers have been removed, the data are no longer considered protected by the HIPAA regulation. Check with your privacy officer for circumstances that require de-identification.

11. Limited data set

limited data set Protected health information from which certain patient identifiers have been removed.

A **limited data set** is protected health information from which certain specified, direct identifiers of individuals and their relatives, household members, and employers have been removed. A limited data set may be used and disclosed for research, health care operations, and public health purposes, provided the recipient enters into an agreement promising specified safeguards for the protected health information within the limited data set.

The HIPAA Privacy Rule does not give patients the express right to sue. Instead, the person must file a written complaint with the secretary of Health and Human Services through the Office for Civil Rights. The HHS secretary then decides whether or not to investigate the complaint. Patients may have other legal standings to sue, under state privacy laws. For example, in the following case, "EMT Liable for Violating Patient's Privacy," a patient sued an emergency medical technician under state law.

security Policies and procedures that protect PHI from unauthorized access.

Standard 3. Security Rule Privacy refers to those policies and procedures health care providers and their business associates put in place to ensure confidentiality of electronic, written, and oral protected health information. **Security** refers to those policies and procedures health care

COURT CASE

EMT Liable for Violating Patient's Privacy

An EMT employed by a volunteer fire department provided emergency treatment to a female patient for a possible drug overdose. The unresponsive patient was transported to a hospital. The EMT returned home and later spoke to a friend, telling her that she had assisted in taking a specific patient to the hospital emergency room for treatment for a possible drug overdose.

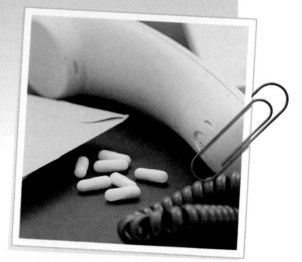

Prior to the emergency, the EMT had never met the patient. However, about two weeks prior to the incident, the EMT had heard about the patient and her medical problems at a social event. The woman who spoke about the patient was apparently a friend, and it was this person whom the EMT telephoned, after the patient's overdose.

The patient sued the EMT and her insurance company, alleging that she had defamed her and violated her privacy by publicizing information concerning her medical condition and making untrue statements indicating that she had attempted suicide. The patient claimed that she had been and was continuing to undergo medical care due to illness, and that the apparent overdose she suffered was a "reaction to medication."

The insurance company claimed the EMT's actions were within the scope of her employment. The EMT argued that she had not acted recklessly or unreasonably in contacting the patient's friend regarding her care.

The EMT offered to settle for $5,000, but the plaintiff refused and the matter went to a jury trial. The jury found that the EMT had violated the plaintiff's right of privacy, as alleged. The jury also awarded the plaintiff/patient $37,909.86 in compensatory damages and attorney fees.

The EMT and her insurance company appealed. An appeals court upheld the judgment of the lower court.

Source: Pachowitz v. Ledoux, 2003 WL 21221823 (Wis. App., May 28, 2003).

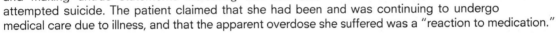

providers and their business associates use to protect electronically transmitted and stored PHI from unauthorized access.

Maintaining security of electronic data is complex, and specific technical knowledge and experience is required to implement the requirements of this rule. All health care providers must conduct security risk assessment surveys to determine their specific vulnerabilities, and to determine the appropriate responses. Security aspects that must be considered include

- Has a security officer for the practice been appointed?
- Are passwords that allow access to electronic information protected?
- Risk assessment should include evaluating how each person protects the password.
- Passwords should not be posted for all to see.
- Passwords should not be unnecessarily divulged to others.
- Are appropriate security measures, such as firewalls, encryption, and antivirus software in place, and are they checked and updated regularly?

Some covered entities and their business associates use private, secure networks not subject to the security problems on the Internet. Other entities

firewalls Hardware, software, or both designed to prevent unauthorized persons from accessing electronic information.

encryption The scrambling or encoding of information before sending it electronically.

and associates use the Internet, but they use **firewalls** (hardware or software designed to keep out unauthorized users) and encryption software to keep information private. **Encryption** software translates information into a code that can be decoded by the recipient but cannot be read by unauthorized viewers.

- Are security measures "reasonable and appropriate" for the health care practice and are they periodically reviewed?

- Have security breaches occurred in the past? If so, what caused the breaches, and have causes been remedied?

- Are security measures in place for business associates that have access to PHI?

- Have staff members been trained in maintaining security of electronic information?

- Are internal sanctions in place for security breaches, and have staff members been informed of such sanctions?

As stated earlier, the implementation of the HIPAA Security Rule can be a technically daunting task. It is best to involve the appropriate technical person or department as early as possible in the process, to ensure that the appropriate security level has been achieved and documented.

Standard 4. National Identifier Standards The purpose of the National Identifier Standards is to provide unique identifiers (addresses) for electronic transmissions. Just as Web sites you visit on the Internet have unique "addresses," called uniform resource locators (URLs), this standard gives certain health care–related entities identifying numerical or alphanumerical addresses. The standard was fully implemented as of May 2008.

These identifiers are kept in a central databank and include unique "addresses" for employers, providers, and health plans.

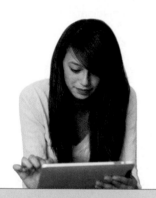

check your **progress**

12. Briefly summarize the four HIPAA standards.

13. Which of the four standards is most concerned with confidentiality of medical records?

14. What are the two required disclosures of health care information that HIPAA mandates?

15. Which HIPAA standard addresses the transmission of electronic health information?

16. You are a hospital nurse, and a patient's family member calls to ask if Mr. Smith is a patient on your floor. How do you respond? Which of the previously described HIPAA standards apply to this situation?

LO 8.3
Discuss the special requirements for disclosing protected health information.

Special Requirements for Disclosing Protected Health Information

As discussed earlier, each use and disclosure of PHI must fall within 1 of the 11 permissions. However, before using or disclosing PHI you must also review any special restrictions that were agreed to and requirements for disclosing information for certain purposes, such as marketing or fund-raising. These special requirements follow.

1. Verification

Ask any person who requests access to PHI to show identification if the request is made in person. If a person asks over the telephone for you to fax PHI and you don't know that person, use common sense. If a patient is making the request, ask for information that you can verify by checking the medical record. If an outside company representative, such as an insurance employee, is making the request, say that you will return the call, and call the insurance office's business telephone number (not a number the caller gave you) to verify that the employee works there. Once you have verified that a patient has made the request, or that the request is legitimate, call the receiving office to say that you are faxing PHI. Fax only the information the patient has requested from the medical record. After you send the fax, request confirmation that it was received. Note the request in the patient's record.

2. Minimum Necessary

This refers to the limited amount of patient data that may be disclosed as required by circumstances. For example, within a medical office a receptionist may need to know only that a patient's insurance information is up to date. An insurance clerk may need to know only a patient's insurance coverage. A billing clerk may need to know only the patient's copay and related contact information. The insurance company needs to access only those portions of the medical record that concern the reason for a patient's visit. (The company does not need the entire medical record, for instance, to pay for a child's immunization visit.)

When responding to requests to provide PHI, remember to provide only the information the patient has requested and to provide only the information necessary for workplace duties to be fulfilled. Everyone requesting information does not need to see a patient's entire medical record. If a patient has requested, in writing, that certain individuals not be allowed access to his or her PHI, you must honor the request. Therefore, before disclosing PHI, check the patient's record for special requirements. Always use the "minimum necessary" standard when disclosing PHI.

3. Marketing

Pharmaceutical and survey companies and other organizations may request patient information to target marketing efforts toward certain patient groups or to communicate general health information. These disclosures are generally not allowed without a patient authorization.

Communications such as mammogram reminder mailings, newsletters about childhood vaccinations, or news about health fairs and classes are not considered marketing and may be conducted without a patient authorization, although if a patient requests that you stop such communications, you should honor the request. If you have the patient's authorization to send additional marketing materials, you may do so. These authorizations are commonly granted at the time of treatment, but you may not make treatment dependent on the patient's signing the authorization. Consult your privacy officer before using patient lists for nontreatment, payment, or health care operations communications.

4. Psychotherapy Notes

HIPAA defines *psychotherapy notes* as those notes that are

- Recorded by a health care provider who is a mental health professional documenting or analyzing the contents of conversation during a private counseling session or a group, joint, or family counseling session.
- Maintained separately from the medical record.

verification The requirement under HIPAA to verify any request as legitimate before protected health information is released.

minimum necessary Term referring to the limited amount of patient information that may be disclosed, depending on circumstances.

Protected psychotherapy notes do *not* include

- Medication prescription and monitoring.
- Counseling session start and stop times.
- The modalities and frequencies of treatment furnished.
- Results of clinical tests.
- Any summary of diagnosis, functional status, the treatment plan, symptoms, prognosis, and progress to date.

Health care providers may *not* use or disclose psychotherapy notes for any purpose, including most treatment, payment, or health care operations, without written authorization from the patient. Exceptions include

- The person who originated the notes wants to review them.
- Counseling training programs want to use PHI to help trainees improve their skills.
- The notes are used as a defense in a legal action or other proceedings brought by the patient.
- The secretary of HHS wants to see them.
- Use or disclosure is required by law.
- A health care practitioner needs to report a serious threat to health or safety, under specific conditions.

Consult your privacy officer for guidance if you are asked to disclose psychotherapy notes.

5. **Policies and Procedures Consistent with Notice of Privacy Practices**

   HIPAA requires health care providers to have in place written policies and procedures on how to handle privacy. These internal policies and procedures must be consistent with the written privacy notification provided to every patient. If you work in a dentist's office, for example, and you will send appointment reminders to patients, the practice's privacy notification must state that the reminders will be sent. HIPAA compliance officers and privacy officers can provide advice on how to implement consistent privacy policies and notifications.

6. **State Laws**

   All HIPAA compliance policies and procedures must be consistent with both state and federal laws. If state and federal laws conflict, you must follow either the law that offers the greater privacy protection or that which offers more patient rights. If a state law is more stringent or offers more patient rights than federal laws, the state law must be followed. Conversely, if HIPAA conflicts with state laws, and HIPAA is more limiting or grants more patient rights, follow the HIPAA regulations. Consult HIPAA compliance officers, privacy officers, and attorneys to develop consent forms compatible with laws in your state.

The ARRA of 2009 added new privacy requirements and guidelines:

- Additional privacy rights for individuals.
  - Practices can forgo the filing of a claim for payment with group health plans if the patient pays out-of-pocket for health care service.
  - Individuals may request and receive information in electronic format at a reasonable cost if it is maintained as an EHR.
  - Individuals may receive an accounting of PHI disclosures made by covered entities or business associates during the previous three years.

- Determination of whether a breach of PHI has occurred.

  - A breach is defined as the unauthorized acquisition, access, use, or disclosure of PHI.

  - Notifications to individuals, media, and HHS when privacy of PHI has been breached.

    - Breach notifications must be in plain, reasonable language.

    - Breach notifications must be sent to next of kin if the patient has expired.

    - Duplicate breach notifications should not be sent from both a covered entity and a business associate.

- Workforce training and complaints.

  - Covered entities and business associates must train employees in HIPAA privacy requirements, must develop and document policies and procedures, must have sanctions for noncompliance, and must require covered entities to refrain from intimidation or retaliation.

- How to render PHI unusable, unreadable, or indecipherable to unauthorized individuals.

  - Electronic PHI is secure only if encrypted.

  - Nonelectronic PHI that is destroyed must be shredded or otherwise rendered unusable.

ARRA also added to HIPAA's enforcement and penalties requirements:

- Covered entities and business associates can be fined for violations they are unaware of.

- Business associates are directly liable under the HIPAA security standard.

- The total amount of fines that can be levied in 1 year was raised.

  - HHS may impose civil penalties ranging from $100 to $50,000 for each offense, and up to a cumulative amount of $1,500,000 in 1 year.

  - State attorneys general can also bring civil actions in federal court.

  - The U.S. Department of Justice may enforce criminal sanctions that involve fines as well as prison terms. Dependent on the intent of the defendant, violations of the Privacy Rule may be misdemeanours or felonies. Misdemeanors—breaches committed without malicious intent—are punishable by a maximum fine of $50,000 and/or a prison term of 1 year. Felonies—breaches committed with ill will or misrepresentation—are punishable by a maximum fine of $100,000 and 5-year prison terms. Violators who obtain PHI with the intent to sell the information or otherwise use it for personal gain or malicious purposes are subject to prosecution for a felony, with penalties of up to $250,000 fines and prison terms of up to 10 years.

While HHS received 19,420 privacy violation complaints between April 2003 and June 2006, no fines were levied. However, since the HIPAA Privacy Rule was implemented in 2003, criminal prosecutions have been brought against Privacy Rule violators and fines have been levied.

In 2008, Anne Pressly—a news anchor for a Little Rock, Arkansas, television station—was brutally attacked in her home. Her mother found her, and she was rushed to St. Vincent Medical Center in Little Rock, but she died five days later without regaining consciousness.

The murder received extensive media coverage, and out of curiosity three St. Vincent employees accessed Pressly's medical records. The breach was discovered, and all three employees—a doctor, an account representative, and an emergency room unit coordinator—pled guilty to misdemeanor violations of the HIPAA Privacy Rule. The doctor was fined $5,000 and sentenced to 50 hours of community service educating others on maintaining patient privacy. The account representative was fined $2,500; the emergency room employee paid $1,500 in fines. St. Vincent Medical Center suspended and disciplined the doctor and fired the other two employees.

Other criminal prosecutions for HIPAA privacy breaches have included a nurse and her husband, who illegally obtained PHI and then threatened the patient with misuse of the information, and a disgruntled researcher from China, working at UCLA, who accessed his supervisor's and coworker's medical records apparently out of spite and then moved on to access medical records of celebrities including Drew Barrymore, Tom Hanks, and Cameron Diaz. The nurse pled guilty to wrongful disclosure of PHI for personal gain and was sentenced to two years of probation and 100 hours of community service. (Charges against her husband were dropped.) She was also fired from her job and faced a nursing board hearing. The UCLA researcher was sentenced to four months in a federal prison.

In a press release announcing the defendants' guilty pleas in the Pressly matter, Jane Duke, the U.S. attorney who prosecuted the case, stated, "The HIPAA privacy protections are real, and we hope that through vigorous enforcement of HIPAA's right-to-privacy protections and swift prosecution of those who violate HIPAA, we can deter those in the medical industry who have access to protected health information from searching others' medical records merely to satisfy their own curiosity."

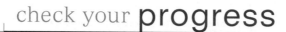

check your **progress**

17. You are the person responsible for releasing patients' health information to those who submit requests. What will you do first when a person claiming to be an insurance company representative asks for a patient's medical records?

18. Define the term *minimum necessary* as it applies to the release of medical records.

19. Can a patient sue over professed privacy violations as defined in HIPAA? Explain your answer.

20. How did ARRA of 2009 affect patient privacy requirements as defined by HIPAA?

21. You are a nursing assistant in a private hospital, and you recognize the patient "James Smith" as a popular television star whose name is *not* James Smith. You hear your coworker, a nurse, revealing this information over the telephone. What will you do?

LO 8.4

Discuss the patient rights defined by HIPAA.

Patient Rights

HIPAA has also put in writing six important patient rights that must be explained in health care provider privacy notifications, and health care providers may not ask patients to waive their rights. These rights are found in Table 8-2. Table 8-3 lists ways for patients to protect their health care information.

Providers' HIPAA compliance and privacy officers are best qualified to answer specific questions about HIPAA and medical privacy. Other sources include the following Web sites and publications.

Web Sites

www.hhs.gov/ocr/hipaa

www.hhs.gov/news/facts/privacy.html

www.healthprivacy.org

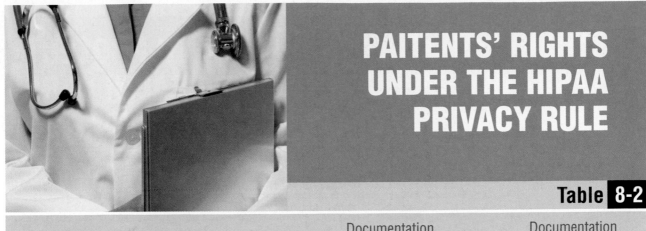

PAITENTS' RIGHTS UNDER THE HIPAA PRIVACY RULE

Table 8-2

Patient Right	Comments	Documentation Required	Documentation Recommended
Access to medical records and the right to copy them	Access to records is guaranteed under HIPAA, but there are some limitations, as mentioned	No	Yes
Request for amendment to designated record set	A patient has the right to request amendments to his or her PHI or other personal information. Unless a provider has grounds to deny the request, amendments must be made	Yes	—
Request for an accounting of disclosures of PHI	You are required to account for certain disclosures during the past three years. Check with your privacy officer for a list. You have up to 60 days to provide the disclosure list	Yes. Always keep a record of the appropriate disclosures, and make a copy of the disclosure report for the patient's file	—
Request to be contacted at an alternate location	Patients can request to have you contact them at places other than work or home. You can deny the request if you cannot reasonably comply	Yes. Obtain a request from the patient in writing. Note in the patient's electronic medical record and in a paper communication for staff members who do not have access to the patient's electronic medical record. Document reasons for denying the request if it is denied	—
Requests for further restrictions on who has access to PHI	A patient can request that certain persons or entities do not have access to his or her medical record. You may deny the request if you cannot reasonably comply	Yes. Ask the patient to complete an opt-out form that is then filed with electronic and paper records. Document reasons for denying the request if it is denied	—
Right to file a complaint	Enforcement of the Privacy Rule is complaint-driven. Patients should be encouraged to work first with the provider. Retaliation is prohibited	Yes. Refer the complaint to the privacy officer. Document the complaint in a privacy complaint log. Evaluate the complaint and determine how best to solve it	—

www.ama-assn.org/ama/pub/category/4234.html (Or at www.ama-assn.org, do a search for HIPAA to reach the current page.)

www.hipaa.com

Publications

Carter, Patricia I. *HIPAA Compliance Handbook, 2010 Edition.* Gaithersburg, MD: Aspen Publishers, 2010.

Hartley, Carolyn P., and Edward D. Jones III. *HIPAA Plain & Simple: A Compliance Guide for Health Care Professionals.* Chicago: AMA Press, 2004.

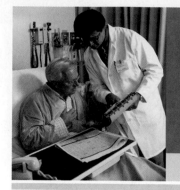

HOW TO PROTECT YOUR HEALTH CARE INFORMATION

Table 8-3

Read notices of privacy practices carefully to become aware of the possible uses and disclosures of your information

- Tell your health care provider your confidentiality concerns
- Ask how large health care organizations share your information

Read authorization forms carefully before you sign; edit them to limit the sharing of information if you wish. Initial and date your revisions

Register your objection to disclosures you consider inappropriate. You can file a complaint with the provider, plan, or Department of Health and Human Services

Request a copy of your medical record, and review it carefully to be sure the information is correct. You can request amendments or corrections

Be cautious when visiting Web sites. If you participate in surveys or health screenings on medical information Web sites, look for and read privacy policies. Don't participate if you don't know how the information will be used and who will have access to it

Request a copy of your file from the Medical Information Bureau (MIB). MIB is an organization of insurance companies that compiles reports on individuals with serious medical conditions or other factors that could affect longevity, such as participating in dangerous sports. If MIB has a file on someone, that person has a right to see and correct misinformation in the file. To obtain a copy of your file, if one exists, contact MIB Inc., 50 Braintree Hill Park, Suite 400, Braintree, MA 02184-8734; (866) 692-6901; www.mib.com

Educate yourself about medical privacy issues

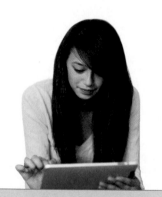

check your progress

22. You are a medical assistant working in a practice that includes several physicians. A patient asks you for a copy of her medical records. How do you respond?

23. You work in the medical records department of the medical office described in question 21. A patient has read his medical record, and he asks you to make changes. How do you respond?

24. A patient in the same medical office asks the records department for a list of all those who have received her PHI over the last three years. Can the records department comply with this request? Explain your answer.

25. You are a physician assistant in the Wellness Clinic. A patient with a history of mental health disorders asks to see his medical record. How do you reply?

26. A patient in a medical office tells the office receptionist she wants to file a complaint. What procedure should be followed?

Recognizing and Dispelling Myths about HIPAA

LO 8.5

Recognize and dispel some of the more prevalent myths concerning HIPAA.

For fear of government prosecution, HIPAA compliance overkill has been a problem in some cases. Myths and misinterpretations often must be dispelled as health care providers implement HIPAA standards and rules. For example, it is not true in all cases that health care providers cannot issue the names of hospital patients and patient condition updates to family members. Nor is it true that health care providers cannot correspond about a patient's care, or that police 911 dispatchers cannot give EMTs a patient's name. Here are a few frequently asked questions about HIPAA provisions that can help dispel myths.

Q: May one physician office send a patient's medical records to another physician office without the patient's consent?

A: Yes.

Q: Does the HIPAA Privacy Rule prohibit or discourage doctor–patient e-mails?

A: Health care practitioners can continue to correspond with patients via e-mail, but appropriate electronic safeguards must be in place.

Q: May an employer access your health information without your permission?

A: No.

Q: What if the employer has paid for the health care administered?

A: Still cannot access without your written permission.

Q: Can health records affect your credit rating?

A: Yes. If you don't pay medical bills, your credit rating could suffer.

Q: May a patient be listed in a hospital's directory without the patient's consent, and may the directory be shared with the public?

A: The HIPAA Privacy Rule allows hospitals to continue providing directory information to the public, unless the patient has specifically chosen not to be included.

Q: May clergy members learn whether members of their congregation or religious affiliation are hospitalized?

A: Hospitals may continue disclosing directory information to members of the clergy, unless the patient has objected to such disclosure.

Q: Is a hospital allowed to share patient information with the patient's family without the patient's express consent?

A: Providers can disclose information to individuals identified by the patient as entitled to receive the information.

Q: May a patient's family member pick up prescriptions for the patient?

A: Yes. The Privacy Rule allows family members or others to "pick up filled prescriptions, medical supplies, X-rays, or other similar forms of protected health information."

Q: If a patient refuses to sign an acknowledgment stating that he or she received the health care provider's Notice of Privacy Practices, must the health care provider refuse to provide services?

A: The Privacy Rule gives the patient a "right to notice" of privacy practices for protecting identifying health information. It requires that providers make a "good faith effort" to have patients acknowledge receipt of the notice, but the law does not give health care practitioners the right to refuse treatment to people who do not sign the acknowledgment.

Q: May the media access public information from hospitals about accident or crime victims?

A: Certain information can be made public, unless the patient specifically opts out.

Q: If I need emergency assistance from the police or fire department, is the 911 dispatcher prohibited from giving my name to rescue units or EMTs?

A: No. Names and addresses should be given to rescue or EMT staff for help in locating patients and treating their medical problems as quickly as possible.

Q: Do HIPAA privacy requirements cover privacy and security for all medical records?

A: Health care providers and facilities, insurers, and certain business associates are subject to HIPAA privacy regulations. However, others may have access to PHI who are not regulated by HIPAA. For example, some Internet-based services offer to store PHI, usually for a fee, for quick access in emergencies. Such services are presently not subject to HIPAA privacy rules.

While HIPAA legislation is complicated, all health care practitioners should become familiar with its provisions. When in doubt about whether or not an action violates the law, medical providers should have access to a HIPAA compliance and privacy officer with whom they can consult.

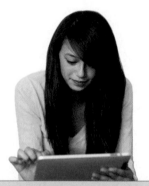

check your **progress**

Check mark the following statements that are not allowed or are not true under HIPAA regulations.

_____ 27. Dr. Goodhealth sends Mr. Jones's medical record to Dr. Wellness without obtaining Mr. Jones's consent.

_____ 28. A prospective employer wants to access a job applicant's medical record, but without her knowledge or consent.

_____ 29. Your credit rating does not suffer when you fail to pay your medical bills.

_____ 30. A hospital patient is listed in the facility's directory, but the patient has not consented to the listing.

_____ 31. A patient's family member picks up the patient's prescriptions from the hospital pharmacy.

_____ 32. A medical assistant calls a patient's name to see the doctor, and others in the waiting room can hear.

CHAPTER SUMMARY

LO 8.1 What considerations do federal and state privacy laws share?

- Information collected and stored about individuals should be limited to what is necessary to carry out the functions of the business or government agency collecting the information.
- Access to personal information should be limited to those employees who must use the information in performing their jobs.
- Personal information cannot be released outside the organization collecting it unless authorization is obtained from the subject.
- When information is collected about a person, that person should know that the information is being collected and should have the opportunity to check the information for accuracy.

Which federal laws most extensively regulate health care, including privacy?

- Health Insurance Portability and Accountability Act (HIPAA) of 1996.
- American Recovery and Reinvestment Act (ARRA) of 2009.
  - Title XIII, called the Health Information Technology for Economic and Clinical Health (HITECH) Act.
- Patient Protection and Affordable Care Act (PPACA) of 2010.
- Health Care and Education Reconciliation Act (HCERA) of 2010.

LO 8.2 Which HIPAA terms are health care practitioners most likely to routinely use?

- Business associate.
- Covered entity.
- Covered transaction.
- De-identify.
- Designated record set.
- Electronic data interchange (EDI).
- Electronic transmission.
- Encryption.
- Limited data set.
- Minimum necessary.
- Notice of Privacy Practices.
- Patient identifiers.
- Permission.
- Protected health information.

What are the four HIPAA standards and rules?

- Transactions and Code Sets: A transaction refers to the transmission of information between two parties to carry out financial or administrative activities. A code set is any set of codes used to encode data elements, such as tables of terms, medical concepts, medical diagnostic codes, or medical procedure codes.

- Privacy Rule: Policies and procedures health care providers and their business associates put in place to ensure confidentiality of electronic, written, and oral protected health information.

- Security Rule: Security refers to those policies and procedures health care providers and their business associates use to protect electronically transmitted and stored PHI from unauthorized access

- National Identifier Standards: Provide unique identifiers (addresses) for electronic transmissions

LO 8.3 What special requirements does HIPAA mandate for disclosing protected health information?

- Permissions are required for releasing PHI.

- There are special requirements for disclosing PHI.

- There are civil and criminal penalties for unauthorized disclosure of PHI.

- Patients have specific rights under HIPAA which include

  - The right to obtain one's own medical records (with some exceptions).

  - The right to request changes to one's own medical records.

  - The right to request a list of disclosures over the past three years.

  - The right to request notifications at alternative locations.

  - The right to restrict access.

  - The right to file a complaint.

What recent legislation significantly changed HIPAA privacy, security, and enforcement rules?

- American Recovery and Reinvestment Act (ARRA) of 2009.

  - Title XIII, called the Health Information Technology for Economic and Clinical Health (HITECH) Act.

LO 8.4 What patient rights does HIPAA define?

- Access to medical records and the right to copy them.

- Request for amendment to designated record set.

- Request for an accounting of disclosures of PHI.

- Request to be contacted at an alternate location.

- Requests for further restrictions on who has access to PHI.

- Right to file a complaint.

How can you protect the privacy of your own medical records?

- Read notices of privacy practices carefully.

- Tell your health care provider your confidentiality concerns.

- Ask how large health care organizations share your information.

- Read authorization forms carefully before you sign.

- Register your objection to disclosures you consider inappropriate.

- Request a copy of your medical record, and review it carefully to be sure the information is correct.

- Be cautious when visiting Web sites.

- Request a copy of your file from the Medical Information Bureau (MIB).

- Educate yourself about medical privacy issues.

LO 8.5 What is the truth about some common HIPAA myths?

- Physicians may exchange information about a patient without written authorization.

- Doctor–patient e-mails are permitted, as long as proper security is in place.

- Employers may not access employees' PHI without patients' written authorization, even if the employer is the health care payer.

- Failure to pay medical bills can affect one's credit rating.

- Patients must give consent before being listed in a hospital directory.

- Hospital directories may be available to the public, with patients' consent.

- Clergy members can learn of congregation members' hospitalization, but only with patients' authorization.

- Hospitals can share patient information with designated family members.

- Family members can pick up prescriptions, X-rays, and other similar forms of PHI for patients.

[ETHICS ISSUES Privacy Law and HIPAA]

Laurinda Beebe Harman, PhD, RHIA, Associate Professor and Chair, Department of Health Information Management (HIM), at Temple University in Philadelphia, is editor of a 2006 text for health care students and practitioners, titled *Ethical Challenges in the Management of Health Information*, 2nd edition.

"There are many ethical issues that health care providers and HIM practitioners face," says Harman, "including those related to coding, quality review, research, public health, managed care, clinical care, the electronic health record, adoption, genetic and behavioral health." Health care practitioners also face many ethical issues in the special roles they assume, Harman continues, "including management, entrepreneurship, advocacy, and working with vendors. The legal system is a necessary but often insufficient resource when facing these issues."

For example, although HIPAA spells out specific requirements for privacy and confidentiality of medical records, like any law it cannot anticipate or address every possible situation. "It is within these voids that ethics must prevail and guide our decisions. . . . There must be a constant balancing between protecting privacy and releasing information, in accordance with federal privacy legislation, to authorized users so that business functions that support health care can be accomplished."

Furthermore, Harman states, "Several important criteria should be used when evaluating requests for the release of information, including the 'need-to-know' (minimum necessary) criterion."

Ethics ISSUE 1: HIPAA has made it illegal, under threat of penalty, for health care practitioners to disclose confidential health information about patients to unauthorized sources.

Discussion Questions

1. Sharon, a second-year nursing student, is completing a surgical rotation in a community hospital. At the breakfast table, Sharon's husband asks her to find out what is wrong with one of his employees, who has been hospitalized for several days. He is interested in knowing when the man may be able to return to work. Is it ethical for Sharon to give her husband this information? Explain your answer.

_____

_____

2. What should health care practitioners do when family members or friends ask them for information about others that they have discovered in the course of their employment?

_____

_____

Ethics ISSUE 2: HIPAA requires health care providers to issue privacy notices to patients.

Discussion Question

1. You are the medical office employee responsible for giving patients your employer's privacy notice. Even though you have explained why an elderly patient has been given the privacy notice, he complains about yet another "health care form" and refuses to read it. How will you respond?

_____

_____

Ethics ISSUE 3: Some sources distinguish between *privacy* in health care and *confidentiality*. According to Harman, privacy refers to the right of an individual to be left alone and to the fact that patients must authorize release of information. Confidentiality refers to limiting disclosure to authorized persons and ensuring protection of records documenting communication between providers and patients.

Discussion Questions

1. Why are privacy and confidentiality so important to patients and to health care practitioners?

_____

_____

2. With the implementation of HIPAA, the extensive federal law mandating certain privacy and security precautions, is privacy for protected health information now guaranteed? Explain your answer.

_____

_____

3. The health care practitioners in the following text have followed the letter of HIPAA law. Have they also acted ethically? Explain why or why not.

   A patient asks to see her medical records, and a medical office records assistant complies, but slams down the records in front of the patient and mutters about being "too busy" for this service.

   A physician does not refuse to see a patient who declares that he will not complete his notification preference form, but his abrupt manner discourages the patient from continuing to see the physician.

   A patient asks for a list of disclosures his physician has made of his health information within the past six years, and he is politely asked to submit his request in writing.

   The person responsible for faxing a patient's protected health information from one physician office to another sends the information to the wrong fax number.

_____

_____

Ethics ISSUE 4: Under HIPAA, permissions are required for releasing PHI.

Discussion Questions

1. John works as an LPN at a Hollywood hospital. He was passing out meds to the patients on his floor and noticed that the patient in Room 402, named Jason Wilson, was really Tom Cruise, a famous actor. John then called home and told his wife, "Tom Cruise is in the hospital!" Is John's statement a HIPAA violation?

_____

_____

2. Can Tom Cruise sue for punitive damages?

_____

_____

Go to **www.mhhe.com/judson6e** to practice your case review skills. Then read on for more information.

code set

covered entities

covered transaction

de-identify

designated record set

electronic data inter-
change (EDI)

electronic transmission

encryption

firewalls

Health Insurance
Portability and
Accountability Act
(HIPAA)

limited data set

minimum necessary

Notice of Privacy Prac-
tices (NPP)

permission

privacy

protected health
information (PHI)

rule

security

standard

state preemption

transaction

treatment, payment,
and health care
operations (TPO)

verification

[CHAPTER 8 REVIEW]

Applying Knowledge

LO 8.1

Circle the correct answer for each of the following questions.

1. Which of the following statements is true?
   a. The U.S. Constitution, under Article 2, Section 8, specifically protects citizens' privacy.
   b. Privacy is protected by the Second Amendment of the U.S. Constitution.
   c. The U.S. Constitution does not specifically protect citizens' privacy.
   d. None of the above is true.

2. Which of the following amendments to the U.S. Constitution has (have) particular implications in science, medicine, and the delivery of health care?
   a. Tenth Amendment
   b. First, Third, and Fourth Amendments
   c. First, Second, and Third Amendments
   d. Fourth, Fifth, and Sixth Amendments

LO 8.2

Fill in the blanks or answer the following questions in the spaces provided.

3. HIPAA stands for _____.

4. The department of the federal government responsible for supervising HIPAA compliance and implementation is _____.

5. Patient complaints about privacy must be directed to which government agency?

_____

_____

6. What is the determining factor in deciding whether or not health care providers are considered *covered entities* under HIPAA?

_____

_____

7. What is an *electronic transmission*, and how and why does HIPAA address it?

_____

_____

8. A document that informs patients on how a health care provider intends to use and disclose patient information and also informs patients of their rights is called _____.

9. Protected health information (PHI) refers to _____.

10. If a state law and HIPAA's federal law disagree, which law should you follow?

_____

_____

11. The primary reason for the Security Rule is _____.

Circle the correct answer for each of the following questions.

12. A *business associate* is
    a. A person, group, or organization outside the medical practice that has a HIPAA-approved reason to see protected health information
    b. A health care practitioner's financial advisor
    c. Anyone who sells products related to health care
    d. None of the above

LO 8.3

13. Covered entities may:
    a. be found guilty of criminal charges when violating patient confidentiality
    b. be fined up to $1.5 million cumulative damages in civil penalties
    c. be fined for violations they were unaware of at the time they occurred
    d. All of the above

14. If a patient complains that his privacy was breached, what should you ask that he do?
    a. Call a lawyer.
    b. Speak to your privacy officer to try to handle the complaint in the office.
    c. Immediately file a complaint with the Office for Civil Rights.
    d. Discuss the problem with someone else in the office.

15. Which of the following are the privacy officer's responsibilities?
    a. Researching the Privacy Rule
    b. Helping develop the Notice of Privacy Practices
    c. Training staff on privacy policies and procedures
    d. All of the above

16. Which of the following is *not* covered by HIPAA's Security Rule?
    a. The content of all documents pertaining to patient privacy
    b. Maintaining electronic security for networked computers
    c. Using HIPAA standards for electronic transmission of protected health information
    d. None of the above

17. Which of the following is *not* considered marketing under HIPAA provisions?
    a. A pharmaceutical company wants to send special mailings to a provider's diabetic patients to announce a new blood sugar testing device.
    b. A reminder to female patients when their mammograms should be scheduled.
    c. Cholesterol screening results sent to patients through the mail.
    d. None of the above.

18. Which of the following is *not* a violation of HIPAA's Privacy Rule?
    a. You call across a crowded waiting room to tell a patient he has forgotten his prescription for Dilantin, a drug used to control seizures.
    b. You are a medical assistant for a physician's private practice, and you tell a friend, who is a bank teller, that a mutual friend has seen your employer and is pregnant.
    c. A telephone caller identifies himself as an insurance plan representative and requests PHI. You do not know the caller, but you comply.
    d. All of the above are violations of HIPAA's Privacy Rule.

19. An unauthorized person (a computer hacker) manages to access the computers in the hospital where you work and downloads information. Who is the most likely person to handle the disaster?
    a. The privacy officer
    b. The hospital administrator
    c. The security officer
    d. The medical records supervisor

20. Which of the following is true under HIPAA?
    a. HIPAA language states unequivocally that patients have no standing to sue under the law.
    b. Patients must submit complaints to the secretary of Health and Human Services through the Office for Civil Rights.
    c. Only a court of law can hear patient complaints.
    d. None of the above.

21. HIPPA's Privacy Rule protects PHI
    a. Only in electronic form
    b. Only in written form
    c. Only in spoken form
    d. In all of the above forms

22. Which statement is *not* true of HIPAA?
    a. HIPAA requires that health care practitioners change a medical record if a patient complains.
    b. If a patients asks to see his or her medical record, the request must be honored.
    c. Health care practitioners must supply patients who ask with a list of those who have received copies of the patient's medical record.
    d. Under HIPAA, any health care facility that transmits protected health information electronically is a covered entity.

23. Which of the following laws made extensive changes to the HIPAA Privacy Rule?
    a. Red flags rule
    b. American Recovery and Reinvestment Act (ARRA)
    c. Patient Protection and Affordable Care Act (PPACA)
    d. Health Care and Education Reconciliation Act (HCERA)

24. Which of the following is true of current medical records privacy law?
    a. Patients can sue in federal court if PHI is breached.
    b. Only federal law covers medical information privacy.
    c. Penalties can be levied against covered entities and business associates for PHI breaches they are unaware of.
    d. There are no criminal penalties for PHI breaches.

Match each definition with the correct term by writing the letter in the space provided.

_____ 24. The HIPAA-mandated standard for electronic transmissions.

_____ 25. A valid reason to disclose protected health information.

_____ 26. This person evaluates, manages, and reports on the security of a health provider's electronic data.

_____ 27. A means of protecting data transmitted over the Internet.

_____ 28. Covered entities.

_____ 29. Covered transactions.

_____ 30. Refers to providing only as much patient information as needed for a request or to conduct health care business.

_____ 31. One of two types of PHI access mandated by HIPAA.

_____ 32. One of a patient's six rights mandated by HIPAA.

_____ 33. To remove patient-identifying information from PHI.

a. File a complaint

b. Encryption

c. Physicians and pharmacists

d. Minimum necessary

e. De-identify

f. Billing patients and filing insurance claims

g. HIPAA representatives ask to see PHI

h. Security officer

i. Privacy officer

j. Permission

k. Electronic data interchange (EDI)

LO 8.4

Circle the correct answer for each of the following questions.

35. Which of the following patient rights is *not* conferred by HIPAA?
    a. The right to sue in federal court over a breach of PHI
    b. The right to submit a complaint over a breach of PHI
    c. The right to request changes to one's own medical record
    d. The right to designate an alternative means of notification

36. Which of the following is *not* a way for you to protect the privacy of your own medical records?
    a. Read Notices of Privacy Practices and be sure you understand them.
    b. Always store your medical records on Web sites expressly for that purpose.
    c. Review your medical records periodically for errors.
    d. Ask to see a list of those to whom your records have been released.

LO 8.5

37. Which of the following statements is true under HIPAA rules?
    a. Doctors and patients are prohibited from communicating by e-mail.
    b. Patients are no longer permitted to sign in for doctors' appointments.
    c. Members of the clergy may no longer ask for names of church members who are hospitalized.
    d. Family members can pick up prescriptions for patients.

[CASE STUDIES]

Use your critical thinking skills to answer the questions that follow each case study.

LO 8.2 and LO 8.3

Mona frequently travels for her job, and even when she is in town, she's usually reached most easily on her cell phone. She has three teenagers at home and doesn't want them to pick up her health care messages. She also wants her medical bills sent to her work address.

38. What should Mona's health care provider do to accommodate her requests?

_____

_____

Lewis received a basketball scholarship to attend college, and he signed a form giving the university health service permission to access his health care records. Lewis now wants to know what is included in his health care records.

39. What should Lewis's health care provider do?

_____

_____

Shirley, an EMT, is off duty and is driving her private vehicle on the interstate in a snowstorm. The car ahead of Shirley hits an icy patch and skids off the road, overturning as it hits the ditch. Shirley stops to help and dials 911 on her cell phone. The lone woman in the wrecked car has scratches and bruises and an obviously broken arm. While Shirley is helping the woman, a news van stops and a television reporter films the wreck for the evening news. The injured driver refuses to answer questions, so the reporter turns to Shirley, who knows the injured driver's name.

40. May Shirley tell the television reporter the injured woman's name without violating federal law? Why or why not?

_____

_____

41. Rescue services arrive while the television reporter is there. Can the ambulance attendants, who are also EMTs, tell the television reporter the apparent extent of the woman's injuries? Why or why not?

_____

_____

You are a nurse and a teenaged patient's mother tells you she wants access to her daughter's medical records.

42. What will you do?

_____

_____

INTERNET ACTIVITIES LO 8.2, LO 8.3, and LO 8.4

Complete the activities and answer the questions that follow.

43. Visit **www.regreform.hhs.gov/hipaaquiz_0204171/sld001.htm** and take the privacy quiz. Answers are provided immediately after the questions, but which, if any, of the answers most surprised you and why?

_____

44. Visit **www.hipaa.com**. Access the HIPAA Key Dates Timeline and click on "Today." What HIPAA compliance deadlines are coming up soon or have passed within the last year? Prepare a list of five questions you would most like to have answered about HIPAA compliance, standards, or rules. Search this site for answers. If answers were found, briefly summarize them. If any of your questions are still unanswered, where might you look for answers?

_____

_____

[RESOURCES]

Center for Democracy & Technology. "Summary of Privacy Provisions of ARRA 2009." 1634 I Street NW, Suite 1100, Washington, DC 20006, March 12, 2009, **www.cdt.org**.

Harman, Laurinda B. "Privacy and Confidentiality." In *Ethical Challenges in the Management of Health Information*, 2nd ed., ed. Laurie A. Rinehart-Thompson and Laurinda B. Harman. Sudbury, MA: Jones & Bartlett, 2006, Chapter 3.

Hartley, Carolyn P., and Edward D. Jones III. HIPAA *Plain & Simple: A Compliance Guide for Health Care Professionals*. Chicago: AMA Press, 2004.

McLendon, Kelly. "HIPAA Privacy Summary." Health Information Xperts, P.O. Box 758, Titusville, FL 32781, 321-268-0320, **www.hixperts.com**.

Smith, Robert Ellis. *Compilation of State and Federal Privacy Laws*. Privacy Journal, 2002, with a 2010 supplement.

Telephone interview, October 24, 2007, with Laurinda B. Harman, Temple University, Philadelphia, PA.

Torrey, Trisha. "10 Myths About HIPAA, Patients, and Medical Records Privacy." Ask.com Guide, **http://patients.about.com/od/yourmedical-records/ss/hipaamyths.htm**, updated March 15, 2009.

HIPAA enactment dates Web site:

www.hipaa.com.

Quote from Jane Duke:

U.S. Department of Justice, Press Release dated July 20, 2009, "Doctor and Two Former Hospital Employees Plead Guilty to HIPAA Violation."

Statistics for privacy complaints and information about criminal prosecutions:

Seitz, Esther. "Privacy (or Piracy) or Medical Records: HIPAA and Its Enforcement." *Journal of the National Medical Association* 102, no. 8 (August 2010), pp. 745–748.

part three

Professional, Social, and Interpersonal Health Care Issues

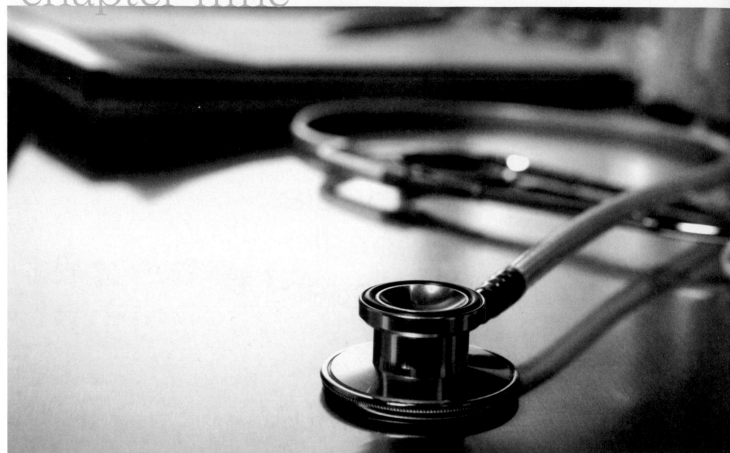

PHYSICIANS' PUBLIC DUTIES AND RESPONSIBILITIES

Learning Outcomes

After studying this chapter, you should be able to:

LO 9.1 List at least four vital events for which statistics are collected by the government.

LO 9.2 Discuss the procedures for filing birth and death certificates.

LO 9.3 Explain the purpose of public health statutes.

LO 9.4 Cite examples of reportable diseases and injuries, and explain how they are reported.

LO 9.5 Discuss federal drug regulations, including the Controlled Substances Act.

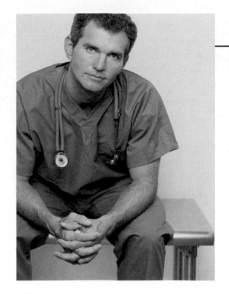

JASON, RN, BSN, is a public health nurse working for sections of three counties in the rural Northwest. "My duties range from home visits for parenting education, to foster child care, to the mainstays of public health—communicable disease investigation and reporting—and everything in between. In fact, once during a home visit I even delivered a baby—it was a boy," Jason says. "I enjoy the autonomy I have in my job, and I've established good rapport with the families I see regularly."

The ability to establish rapport is important, Jason explains, when he contacts individuals who have been diagnosed with a reportable disease, such as a sexually transmitted disease (STD), also referred to as a sexually transmitted infection (STI) and their contacts. "We have a fairly high percentage of STIs in my area, and I'm often persuading people to give me the names of those with whom they have been intimate, so I can let those individuals know that they should see a doctor."

The information is kept confidential, of course, Jason continues, "but it's still a hard subject to approach. Most people are cooperative, but there are a few who don't want to talk to me. That's when my job really becomes difficult."

From Jason's perspective, his job involves helping keep families within his practice area healthy, and also helping hold down the spread of a contagious infection or disease once patients are diagnosed. His investigative work as a public health nurse is mandated by state law, but the process can be difficult and can feel intrusive. Nevertheless, Jason does his best to see that the people in his area are protected.

From the perspective of Jason's patients who learn they have a reportable, contagious condition, his visit is probably stressful. Those who are concerned for loved ones or others with whom they have had contact, however, are generally willing to provide names of individuals he can contact.

From the perspective of public health authorities, nurses like Jason not only see patients in their homes, where health problems often arise, but they also keep contagious disease from becoming epidemic, and they help get vital treatment to those who have been exposed to infectious diseases.

If it were your job to solicit information from a person with a communicable disease, how would you proceed?

What factors are involved in "establishing rapport" with patients?

Vital Statistics

To assess population trends and needs, state and federal governments collect **vital statistics.** Vital events for which statistics are collected include live births, deaths, fetal deaths, marriages, divorces, induced terminations of pregnancy, and any change in civil status that occurs during an individual's lifetime. Health care practitioners help in gathering this information and in filling out forms for filing with the appropriate state and federal agencies.

The information provided through the reporting of vital statistics is useful to educational institutions, governmental agencies, research scientists,

LO 9.1

List at least four vital events for which statistics are collected by the government.

private industry, and many other organizations and individuals. For example, the recording of vital statistics allows for tracking population composition and growth, measuring educational standards, and monitoring communicable diseases and other community and environmental health problems. Health care practitioners play an important role in collecting and recording valuable health data required by law; therefore, it is important that they know the correct methods and procedures for reporting public health information.

LO 9.2
Discuss the procedures for filing birth and death certificates.

Records for Births and Deaths

Birth and death certificates are permanent legal records, and a copy of a person's birth certificate is required to obtain certain government documents, such as a passport, driver's license, voter registration card, or Social Security card. Guidelines for completing the forms are as follows:

- Type or legibly print all entries. In some states, only black ink may be used.

- Leave no entries blank. Each state has specific requirements for recording information.

- Avoid corrections and erasures.

- Where requested, provide signatures. Do not use rubber stamps or initials in place of signatures.

- File only originals with state registrars.

- Verify the spelling of names.

- Avoid abbreviations, except those recommended in instructions for specific items.

- Refer any problems to the appropriate state officials.

Births

All live births must be reported to the state registrar. Figure 9-1 illustrates a sample birth certificate. In some states, separate birth and death certificates must be filed for stillbirths, while in others there are special forms for stillbirths that include both birth and death information. Generally, birth and death certificates are not required for fetal deaths in which the fetus has not passed the 20th week of gestation.

Hospitals file birth certificates for babies born to mothers who have been admitted as patients. The attending physician must verify all medical information. For nonhospital births, the person in attendance is responsible for filing the birth certificate. (Jason, the public health nurse in the chapter's opening scenario, filed the birth certificate for the birth he attended.)

Deaths

After a person is pronounced dead, the attending physician must complete the medical portion of the certificate of death, which generally includes the following information:

- Disease, injury, and/or complication that caused the death and how long the decedent was treated for this condition before death occurred.

DO NOT WRITE IN MARGIN RESERVED FOR ODH DATA CODING

a. _____
b. _____
c. _____

CHILD

d. _____
e. _____
f. _____
g. _____
h. _____

ATTENDANT

MOTHER

FATHER

INFORMANT

Ohio Department of Health
VITAL STATISTICS
CERTIFICATE OF LIVE BIRTH
TYPE OR PRINT IN PERMANENT BLACK INK

Reg. Dist. No. _____
Primary Reg. Dist. No. _____
Registrar's No. _____

Birth No. 134____

| 1. CHILD NAME | First | Middle | Last | 2.SEX | 3a. DATE OF BIRTH (Month, Day, Year) | 3b. TIME OF BIRTH M |

| 4a. FACILITY NAME (If not institution, give street and number) | 4b. CITY, VILLAGE, OR LOCATION OF BIRTH | 4c. COUNTY OF BIRTH |

5. PLACE OF BIRTH ☐ Hospital ☐ Freestanding Birthing Center ☐ Clinic/Doctor's Office ☐ Residence ☐ Other (Specify)

| 6. REGISTRAR'S SIGNATURE | 7. DATE FILED BY REGISTRAR (Month, Day, Year) |

| 8a. I certify that the above named child was born alive at the place and time and on the date stated above. SIGNATURE ► | 8b. DATE SIGNED | 8c. ATTENDANT ☐ M.D. ☐ D.O. ☐ C.N.M. ☐ OTHER MIDWIFE ☐ OTHER (Specify) |

| 8d. ATTENDANT - NAME (Type or Print) | 8e. MAILING ADDRESS (Street or R.F.D. No., City or Village, State, Zip) |

| 9a. MOTHER'S NAME (First, Middle, Last) | 9b. MAIDEN NAME | 10a. DATE OF BIRTH (Month, Day, Year) | 10b. AGE |

| 11. BIRTHPLACE (State or Foreign Country) | 12a. RESIDENCE - STATE | 12. COUNTY | 12c. CITY, TOWN, OR LOCATION |

| 12d. STREET AND NUMBER | 12e. INSIDE CITY LIMITS? ☐ Yes ☐ No | 13. MOTHER'S MAILING ADDRESS (If same as residence, enter zip code only) |

| 14. FATHER'S NAME (First, Middle, Last) | 15a. DATE OF BIRTH (Month, Day, Year) | 15b. AGE | 16. BIRTHPLACE (State or Foreign Country) |

17. I certify that the personal information provided on this certificate is correct to the best of my knowledge and belief. (ENTER INFORMANT'S NAME OR WHEN REQUIRED BY LAW, PARENTS' SIGNATURES)

INFORMATION FOR MEDICAL AND HEALTH USE ONLY

MOTHER
FATHER

18. OF HISPANIC ORIGIN? (Specify NO or Yes - if yes, specify Cuban, Mexican, Puerto Rican, etc.)	19. RACE American Indian, Black, White, etc. (Specify below)	20. EDUCATION (Specify only highest grade completed)		21. OCCUPATION AND BUSINESS/INDUSTRY (Worked during last year)	
		Elementary / Secondary (0-12)	College (1-4 or 5+)	Occupation	Business/Industry
18a. ☐ NO ☐ YES Specify:	19a.	20a.		21a.	21b.
18B. ☐ NO ☐ YES Specify:	19b.	20b.		21c.	21d.

VOID

i. _____
j. _____
k. _____
l. _____
m. _____
n. _____
o. _____
p. _____
q. _____
r. _____
s. _____
t. _____
u. _____
v. _____
w. _____
x. _____
y. _____
z. _____
aa. _____
bb. _____
cc. _____
dd. _____
ee. _____
ff. _____
gg. _____
hh. _____
ii. _____
jj. _____
kk. _____
mm. _____

| 22. PREGNANCY HISTORY (Complete each section) | | 23. MOTHER MARRIED? (At birth, conception, or any time between) (Yes or No) | 24. DATE LAST NORMAL MENSES BEGAN (Month, Day, Year) |
| LIVE BIRTHS (Do not include this child) | OTHER TERMINATIONS (Spontaneous and induced at any time after conception) | | 26a. TOTAL PRENATAL VISITS (If none, so state) |

| 22a. NOW LIVING NUMBER ☐ NONE | 22b. NOW DEAD NUMBER ☐ NONE | 22d. NUMBER ☐ NONE | 25. MONTH OF PREGNANCY PRENATAL CARE BEGAN First, Second, Third, etc. (Specify) | 26b. CITY | 26c. COUNTY |
| | | | 27. BIRTH WEIGHT IN GRAMS | 28. CLINICAL ESTIMATE OF GESTATION (Weeks) | |

| 22c. DATE OF LAST BIRTH (Month, Year) | 22e. DATE OF LAST OTHER TERMINATION (Month, Year) | 29a. PLURALITY - Single, Twin, Triplet, etc. (Specify) | 29b. IF NOT SINGLE BIRTH - Born First, Second, Third, etc (Specify) |

30. APGAR SCORE	31a. MOTHER TRANSFERRED PRIOR TO DELIVERY? ☐ No ☐ Yes Yes, If yes, enter name of facility and city transferred FROM
30a.1 MINUTE	30b. 5 MINUTES	31b. FACILITY NAME	31c. CITY
		31d. INFANT TRASFERRED? ☐ No ☐ Yes Yes, If yes, enter name of facility and city transferred TO.
		31e. FACILITY NAME	31f. CITY

MULTIPLE BIRTHS
Enter State File Number for Mate(s)
LIVE BIRTH(S)

FETAL DEATH (S)

32a. MEDICAL RISK FACTORS FOR THIS PREGNANCY (Check all that apply)

Anemia (Hct. <30/Hgb. <10) - - - - - - - - - - 01 ☐
Cardiac disease - - - - - - - - - - - - - - - - 02 ☐
Acute or chronic lung disease - - - - - - - - - 03 ☐
Diabetes - - - - - - - - - - - - - - - - - - - 04 ☐
Genital herpes - - - - - - - - - - - - - - - - 05 ☐
Hydramnios/Oligohydramnios - - - - - - - - - 06 ☐
Hemoglobinopathy - - - - - - - - - - - - - - - 07 ☐
Hypertension, chronic - - - - - - - - - - - - - 08 ☐
Hypertension, pregnancy-associated - - - - - - 09 ☐
Eclampsia - - - - - - - - - - - - - - - - - - - 10 ☐
Incompetent cervix - - - - - - - - - - - - - - - 11 ☐
Previous infant 4000 + grams - - - - - - - - - 12 ☐
Previous preterm or small-for-gestational-age infant 13 ☐
Renal disease - - - - - - - - - - - - - - - - - 14 ☐
Rh sensitization - - - - - - - - - - - - - - - - 15 ☐
Uterine bleeding - - - - - - - - - - - - - - - - 16 ☐
None - 00 ☐
Other (Specify) - - - - - - - - - - - - - - - - 17 ☐

32b. OTHER RISK FACTORS FOR THIS PREGNANCY (Complete all items)
Tobacco use during pregnancy _____ Yes No
Average number cigarettes per day _____
Alcohol during pregnancy _____ Yes No
Average number drinks per week _____
Weight gained during pregnancy _____ lbs.
Pre-Pregnancy weight _____ lbs.

33. OBSTETRIC PROCEDURES (Check all that apply)
Amniocentesis - - - - - - - - - - - - - - - - - 01 ☐
Electronic fetal monitoring - - - - - - - - - - - 02 ☐
Induction of labor - - - - - - - - - - - - - - - 03 ☐
Stimulation of labor - - - - - - - - - - - - - - 04 ☐
Tocolysis - - - - - - - - - - - - - - - - - - - 05 ☐
Ultrasound - - - - - - - - - - - - - - - - - - 06 ☐
None - 00 ☐
Other (Specify) - - - - - - - - - - - - - - - - 07 ☐

34. COMPLICATIONS OF LABOR AND/OR DELIVERY (Check all that apply)

Fabrile (>100°F. or 38° C.) - - - - - - - - - - 01 ☐
Meconium, moderate/heavy - - - - - - - - - - 02 ☐
Premature rupture of membrane (>12hours) - - 03 ☐
Abruptio placenta - - - - - - - - - - - - - - - 04 ☐
Placenta previa - - - - - - - - - - - - - - - - 05 ☐
Other excessive bleeding - - - - - - - - - - - 06 ☐
Seizures druing labor - - - - - - - - - - - - - 07 ☐
Precipitous labor (< 3 hours) - - - - - - - - - 08 ☐
Prolonged labor (> 20 hours) - - - - - - - - - 09 ☐
Dysfunctional labor - - - - - - - - - - - - - - 10 ☐
Breech/Malpresentation - - - - - - - - - - - - 11 ☐
Cephalopelvic disproportion - - - - - - - - - - 12 ☐
Cord prolapse - - - - - - - - - - - - - - - - - 13 ☐
Anesthetic complications - - - - - - - - - - - 14 ☐
Fetal distress - - - - - - - - - - - - - - - - - 15 ☐
None - 00 ☐
Other (Specify) - - - - - - - - - - - - - - - - 16 ☐

35. METHOD OF DELIVERY (Check all that apply)
Vaginal - 01 ☐
Vaginal birth after previous C-section - - - - - 02 ☐
Primary C-section - - - - - - - - - - - - - - - 03 ☐
Repeat C-section - - - - - - - - - - - - - - - 04 ☐
Forceps - 05 ☐
Vacuum - 06 ☐

36. ABNORMAL CONDITIONS OF THE NEWBORN (Check all that apply)
Anemia (Hct. <39/Hgb. < 13) - - - - - - - - - 01 ☐
Birth injury - - - - - - - - - - - - - - - - - - 02 ☐
Fetal alcohol syndrome - - - - - - - - - - - - 03 ☐
Hyaline membrane disease/RDS - - - - - - - - 04 ☐
Meconium aspiration syndrome - - - - - - - - 05 ☐
Assisted ventilation < 30 min - - - - - - - - - 06 ☐
Assisted ventilation ≥ 30 min - - - - - - - - - 07 ☐
Seizures - - - - - - - - - - - - - - - - - - - 08 ☐
None - 00 ☐
Other (Specify) - - - - - - - - - - - - - - - - 09 ☐

37. CONGENITAL ANOMALIES OF CHILD (Check all that apply)

Anencephalus - - - - - - - - - - - - - - - - - 01 ☐
Spina bifida/Meningocele - - - - - - - - - - - 02 ☐
Hydrocephalus - - - - - - - - - - - - - - - - - 03 ☐
Microcephalus - - - - - - - - - - - - - - - - - 04 ☐
Other central nervous system anomalies (Specify) - - - - - - - - - - - - - - - - - - - 05 ☐
Heart malformations - - - - - - - - - - - - - - 06 ☐
Other circulator / respiratory anomalies (Specify) - - - - - - - - - - - - - - - - - - - 07 ☐
Rectal atresia / stenosis - - - - - - - - - - - - 08 ☐
Tracheo-esophageal fistula / Esophageal atresia 09 ☐
Omphalocele / Gastroschisis - - - - - - - - - - 10 ☐
Other gastrointestinal anomalies (Specify) - - - - - - - - - - - - - - - - - - - 11 ☐
Malformed genitalia - - - - - - - - - - - - - - 12 ☐
Rental agenesis - - - - - - - - - - - - - - - - 13 ☐
Other urogenital anomalies (Specify) - - - - - - - - - - - - - - - - - - - 14 ☐
Cleft lip / palate - - - - - - - - - - - - - - - - 15 ☐
Polydactyly / Syndactyly / Adactyly - - - - - - 16 ☐
Club foot - - - - - - - - - - - - - - - - - - - 17 ☐
Diaphragmatic hernia - - - - - - - - - - - - - 18 ☐
Other musculoskeletal / integumental anomalies (Specify) - - - - - - - - - - - - - - - - - - - 19 ☐
Down's syndrome - - - - - - - - - - - - - - - 20 ☐
Other chromosomal anomalies (Specify) - - - - - - - - - - - - - - - - - - - 21 ☐
None - 00 ☐
Other (Specify) - - - - - - - - - - - - - - - - 22 ☐

37a. PARENT(S) REQUEST ISSUANCE OF A SOCIAL SECURITY NUMBER FOR THIS CHILD
☐

| 38. NAME OF PROPHYLACTIC USED IN EYES OF CHILD | 39. DATE OF APPROVED TEST FOR SYPHILIS, IF NONE, STATE REASON | 40. DATE OF APPROVED TEST FOR GONORRHEA, IF NONE, STATE REASON |

HEA 2703
5112.06 (REV 7/92)

- Date and time of death.

- Place of death.

- If decedent was female, presence or absence of pregnancy.

- Whether or not an autopsy was performed. An **autopsy** is a postmortem examination to determine the cause of death or to obtain physiological evidence, as in the case of a suspicious death.

autopsy A postmortem examination to determine the cause of death or to obtain physiological evidence, as in the case of a suspicious death.

In most states it is against the law for an attending physician to sign a death certificate if the death was

- Possibly due to criminal causes.

- Not attended by a physician within a specified length of time before death.

- Due to causes undetermined by the physician.

- Violent or otherwise suspicious.

If any of these situations exist, a coroner or medical examiner must sign the death certificate. If a death occurs under suspicious circumstances, permission from next of kin is *not* needed for an autopsy to be performed. If the death did not occur under suspicious circumstances, however, consent from next of kin or a legally responsible party must be obtained for an autopsy to be performed.

When death has occurred under normal circumstances, after authorization has been obtained from the next of kin or from a legally responsible party, the body can be removed to a funeral home. In many states, the death certificate must be signed within 24 to 72 hours. The *mortician* or *undertaker* (person trained to attend to the dead) files the death certificate with the state. (See Figure 9-2 for a sample death certificate.)

If the deceased has not been under a physician's care at the time of death, the appropriate county health officer—usually the coroner or medical examiner—is responsible for completing the death certificate. A **coroner** is a public official who investigates and holds inquests over those who die from unknown or violent causes. He or she may or may not be a physician, depending on state law.

coroner A public official who investigates and holds inquests over those who die from unknown or violent causes; he or she may or may not be a physician, depending on state law.

The purpose of a coroner's inquest is to gather evidence that may be used by the police in the investigation of a violent or suspicious death. It is not a trial, but it is a criminal proceeding, in the nature of a preliminary investigation.

Some states employ a medical examiner instead of a coroner. A **medical examiner** is a physician, frequently a pathologist, who investigates suspicious or unexplained deaths in a community. As a physician, the medical examiner can order and perform autopsies.

medical examiner A physician who investigates suspicious or unexplained deaths.

Forensic Medicine

Forensics is a division of medicine that incorporates law and medicine and involves medical issues or medical proof at trials having to do with malpractice, crimes, and accidents. Forensic scientists investigate crime scenes and present medical proof at trials and hearings. Crime scene investigators are specifically trained to determine cause of death or injury and to help identify a criminal, a victim, and others involved in crimes. Specialists in forensic medicine study such subjects as forensic pharmacology, doping control, postmortem toxicology, blood spatter interpretation, DNA (deoxyribonucleic acid) analytical techniques, and expert testimony procedures. They work for police departments and other criminal investigative bureaus,

forensics A division of medicine that incorporates law and medicine and involves medical issues or medical proof at trials having to do with malpractice, crimes, and accidents.

Figure 9-2 A Sample Death Certificate

Ohio Department of Health
VITAL STATISTICS
CERTIFICATE OF DEATH

DO NOT WRITE IN MARGIN RESERVED FOR ODH DATA CODING

a. _____
b. _____
c. _____
d. _____
e. _____

Reg. Dist. No. _____
Primary Reg. Dist. No. _____

State File No. _____
Registrar's No. _____

DECEDENT

1. DECEDENT'S NAME (First, Middle, LAST)

2. SEX

3. DATE OF DEATH (Month, Day, Year)

4. SOCIAL SECURITY NUMBER

5a. AGE - Last Birthday (Years)

5b. UNDER 1 YEAR — Months | Days

5c. UNDER 1 DAY — Hours | Minutes

6. DATE OF BIRTH (Month, Day, Year)

7. BIRTHPLACE (City and State or Foreign Country)

8. WAS DECEDENT EVER IN U.S. ARMED FORCES? ☐ Yes ☐ No

9a. PLACE OF DEATH (Check only one)
HOSPITAL: ☐ Inpatient ☐ ER/Outpatient ☐ DOA   OTHER: ☐ Nursing Home ☐ Residence ☐ Other (Specify)

IF DEATH OCCURRED IN INSTITUTION. GIVE RESIDENCE BEFORE ADMISSION

9b. FACILITY NAME (If not institution, give street and number)

9c. CITY, VILLAGE, TWP., OR LOCATION OF DEATH

9d. COUNTY OF DEATH

10. MARITAL STATUS - Married, Never Married, Widowed, Divorced (Specify)

11. SURVIVING SPOUSE (If wife give maiden name)

12a. DECEDENTS USUAL OCCUPATION (Give kind of work done during most of working life. Don't use retired.)

12b. KIND OF BUSINESS/INDUSTRY

13a. RESIDENCE - STATE

13b. COUNTY

13c. CITY, TOWN, TWP., OR LOCATION

13d. STREET AND NUMBER

13e. INSIDE CITY LIMITS? (Yes or No)

13f. ZIP CODE

14. WAS DECEDENT OF HISPANIC ORGIN? (Specify No or Yes - If yes, specify Cuban, Mexican, Puerto Rican, etc.) ☐ No ☐ Yes Specify

15. RACE - American Indian, Black White, etc. (Specify)

16. DECEDENT'S EDUCATION (Specify only highest grade completed)
Elementary/Secondary (0-12)   College (1-4 or 5+)

PARENTS

17. FATHER'S NAME (First, Middle, Last)

18. MOTHER'S NAME (First, Middle, Maiden Surname)

INFORMANT

19a. INFORMANT'S NAME (Type/Print)

19b. MAILING ADDRESS (Street and Number or Rural Route Number, City or Town, State, Zip Code)

DISPOSITION

20a. METHOD OF DISPOSITION
☐ Burial ☐ Cremation ☐ Remove from State ☐ Donation ☐ Other (Specify)

20b. PLACE OF DISPOSITION (Name of cemetery, crematory, or other place)

20c. LOCATION - City or Town, State

20d. DATE OF DISPOSITION

21a. NAME OF EMBALMER

21b. LICENSE NUMBER

22a. SIGNATURE OF FUNERAL DIRECTOR OR OTHER PERSON

22b. LICENSE NUMBER (of Licensee)

23. NAME AND ADDRESS OF FACILITY

REGISTRAR

24. REGISTRAR'S SIGNATURE

25. DATE FILED (Month, Day, Year)

26a. SIGNATURE OF PERSON ISSUING PERMIT

26b. DIST. No.

27. DATE PERMIT ISSUED

CERTIFIER

28a. CERTIFIER (Check only one)
☐ CERTIFYING PHYSICIAN
To the best of my knowledge, death occurred at the time, date, and place, and due to the cause(s) and manner as stated.
☐ CORONER
On the basis of examination and/or investigation, in my opinion, death occurred at the time, date, and place, and due to the cause(s) and manner as stated.

28b. TIME OF DEATH M

28c. DATE PRONOUNCED DEAD (Month, Day, Year)

20d. WAS CASE REFERRED TO CORONER? ☐ Yes ☐ No

28e. SIGNATURE AND TITLE OF CERTIFIER

28f. LICENSE NUMBER

28g. DATE SIGNED (Month, Day, Year)

29. NAME AND ADDRESS OF PERSON WHO COMPLETED CAUSE OF DEATH (Type/Print)

CAUSE OF DEATH

SEE INSTRUCTIONS ON OTHER SIDE

30. PART I. Enter the diseases, injuries, or complications that caused the death. Do not enter the mode of dying, such as cardiac or respiratory arrest, shock, or heart failure. List only one cause on each line. TYPE OR PRINT IN PERMANENT INK

Approximate Interval Between Onset and Death

IMMEDIATE CAUSE (Final disease or condition resulting in death)
a. _____
DUE TO (OR AS A CONSEQUENCE OF):

Sequentially list conditions, if any, leading to immediate cause. Enter UNDERLYING CAUSE (Disease or injury that initiated events resulting in death) LAST
b. _____
DUE TO (OR AS A CONSEQUENCE OF):
c. _____
DUE TO (OR AS A CONSEQUENCE OF):
d. _____

PART II. Other significant conditions contributing to death but not resulting in the underlying cause given in Part I.

31a. WAS AN AUTOPSY PERFORMED? ☐ Yes ☐ No

31.b WERE AUTOPSY FINDINGS AVAILABLE PRIOR TO COMPLETION OF CAUSE OF DEATH? ☐ Yes ☐ No

32. MANNER OF DEATH
☐ Natural ☐ Pending Investigation
☐ Accident
☐ Suicide ☐ Could not be Determined
☐ Homicide

33a. DATE OF INJURY (Month, Day, Year)

33b. TIME OF INJURY M

33c. INJURY AT WORK? ☐ Yes ☐ No

33d. DESCRIBE HOW INJURY OCCURRED

33e. PLACE OF INJURY - At home, farm, street, factory, office, building, etc. (Specify)

33f. LOCATION (Street and Number or Rural Route Number, City or Town, State)

TYPE OR PRINT IN PERMANENT INK

f. _____
g. _____
h. _____
i. _____
j. _____
k. _____
l. _____
m. _____
n. _____
o. _____
p. _____
q. _____
r. _____
s. _____
t. _____
u. _____

HEA 2717
5152.06 Rev. 2/89

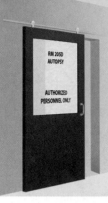

When a prisoner was executed in Tennessee on December 2, 2009, an autopsy was scheduled, since Tennessee state law mandates that autopsies be performed for all apparent "homicides" and "unnatural" deaths. The execution was not technically a "homicide," but it was an "unnatural" death, since the prisoner was healthy at the time of execution. Before he was executed, the prisoner had filed a religious objection to autopsy with his religious advisor, and the objection was also stated in his will. The state claimed it had "a compelling government interest" in performing the autopsy, but the court held for the prisoner's wife, who filed on his behalf under Tennessee's "Preservation of Religious Freedom" statute, asking for an injunction to prevent the autopsy from proceeding. The injunction was granted and the autopsy was not performed.

Source: Johnson v. Levy et al., No. M2009-02596-COA-R3-CV, Tennessee Court of Appeals, Nashville 2010.

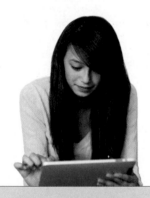

medical examiners' offices, universities, and other facilities and government agencies.

In the case, "Routine Autopsy Overruled," notice how one state law, which mandates when autopsies are routinely performed, is superseded by another protecting religious freedom.

check your **progress**

1. Define *vital statistics.*

2. Define *autopsy.*

3. Define *coroner.*

4. Define *medical examiner.*

5. Define *forensics.*

6. Where are birth certificates and death certificates filed?

7. Birth certificates must be filed for _____.
   Requirements vary with states for _____.

8. Name three circumstances in which an attending physician may not legally complete a death certificate.

Public Health Statutes

LO 9.3

Explain the purpose of public health statutes.

The power of the states to initiate public health statutes is inferred from the Tenth Amendment to the U.S. Constitution, included in the Bill of Rights. The amendment states: "The powers not delegated to the United States by the Constitution, nor prohibited by it to the States, are reserved to the States, respectively, or to the people." In other words, states retain police powers and all other powers not expressively granted to the federal government—a practice referred to as **federalism**—the sharing of power among national, state, and local governments.

In all states, public health statues help guarantee the health and well-being of citizens. As part of public health law, physicians or other health care practitioners must report births, deaths, certain communicable diseases, specific injuries, and child and drug abuse to the appropriate local, state, and federal authorities. Public health statutes vary with states concerning the reporting of fetal deaths and stillbirths, time limits for filing reports, and the manner in which information must be recorded. However, all provide for

federalism The sharing of power among national, state, and local governments.

- Guarding against unsanitary conditions in public facilities.

- Inspecting establishments where food and drink are processed and sold.

- Exterminating pests and vermin that can spread disease.

- Checking water quality.

- Setting up measures of control for certain diseases.

- Requiring physicians, school nurses, and other health care workers to file certain reports for the protection of citizens.

Since enforcing public health laws is vital to the health of individuals within communities, the states have enforcement power granted through each state's constitution. For example, the state can

- Require investigations be conducted in infectious disease outbreaks.

- Make childhood vaccinations a condition for school entry.

- Ban the distribution of free cigarette samples around schools or in areas where children congregate.

- Institute smoking bans or restrictions.

- Involuntarily detain (quarantine) individuals who have certain infectious diseases.

- Seize and/or destroy property to contain the threat of toxic substances.

Table 9-1 shows how laws affect public health issues.

Reportable Diseases and Injuries

LO 9.4
Cite examples of reportable diseases and injuries, and explain how they are reported.

Under each state's public health statutes, physicians, other health care practitioners, and anyone who has knowledge of a case must report to county or state health agencies the occurrence of certain diseases that, if left unchecked, could threaten the health and well-being of the population.

The list of reportable diseases is long and varies with the state. Requirements for reporting—such as time lapses and whether to report by telephone, mail, or online—also vary, so medical office personnel should be familiar with the specific requirements for reporting communicable diseases in their county and state of employment. Requirements for reporting and forms for reporting by mail are available from county and state health departments, either by mail or, in most cases, online. Those communicable diseases most likely to have mandated reporting by state statutes are diphtheria, cholera, meningococcal meningitis, plague, smallpox, tuberculosis, anthrax, HIV and AIDS, brucellosis, infectious and serum hepatitis,

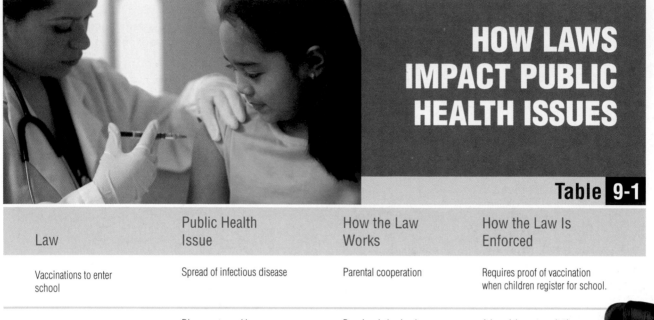

HOW LAWS IMPACT PUBLIC HEALTH ISSUES

Table 9-1

Law	Public Health Issue	How the Law Works	How the Law Is Enforced
Vaccinations to enter school	Spread of infectious disease	Parental cooperation	Requires proof of vaccination when children register for school.
Smoking bans/restrictions	Diseases caused by exposure to tobacco smoke	Requires behavioral changes	Admonishment or citations for noncompliance.
Child safety seat laws	Accidental injuries/death in children	Requires behavioral changes	Citations for noncompliance.
Fluoridation of public water supply	Dental caries	Requires no action on the part of individuals	Periodic checking of public water supply.
Spraying a community for mosquito control	Spread of infectious disease	Requires no action on the part of individuals	City government orders and pays for spraying.
Requiring pasteurization of milk sold for public consumption	Spread of infectious disease	Requires no action on the part of individuals	Milk is tested for pathogens before it is sold.
Restaurant inspections	Spread of food poisoning or other disease	Requires no action on the part of individuals	Local health department routinely inspects restaurants.
Food supply inspections	Spread of food poisoning or other disease	Requires no action on the part of individuals	FDA inspectors can initiate civil action, as well as criminal prosecution.

Source: Adapted from CDC's Public Health Law 101, Lesson 1, "Key Concepts of U.S. Law in Public Health Practice," PPt Slide 11. **www2.cdc.gov/phlp/phl101/**.

leprosy, malaria, rubeola, poliomyelitis, psittacosis, rheumatic fever, rubella, typhoid fever, trichinosis, and tetanus. Other diseases that may have mandated reporting if a higher than normal incidence occurs are influenza and streptococcal and staphylococcal infections.

Certain sexually transmitted infections (STIs) must be reported whenever diagnosed. *Sexually transmitted infection* is a general term that refers to any disease transmitted through sexual contact. Many STIs are transmitted through genital contact, which may or may not include sexual intercourse. For example, practicing oral sex can transmit gonorrhea from the genitals of one partner to the mouth and throat region of the other.

Reportable STIs differ with states but generally include gonorrhea, syphilis, chlamydia, lymphogranuloma venereum (Figure 9-3), chancroid, granuloma inguinale (genital warts), scabies, pubic lice, and trichomoniasis. Public health practitioners use reported cases to find and treat others who may have been infected through sexual contact with the named individual.

Most of the 50 states now have laws that require individuals infected with HIV to notify past and present sexual partners. The case, "State Law Mandates Notification," illustrates how Georgia's HIV notification law was tested in court in 2008.

On April 4, 2003, at the request of the Centers for Disease Control, President George W. Bush signed Executive Order 13295, adding severe acute respiratory syndrome (SARS), a form of viral pneumonia, to the list of communicable diseases for which federal isolation and quarantine are authorized. Thus, SARS joined cholera, diphtheria, infectious tuberculosis, plague, smallpox, yellow fever, and viral hemorrhagic fevers as communicable diseases detainable by the federal government.

Reporting requirements for communicable diseases are usually more stringent for patients who are employed in restaurants, cafeterias, day care centers, schools, health care facilities, and other places where contagion can be rampant.

Through extensive vaccination programs, many communicable diseases that decimated world populations in the past have largely been eradicated. In the United States, for example, smallpox has disappeared, and very few cases of poliomyelitis, typhoid fever, diphtheria, or measles are reported annually.

In some states, certain noncommunicable diseases must also be reported, to allow public health officials to track causes and/or treatment or to otherwise protect the public's health and safety. These diseases include cancer (to determine environmental causes); congenital metabolic disorders in

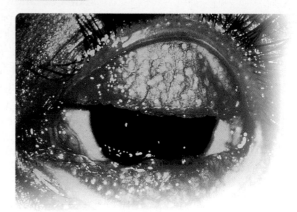

> **Figure 9-3**

" **Primary ocular chlamydial infection** of the eye. STDs (also called STIs) are often systemic infections. "

COURT CASE

State Law Mandates Notification of Sexual Partners by HIV Carrier

A woman convicted of reckless conduct for failing to notify a sexual partner that she was HIV positive appealed her conviction on grounds that her partner knew of her HIV status before she met him, because it was reported in the newspaper. The plaintiff who brought the original suit said he did not know of the woman's HIV status before they were intimate. Since Georgia state law requires individuals with HIV-positive test results or AIDS to notify sexual partners before intimacy, the woman's conviction was upheld by the appeals court. She was sentenced as a recidivist to the maximum of 10 years, with the first 8 years to serve in confinement and the 2 remaining years on probation.

Source: Ginn v. State, 293 Ga. App. 757; 667 S.W.2d 712; 2008 Ga. App.

In your opinion, should state laws require HIV-positive individuals to tell sexual partners of their HIV status?

What is the prevailing reason for such laws?

newborns, such as phenylketonuria, congenital hypothyroidism, and galactosemia (to allow for prompt treatment); epilepsy and some other diseases that cause lapse of consciousness (to determine eligibility to drive a vehicle); and pesticide poisoning.

The National Childhood Vaccine Injury Act of 1986

Parents usually begin programs of vaccination against certain communicable diseases for their children when they are infants. When children reach school age, most states ask for proof of vaccination for children entering the public school system for the first time. Since a small percentage of vaccinated children suffer adverse effects from the vaccine administered, parents or guardians are informed of risks associated with each vaccine and must sign consent forms allowing health care practitioners to **administer** the vaccine (see Figure 9-4).

administer   To instill a drug into the body of a patient.

> **Figure 9-4**   Sample Vaccination Consent Form

Patient Name _____

Clinic Name / Address

Address _____

Birth Date _____

Patient's Name _____

Phone Number _____ Physician _____

Health care providers, health care facilities, federal or state agencies, welfare agencies, schools, or family day care facilities may have access to this information. Immunization records remain confidential, and any person who fails to protect the confidentiality of this information is guilty of a Class 1 misdemeanor.

REFUSAL TO RELEASE INFORMATION: I have read or had explained to me the immunization information system. I understand the benefits of allowing my child's immunization record to be shared with other primary care providers and public health officials. However, I choose NOT to have my child's immunization record shared with other providers.

Signature (parent or legal guardian if minor): _____ Date: _____

Reviewed with parent by (initials): _____ Date: _____

Vaccine	Date Given	Vaccine Mfg.	Vaccine Lot No.	Site Given	*Initials	Parent/Guardian Sig.@
DT DTP DTaP 1						
DT DTP DTaP 2						
DT DTP DTaP 3						
DT DTP DTaP 4						
DT DTP DTaP 5						
MMR 1						
MMR 2						
*Hep B-P 1						
Hep B-P 2						
Hep B-P 3						
*Hep B-H 1						
Hep B-H 2						
Hep B-H 3						
OPV EIPV 1						
OPV EIPV 2						
OPV EIPV 3						
OPV EIPV 4						
OPV EIPV 5						

*Initials: Initials indicate VIS were provided and vaccine administered.

Signature of Vaccine Administrator

_____

@ I have been provided a copy of, and have read or have had explained to me, information about the diseases and the vaccines listed above. I have had a chance to ask questions that were answered to my satisfaction. I believe I understand the benefits and risks of the vaccines cited and ask that the vaccine(s) listed above be given to me or the person named above (for whom I am authorized to make this request).

The **National Childhood Vaccine Injury Act** of 1986 created the **National Vaccine Injury Compensation Program (VICP).** The reason for creating the VICP system was to relieve vaccine manufacturers and providers from having to pay judgments for vaccine injuries that, in turn, could lead to a shortage of vaccines due to the disincentive of legal liability. The VICP is a no-fault system designed to compensate those individuals, or families of individuals, who have been injured by childhood vaccines. The program serves as an alternative to suing vaccine manufacturers and providers, but does not take away an injured person's right to sue vaccine manufacturers and providers. The U.S. Court of Federal Claims decides who will get compensation as the result of problems caused by vaccines. Sometimes, a person may have a reaction to a vaccine that is not listed on the table (see Table 9-2). In such a case, the person or his or her family would have to prove that a vaccine caused the condition.

The **Smallpox Emergency Personnel Protection Act (SEPPA)** of 2003 established a no-fault program to provide benefits and/or compensation to certain individuals, including health care workers and emergency responders, who are injured as the result of the administration of smallpox countermeasures, including the smallpox vaccine. The program also provides benefits to anyone injured as a result of accidental smallpox inoculation through contact.

Following is a complete list of vaccinations recommended by the American Academy of Pediatrics, the American Academy of Family Practice, and the Advisory Committee on Immunization Practices of the Centers for Disease Control and Prevention (CDC):

- Hepatitis B (HepB or HBV): Four doses as follows: the first soon after birth; the second at 1 month of age; the third at 4 months of age; and the fourth at 6 to 18 months of age.

National Childhood Vaccine Injury Act A federal law passed in 1986 that created a no-fault compensation program for citizens injured or killed by vaccines, as an alternative to suing vaccine manufacturers and providers.

National Vaccine Injury Compensation Program (VICP) A no-fault federal system of compensation for individuals or families of individuals injured by childhood vaccination.

Smallpox Emergency Personnel Protection Act (SEPPA) A no-fault program to provide benefits and/or compensation to certain individuals, including health care workers and emergency responders, who are injured as the result of the administration of smallpox countermeasures, including the smallpox vaccine.

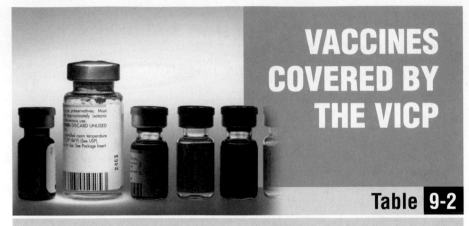

VACCINES COVERED BY THE VICP

Table 9-2

The following vaccines are covered by the VICP

Diphtheria, tetanus, pertussis (DTP, DTaP, Tdap, DT, Td, or TT)

Haemophilus influenzae type b (Hib)

Hepatitis A (HAV)

Hepatitis B (HBV)

Human papillomavirus (HPV)

Influenza (TIV, LAIV) [given each year during the flu season]

Measles, mumps, rubella (MMR, MR, M, R)

Meningococcal (MCV4, MPSV4)

Polio (OPV or IPV)

Pneumococcal conjugate (PCV)

Rotavirus (RV)

Varicella (VZV)

Any combination of the vaccines above

Additional vaccines may be added in the future

Source: **www.hrsa.gov/vaccinecompensation/covered_vaccines.htm.** Check the Web site to see if new vaccines have recently been added to the list.

- Diphtheria, tetanus (lockjaw), and pertussis (whooping cough) (DTP): Five doses administered at 2, 4, and 6 months; at 15 to 18 months; and at 4 to 6 years. Tetanus/diphtheria booster at age 11. Tetanus booster at 10-year intervals thereafter.

- *Haemophilus influenzae* type b (Hib): Administered at age 4 months and again at 2 years.

- Inactivated polio: Four doses: at 2 months, at 4 months, at between 6 and 18 months, and at 4 to 6 years.

- Measles, mumps, and rubella (MMR): Two doses, one administered at 12 to 15 months and the second at 4 to 6 years.

- Varicella (chickenpox): Administered during any doctor's visit at or after 12 to 18 months of age.

- Pneumococcal conjugate vaccine (PCV7): To protect against pneumonia, blood infections, and meningitis (a serious infection of the lining of the brain or spinal cord) caused by the pneumococcus bacterium. Four doses: at 2, 4, and 6 months of age, and at 12 to 15 months. Another form of the vaccine is given to children aged 2 years and over whose immune systems are vulnerable.
- Hepatitis A: Administered to children and adolescents in selected states and regions and to certain high-risk groups.
- Influenza: Administered annually to children aged 6 to 23 months who have certain risk factors, such as asthma, heart disease, sickle cell disease, human immunodeficiency virus (HIV), and diabetes.

Federal law requires that Vaccine Information Statements (VISs), prepared by the CDC, be handed out to recipients, parents, or legal representatives of certain vaccines. The VIS explains risks and benefits of a specific vaccine.

In 2006, the FDA licensed a vaccine for the prevention of infection with the human papillomavirus (HPV), administered via three injections over six months. Certain types of the virus can cause genital warts and other STIs in both sexes and cancer of the cervix in women. Because of the risk of cervical cancer, vaccination is recommended for females aged 9 to 26 years. For optimum protection, the vaccine should be given to girls before they become sexually active.

Vaccination as a Bioethics Issue

Whether or not to have their children vaccinated has become a dilemma for some parents. Since we seldom see diseases such as polio anymore, and some parents have never seen measles, we may tend to fear harmful effects caused by vaccines, rather than the disease itself. For example, several years ago a British physician named Andrew Wakefield noticed that 6 of the 12 children he was treating for a bowel disease also had autism (a brain disorder that appears early in childhood and affects communication, imaginative play, and social interaction). All 12 children Wakefield was treating had received the measles, mumps (Figure 9-6), and rubella (MMR) vaccine. Although the group he observed was small and Wakefield did not conduct a formal study, he published his speculation about a relationship between the MMR vaccine and autism in the British medical journal *The Lancet*. The media disseminated the idea of a relationship between autism and childhood vaccinations, possibly caused by a mercury preservative used in vaccines, and many parents became fearful that vaccinations could cause autism.

Later studies, including an often-cited study by Brent Taylor and colleagues at the Department of Community Child Health, University College, London (published in the June 12, 1999, issue of *The Lancet*), have concluded that there is no relationship between the MMR vaccine and autism. The CDC continues to maintain that there is no relationship, and the American Academy of Pediatrics continues to recommend the MMR vaccine for young children, but some parents remain fearful of vaccinations, even though the use of mercury as a vaccine preservative has been largely discontinued.

In 2007, the General Medical Council (GMC) of Great Britain began an investigation of Andrew Wakefield. After three years, the GMC found Wakefield guilty of professional misconduct, pronounced his research "unethical," and removed his name from the UK's Medical Registry. The council then advised British parents that it was "never too late" to vaccinate their children against measles, mumps, and rubella.

DIPHTHERIA TETANUS & PERTUSSIS **VACCINES**

WHAT YOU NEED TO KNOW

Many Vaccine Information Statements are available in Spanish and other languages. See www.immunize.org/vis.

1. Why get vaccinated?

Diphtheria, tetanus, and pertussis are serious diseases caused by bacteria. Diphtheria and pertussis are spread from person to person. Tetanus enters the body through cuts or wounds.

DIPHTHERIA causes a thick covering in the back of the throat.
   • It can lead to breathing problems, paralysis, heart failure, and even death.

TETANUS (Lockjaw) causes painful tightening of the muscles, usually all over the body.
   • It can lead to "locking" of the jaw so the victim cannot open his mouth or swallow. Tetanus leads to death in up to 2 out of 10 cases.

PERTUSSIS (Whooping Cough) causes coughing spells so bad that it is hard for infants to eat, drink, or breathe. These spells can last for weeks.
   • It can lead to pneumonia, seizures (jerking and staring spells), brain damage, and death.

Diphtheria, tetanus, and pertussis vaccine (DTaP) can help prevent these diseases. Most children who are vaccinated with DTaP will be protected throughout childhood. Many more children would get these diseases if we stopped vaccinating.

DTaP is a safer version of an older vaccine called DTP. DTP is no longer used in the United States.

2. Who should get DTaP vaccine and when?

Children should get 5 doses of DTaP vaccine, one dose at each of the following ages:

▪ 2 months   ▪ 4 months   ▪ 6 months
    ▪ 15-18 months   ▪ 4-6 years

DTaP may be given at the same time as other vaccines.

3. Some children should not get DTaP vaccine or should wait

   • Children with minor illnesses, such as a cold, may be vaccinated. But children who are moderately or severely ill should usually wait until they recover before getting DTaP vaccine.

   • Any child who had a life-threatening allergic reaction after a dose of DTaP should not get another dose.

   • Any child who suffered a brain or nervous system disease within 7 days after a dose of DTaP should not get another dose.

   • Talk with your doctor if your child:

   - had a seizure or collapsed after a dose of DTaP,
   - cried non-stop for 3 hours or more after a dose of DTaP,
   - had a fever over 105°F after a dose of DTaP.

Ask your health care provider for more information. Some of these children

should not get another dose of pertussis vaccine, but may get a vaccine without pertussis, called DT.

4. Older children and adults

DTaP is not licensed for adolescents, adults, or children 7 years of age and older.

But older people still need protection. A vaccine called Tdap is similar to DTaP. A single dose of Tdap is recommended for people 11 through 64 years of age. Another vaccine, called Td, protects against tetanus and diphtheria, but not pertussis. It is recommended every 10 years. There are separate Vaccine Information Statements for these vaccines.
Diphtheria/Tetanus/Pertussis 5/17/2007

5. What are the risks from DTaP vaccine?

Getting diphtheria, tetanus, or pertussis disease is much riskier than getting DTaP vaccine.

However, a vaccine, like any medicine, is capable of causing serious problems, such as severe allergic reactions. The risk of DTaP vaccine causing serious harm, or death, is extremely small.

Mild Problems (Common)

   - Fever (up to about 1 child in 4)
   - Redness or swelling where the shot was given (up to about 1 child in 4)
   - Soreness or tenderness where the shot was given (up to about 1 child in 4)

These problems occur more often after the 4th and 5th doses of the DTaP series than after earlier doses. Sometimes the 4th or 5th dose of DTaP vaccine is followed by swelling of the entire arm or leg in which the shot was given, lasting 1-7 days (up to about 1 child in 30).

Other mild problems include:

   - Fussiness (up to about 1 child in 3)
   - Tiredness or poor appetite (up to about 1 child in 10)
   - Vomiting (up to about 1 child in 50)
     These problems generally occur 1-3 days after the shot.

Moderate Problems (Uncommon)

   - Seizure (jerking or staring) (about 1 child out of 14,000)
   - Non-stop crying, for 3 hours or more (up to about 1 child out of 1,000)
   - High fever, over 105°F (about 1 child out of 16,000)

Severe Problems (Very Rare)

   - Serious allergic reaction (less than 1 out of a million doses)
   - Several other severe problems have been reported after DTaP

vaccine. These include:

- Long-term seizures, coma, or lowered consciousness
- Permanent brain damage.
  These are so rare it is hard to tell if they are caused by the vaccine.

6. What if there is a moderate or severe reaction? What should I look for?

Any unusual conditions, such as a serious allergic reaction, high fever or unusual behavior. Serious allergic reactions are extremely rare with any vaccine. If one were to occur, it would most likely be within a few minutes to a few hours after the shot. Signs can include difficulty breathing, hoarseness or wheezing, hives, paleness, weakness, a fast heart beat or dizziness. If a high fever or seizure were to occur, it would usually be within a week after the shot.

What should I do?

- Call a doctor, or get the person to a doctor right away.
- Tell your doctor what happened, the date and time it happened, and when the vaccination was given.
- Ask your doctor, nurse, or health department to report the reaction by filing a Vaccine Adverse Event Reporting System (VAERS) form. Or you can file this report through the VAERS web site at

---

Controlling fever is especially important for children who have had seizures, for any reason. It is also important if another family member has had seizures. You can reduce fever and pain by giving your child an aspirin-free pain reliever when the shot is given, and for the next 24 hours, following the package instructions.

www.vaers.hhs.gov, or by calling 1-800-922-7967.
VAERS does not provide medical advice

7. The National Vaccine Injury Compensation Program

In the rare event that you or your child has a serious reaction to a vaccine, a federal program has been created to help pay for the care of those who have been harmed.
For details about the National Vaccine Injury Compensation Program, call 1-800-338-2382 or visit the program's website at www.hrsa.gov/vaccinecompensation.

8. How can I learn more?

- Ask your health care provider. They can give you the vaccine package insert or suggest other sources of information.
- Call your local or state health department's immunization program.
- Contact the Centers for Disease Control and Prevention (CDC):
- Call 1-800-232-4636 (1-800-CDC-INFO)
- Visit the National Immunization Program's website at www.cdc.gov/vaccines

U.S. DEPARTMENT OF HEALTH & HUMAN SERVICES
Centers for Disease Control and Prevention

Vaccine Information Statement
DTaP (5/17/07)   42 U.S.C. & 300aa-26

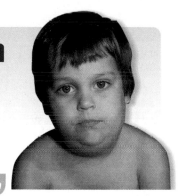

"Swollen parotid glands in a child with mumps.**"**

Children may be declared exempt from vaccination programs on medical grounds, such as HIV infection, organ transplants, or allergies to eggs used to prepare vaccines. Furthermore, since vaccination laws vary with states, in some states it is relatively easy for parents to opt out of vaccinating their children on nonmedical grounds. The downside of vaccination exemption is that children who are not vaccinated, or whose vaccinations are not up to date, are vulnerable to contracting serious infectious diseases that they can then pass on to others. The vaccination issue then becomes a public health concern.

The National Childhood Vaccine Injury Act initiated programs to educate the public about vaccine benefits and risks. The act requires physicians and other health care providers administering vaccines to report adverse events following vaccination and to keep permanent records on vaccines administered and health problems occurring after vaccination. Vaccine administrators are required to document the following in the patient's permanent medical record:

- The date the vaccine was administered.

- The vaccine manufacturer.

- The vaccine lot number.

- The name, address, and title of the health care provider who administered the vaccine.

The Vaccine Adverse Events Reporting System (VAERS), operated by the FDA and CDC, should be notified of any adverse event by the filing of a VAERS reporting form. Health care providers must report the following events:

- Any event listed in the Vaccine Injury Table, available at the Health Resources and Services Administration Web site and from the Health Resources and Services Administration Bureau of Health Professions, 5600 Fishers Lane, Rockville, MD 20857.

- Any contraindicating event listed in the manufacturer's package insert.

Reportable Injuries

In all states, physicians must immediately report to law enforcement officials medical treatment of patients whose injuries resulted from certain acts of violence, such as assault, rape, or domestic violence, so that authorities can investigate the incident. (In most states, spousal abuse is reportable only if the patient says his or her injuries are due to spousal abuse.) Reportable acts of domestic violence include child abuse, spousal abuse, and elder abuse.

Child Abuse Prevention and Treatment Act A federal law passed in 1974 requiring physicians to report cases of child abuse.

Child Abuse To help prevent violence against children, in 1974 Congress passed the **Child Abuse Prevention and Treatment Act,** mandating the reporting of cases of child abuse. All states have enacted legislation making child abuse a crime and requiring that teachers, physicians, and other licensed health care practitioners report child abuse and neglect. The report must immediately be made to the proper authorities—either in person or by telephone—and a written report is generally required within a specified time frame, such as 72 hours. Any individual reporting suspected child abuse is granted absolute immunity from criminal and civil liability resulting from the reported incident. Depending on state law, failure to report suspected cases of child abuse may be a misdemeanor.

Spousal Abuse Unlike cases of child abuse, most state laws do not specifically require a physician to report spousal abuse, unless a spouse states that his or her injuries were the result of spousal abuse. Legal remedies available to battered spouses vary from state to state, but all states have laws protecting victims of domestic abuse. Advocacy programs can explain legal

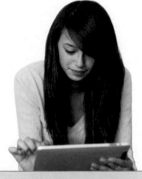

check your **progress**

9. State public health laws generally provide six areas of responsibility, which are

_____ .

10. In your opinion, why have most states passed strict antismoking laws?

11. Check the following areas where public health laws can apply:

_____ Public restaurants

_____ Public swimming pools

_____ Public schools

_____ Private homes where residents have communicable diseases

_____ Private schools

12. What provision has the federal government made for people who sue over vaccinations?

13. Why are certain diseases and injuries reportable to state authorities?

options to victims and can help them cope with the legal system. Courts may issue protective, or restraining, orders, or they may issue injunctions that direct the batterer to stop abusing the victim. In some states, police may be required to arrest batterers under certain conditions. Depending on laws within the jurisdiction and the type of offense committed, a batterer may be criminally prosecuted for assault, battery, harassment, intimidation, rape, or attempted murder.

Elder Abuse The Older Americans Act was signed into law by President Lyndon B. Johnson in 1965. The act created the Administration on Aging and outlined 10 objectives aimed at preserving the rights and dignity of older citizens. The 1987 **Amendments to the Older Americans Act** defines elder abuse, neglect, and exploitation, but does not deal with enforcement. The year 2000 *Amendments to the Older Americans Act* includes a five-year reauthorization for funding, maintains the original 10 objectives, and adds the National Family Caregiver Support Program for addressing the needs of caregivers to elderly individuals. The 2006 amendments to the original Older Americans Act covered a broad range of topics, including aging and disability resource centers, elder justice, elder health, the continuation of an elder justice, elder health, the continuation of a National Family Caregiver Support Program, nutrition, transportation, and other areas of concern for older individuals.

> **Amendments to the Older Americans Act** A 1987 federal act that defines elder abuse, neglect, and exploitation but does not deal with enforcement.

For current information about amendments to the Older Americans Act consult this Web site: **www.aoa.gov/aoaroot/aoa_programs/oaa/index.aspx.**

All 50 states and the District of Columbia have enacted legislation instituting reporting systems to identify domestic and institutional elder abuse, neglect, and exploitation. In most states, reporting suspected elder abuse is mandatory for certain professionals, including physicians. (If not mandated by state law, reporting may be voluntary.) Physical, sexual, and financial

COURT CASE

Spousal Abuse Leads to Criminal Prosecution

A California woman endured several years of abusive behavior from her husband, including injuries for which she was hospitalized. She finally divorced her husband, and received an injunction against him, but he continued to stalk his ex-wife, at one point showing up at her workplace. The woman remarried in early 2004, and her ex-husband then also threatened her husband. He told his ex-wife that if he couldn't have her, "no one would." The defendant was jailed twice, once for assaulting his wife while they were still married, and a second time for stalking. Each time the defendant was released from jail he continued to harass, threaten, and stalk his ex-wife and her husband. The defendant made several explicit death threats over the telephone, and finally showed up at the couple's home, brandishing a knife. When the defendant advanced on his ex-wife's husband, the husband shot him, wounding him in the groin. Police were summoned, and the defendant was tried on several counts involving death threats, stalking, and assault with a deadly weapon. Because of his previous incarcerations, and his alleged unrelenting abuse of his ex-wife, the defendant was sentenced to life in prison with the possibility of parole, after a minimum of 78 years.

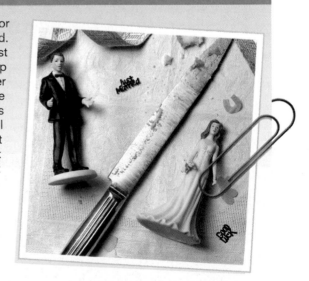

Source: People v. Haller, 174 Cal. App.4th 1080 (2009).

abuses of elderly people are considered crimes in all states. Some forms of emotional abuse and types of neglect may be considered crimes in some states.

In addition to laws regarding child, spousal, and elder abuse, some states have passed laws protecting vulnerable adults, such as individuals who are mentally ill and mentally challenged. Some states also have statutes dealing with the prevention of fetal abuse stemming from sniffing paint and other chemicals, taking drugs, or drinking alcohol while pregnant.

Unborn Victims of Violence Act Also called Laci and Conner's Act, a 2004 federal law that provides for the prosecution of anyone who causes injury to or the death of a fetus in utero.

The Unborn Victims of Violence Act In April 2004, Congress passed and President George W. Bush signed into law the **Unborn Victims of Violence Act,** also called "Laci and Conner's Act," after the December 24, 2002, murder of Laci Peterson, a pregnant woman, and her nine-month-old fetus, Conner. The act provides for the prosecution of anyone who causes injury to or the death of a fetus in utero, in cases where the federal government has jurisdiction. It also states that "the punishment for that separate offense is the same as the punishment provided under Federal law for that conduct had that injury or death occurred to the unborn child's mother." Before this federal law was passed, in most states a person accused of injuring or killing a pregnant woman was tried for offenses against the mother, but not for injuring or killing her fetus as a separate individual. State law determines whether an unborn fetus is considered a "person" in cases where a pregnant woman is assaulted or otherwise injured and, as a result, her unborn baby dies. For example, read the next case, "Is the Death of an Unborn Baby Always Considered a Homicide?"

Identifying Abuse Health care practitioners should be alert for signs of physical abuse, for purposes both of mandatory reporting and of possible

COURT CASE

Is the Death of an Unborn Baby Always Considered a Homicide?

In Colorado, a man being pursued by police during a high-speed car chase collided head-on with a car traveling in the opposite direction. The driver of the other car involved in the collision was a woman who was eight and one-half months pregnant. The woman survived her injuries, but the force of the collision caused an 80 percent abruption of her placenta. Her child was born alive, but died shortly thereafter from asphyxia. The death was ruled a homicide, and the defendant was charged with murder, as well as other charges arising from the car chase. The trial court dismissed the homicide charge, based on Colorado's definition of "person," which specifies (1) the individual is a human being; (2) the individual has already been born; and (3) the individual is alive. The prosecutor appealed the trial court's dismissal of the homicide charge, and the appellate court affirmed the dismissal of that charge, but remanded the defendant to be tried for reckless child abuse resulting in death, and vehicular assault, as well as other charges resulting from the high-speed chase.

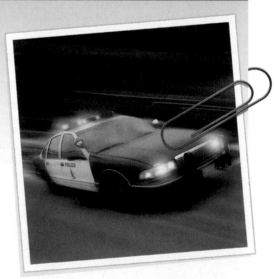

Source: People v. Lage, CO. Ct. App. No. 08CA0617, May 28, 2009.

As of February 2011, 35 states recognized the death of an unborn child, in certain circumstances, as homicide. For the current status of such laws, visit **www.nrlc.org/unborn_victims/Statehomicidelaws092302.html.**

intervention on behalf of the victim. It is imperative, however, that medical personnel not jump to conclusions and make unsubstantiated abuse reports.

Physical signs of abuse may include but are not limited to these:

- Unexplained fractures.
- Repeated injuries, especially those in unusual places or those shaped like objects such as electrical cords, hairbrushes, belt buckles, and so forth.
- Burns with unusual shapes (such as a circle, that may have been caused by a cigarette, or the mark of an object such as an iron).
- Friction burns apparently caused by a rope or cord.
- Bite marks.
- Signs of malnutrition or dehydration, such as extreme weight loss, dry skin, or red-rimmed, sunken eyes.
- Torn or bloody underwear.
- Pain or bruising in the genital area.
- Unexplained venereal disease or other genital infections.

Behavioral signs of abuse may include the following:

- Illogical or unreasonable explanations for injuries.
- Frequently changing physicians and/or missing medical appointments.
- Attempts to hide injuries with heavy makeup or sunglasses.
- Frequent anxiety, depression, or loss of emotional control
- Changes in appetite; problems at school or on the job.

Observation of individuals who accompany the patient may also identify a potential abuser. One might suspect abuse, for example, if, in the presence of additional evidence, an alleged victim of abuse is accompanied by someone who smells of alcohol, exhibits pensive or obsessive behavior, seems unusually or inappropriately emotional, or shows aggressive or otherwise suspicious body language toward the patient.

When a health care practitioner suspects abuse, care and tact must be used in eliciting information from patients. Direct, open-ended questions such as "Has someone harmed you?" may encourage a patient to relate what has caused his or her injuries.

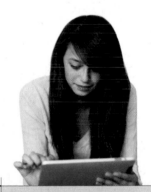

check your **progress**

14. You are a medical assistant in a physician office and you suspect a female patient has been abused. What signs might you look for that could indicate abuse?

15. If you see signs of abuse, but the patient does not admit that she has been abused, how might you proceed?

16. What types of injuries are health care practitioners required to report?

17. As a health care practitioner, should you report abuse if a patient asks you not to? Explain your answer.

18. In your opinion, why does the law require medical providers to report suspected abuse?

Health care practitioners should emphasize to the patient that information offered will be kept confidential, as required by physician–patient confidentiality, except in those cases in which the law mandates reporting abuse. Reporting requirements for abuse should be explained during the patient's first visit. Some sources recommend having patients sign a statement indicating that they understand the reporting requirements and agree with them.

Forcing the issue to encourage an adult to leave a batterer is not always the immediate answer. Similarly, providing hotline numbers, information on safe houses, or handouts about abuse may not be helpful if the batterer is waiting in the reception area for the patient or may later find the material and be further enraged. Instead, many medical facilities have bulletins posted in restrooms, telling patients where to call for help. If tear strips with the telephone number are provided, a victim can tear off the small, easily concealed strip for future reference.

LO 9.5

Discuss federal drug regulations, including the Controlled Substances Act.

Food and Drug Administration (FDA) A federal agency within the Department of Health and Human Services that oversees drug quality and standardization and must approve drugs before they are released for public use.

Drug Enforcement Administration (DEA) A branch of the U.S. Department of Justice that regulates the sale and use of drugs.

Controlled Substances Act The federal law giving authority to the Drug Enforcement Administration to regulate the sale and use of drugs.

prescribe To issue a medical prescription for a patient.

dispense To deliver controlled substances in some type of bottle, box, or other container to a patient.

Drug Regulations

The federal government has jurisdiction over the manufacture and distribution of drugs in the United States. The **Food and Drug Administration (FDA),** an agency within the Department of Health and Human Services, tests and approves drugs before releasing them for public use. This agency also oversees drug quality and standardization.

The FDA also has responsibility for major product recalls—a function vital to maintaining public health. For example, in August 2010 more than a half billion eggs were recalled from stores to prevent the spread of *Salmonella enteritidis* infections linked to the tainted eggs. About 1,500 cases of the infection were reported in the spring of 2010—the largest known outbreak associated with the strain of salmonella found in the eggs. FDA inspectors found widespread food safety violations in the barns of two Iowa egg producers where most of the eggs originated, including flies, maggots, rodents, and overflowing manure pits, and inspectors planned to visit all 600 of the nation's major egg-producing facilities within following months.

Both federal and state governments regulate the sale and use of certain drugs. At the federal level, the **Drug Enforcement Administration (DEA),** a branch of the Department of Justice, regulates the sale and use of drugs by the authority granted in the Comprehensive Drug Abuse Prevention and Control Act of 1970, commonly called the **Controlled Substances Act.**

General regulations mandated by the Controlled Substances Act require physicians who purchase, **prescribe, dispense,** administer, or in any way handle controlled drugs to follow these procedures:

- Register with the Drug Enforcement Administration through a division office. (A list of division offices is available online at the DEA Web site.) The physician will receive a registration number that must appear on all prescriptions for controlled substances and must be renewed periodically for a specified fee. Each DEA number is issued for a specific physician in a specific location. That location is the only one at which the physician may store controlled substances, including salespeople's samples. If a physician practices in more than one state, he or she needs a DEA number for each state. The physician must notify the appropriate state authorities and the DEA whenever he or she moves from a registered location.

- Keep records concerning the administering or dispensing of a controlled drug on file for two years. Such records must include the patient's full name and address, the reason for use of the drug, the date of the order, the name of the drug, the dosage form and quantity of the drug, and whether the drug was administered or dispensed.

- Note on a patient's chart when controlled substances are administered or dispensed.

- Make a written inventory of drug supplies every two years, and keep such records an additional two years.

- Keep drugs in a locked cabinet or safe, and report any thefts immediately to the nearest DEA office and the local police.

The Controlled Substances Act

The Controlled Substances Act is a federal law that regulates drugs under five schedules, based on their potential for abuse and their medical usefulness. If a drug has no potential for abuse, it is not listed as controlled. Table 9-3 lists the five schedules for controlled substances.

Drugs included in Schedule II and IIn require a properly executed, manually signed prescription. No refills are permitted on these prescriptions. All other scheduled drugs (Schedules III through V) may be prescribed on written or oral orders, and refills are generally permitted with certain limitations.

Whenever prescriptions are written for controlled substances, a copy should be filed with the patient's record. When a physician discontinues practice, he or she must return the registration certificate and any unused order forms (preferably marked "void") to the DEA. When it is necessary to dispose of controlled drugs, the physician or employee charged with disposal should contact the nearest field office of the DEA and the responsible state agency for disposal information.

State laws governing controlled substances may be as strict as or stricter than federal laws. Physicians may be required to register with the appropriate state agency as well as the DEA, and must follow all state and federal requirements in prescribing, dispensing, and administering controlled substances. Whenever state and federal regulations differ, the more stringent regulation must be followed. For example, if federal law requires that

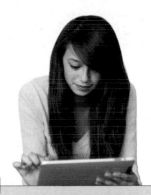

check your **progress**

Use these three terms correctly in the sentences that follow: *prescribe, dispense, administer.*

19. Dr. Wellness will _____ the drug to his patient, Mrs. Doe, when he starts an intravenous injection.

20. Under the law, medical assistants may not _____ drugs for patients but may _____ or _____ them under a physician's direct order.

21. When a pharmacist fills a patient's prescription, he or she then will _____ the drug to the patient.

22. What two federal agencies control the manufacture and standardization of drugs and their sale and use?

23. If state and federal regulations differ concerning the abuse of certain drugs, which law will be applied?

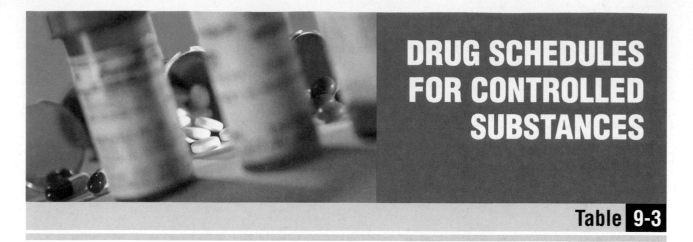

Schedule I

Potential for abuse is high and there is no currently accepted medical use of the drug or substance in the United States. Schedule I substances have been used strictly for research. Potential for abuse is determined by the following criteria:

1. There is evidence that individuals are taking the drug or other substance in amounts sufficient to create a hazard to their health or to the safety of other individuals or to the community;
   or
2. There is significant diversion of the drug or other substance from legitimate drug channels;
   or
3. Individuals are taking the drug or other substance on their own initiative rather than on the basis of medical advice from a practitioner licensed by law to administer such drugs;
   or
4. The drug is a new drug so related in its action to a drug or other substance already listed as having a potential for abuse to make it likely that the drug will have the same potential for abuse as such drugs. Of course, evidence of actual abuse of a substance is indicative that a drug has a potential for abuse.

Examples of Schedule I drugs include heroin, lysergic acid diethylamide (LSD), marijuana, and methaqualone.

Schedule II

Potential for abuse of these narcotic drugs is high, but there are currently accepted medical uses for the drug or substance in the United States, often with severe restrictions. Severe psychological and physical dependence is possible. Examples of Schedule II drugs include morphine, phencyclidine (PCP), cocaine, methadone, and methamphetamine.

A subdivision of Schedule II, called IIn, refers to nonnarcotic drugs with a high potential for abuse. Examples of such drugs include Dexedrine®, Desoxyn®, Preludin®, Ritalin®, and pentobarbital.

Schedule III

The drug or other substance has less potential for abuse than the drugs or other substances in Schedules I and II, and has currently accepted medical uses in the United States.

Abuse of the drug or other substance may lead to moderate or low physical dependence or high psychological dependence. Examples of Schedule III substances include anabolic steroids, codeine and hydrocodone with aspirin or Tylenol®, and some barbiturates. Schedule IIIn refers to nonnarcotic central nervous system depressants. These drugs include glutethimide, methyprylon, and barbiturates not listed in other schedules, as well as anorectant agents (suppositories) not listed elsewhere.

Schedule IV

The drug or other substance has a low potential for abuse relative to the drugs or other substances in Schedule III, and has currently accepted medical uses in the United States.

Abuse of the drug may lead to limited physical dependence or psychological dependence Examples of Schedule IV drugs include Darvon®, Talwin®, Equanil®, Valium®, and Xanax®.

Schedule V

The drug or other substance has a low potential for abuse relative to the drugs or other substances in Schedule IV, and has a currently accepted medical use in the United States.

Abuse of the drug or other substances may lead to limited physical dependence or psychological dependence relative to the drugs or other substances in Schedule IV. Cough medicines with codeine are examples of Schedule V drugs, as well as antitussive, antidiarrheal, and analgesic drugs.

records be held for two years and state law specifies five years, the state law takes precedence.

Since violation of a law dealing with a state-controlled and/or federally controlled substance is a criminal offense and can result in fines, jail sentences, and loss of license to practice medicine, physicians, other health care practitioners, and medical office employees should be familiar with all state and federal narcotics laws.

The role of the medical assistant concerning compliance with DEA regulations is to remind the physician of license renewal dates, to keep accurate records for scheduled drugs, to maintain an accurate inventory and inventory records, and to ensure the security of scheduled drugs kept in the office. This is accomplished by

- Checking to be sure that all controlled substances are kept in a locked cabinet or safe.

- Reminding the physician to keep his or her "black bag" in a safe place.

- Keeping all prescription blanks, especially those used for narcotics, under lock and key.

- Ordering prescription blanks that are serially numbered or otherwise printed to help detect alterations and theft.

- Reporting to the physician any behavior by patients that would suggest an attempt to secure addictive drugs.

- Checking patients' records to verify all prescriptions that may be questioned by a pharmacist.

Physicians and other members of the health care team must be familiar with the laws that govern such threats as communicable disease, physical abuse, and drug abuse because they play a vital role in helping maintain healthy—and ultimately safe—communities.

[CHAPTER SUMMARY]

LO 9.1 What are the vital events for which the government collects statistics?

- Live births.
- Deaths.
- Fetal deaths.
- Marriages.
- Divorces.
- Induced terminations of pregnancy.
- Any change in an individual's civil status.

LO 9.2 What is the correct procedure for completing a birth certificate?

- Type or legibly print all entries.
- Leave no entries blank.

- Avoid corrections and erasures.
- Where requested, provide signatures. Do not use rubber stamps or initials in place of signatures.
- File only originals with state registrars.
- Verify the spelling of names.
- Avoid abbreviations, except those recommended in instructions for specific items.
- Refer any problems to the appropriate state officials.

What information does a death certificate generally include?

- Disease, injury, and/or complication that caused the death and time treated before death.
- Date and time of death.
- Place of death.
- If decedent was female, presence or absence of pregnancy.
- Whether or not an autopsy was performed.

When are autopsies performed?

- When a death is suspicious.
- To determine cause of death, if cause is unknown.

When is a physician not allowed to sign a death certificate?

- When death is possibly due to criminal causes.
- When person is not attended by a physician within a specified length of time before death.
- When death is due to causes undetermined by the physician.
- In cases of violent or otherwise suspicious deaths.

LO 9.3 What provisions do all public health statutes have in common?

- Guard against unsanitary conditions in public facilities.
- Inspect establishments where food and drink are processed and sold.
- Exterminate pests and vermin that can spread disease.
- Check water quality.
- Set up measures of control for certain diseases.
- Require physicians, school nurses, and other health care workers to file certain reports for the protection of citizens.

What are some examples of the authority states have to enforce public health laws?

- Require investigations be conducted in infectious disease outbreaks.
- Make childhood vaccinations a condition for school entry.
- Ban the distribution of free cigarette samples around schools or in areas where children congregate.
- Institute smoking bans or restrictions.
- Involuntarily detain (quarantine) individuals who have certain infectious diseases.
- Seize and/or destroy property to contain the threat of toxic substances.

LO 9.4 Under public health law, what diseases and conditions are generally reported to public health departments?

- Diseases that, if left unchecked, could threaten the health and well-being of the population.
  - Infectious diseases.
  - Sexually transmitted diseases or infections.
- Other diseases that may have mandated reporting if a higher than normal incidence occurs.

Which no-fault federal laws compensate for vaccine injury?

- National Childhood Vaccine Injury Act of 1986.
  - Established National Vaccine Injury Compensation Program (VICP).
  - Smallpox Emergency Personnel Protection Act of 2003.

What information must vaccine administrators document in a patient's medical record?

- The date the vaccine was administered.
- The vaccine manufacturer.
- The vaccine lot number.
- The name, address, and title of the health care provider who administered the vaccine.
- Any adverse event listed in the Vaccine Injury Table.
- Any contraindicating event as listed in the manufacturer's package insert.

What injuries are reportable to the authorities under the auspices of public health?

- Spousal abuse
- Child abuse
- Elder abuse

LO 9.5 What two federal agencies oversee drugs in the United States?

- Food and Drug Administration (FDA).
  - Oversees drug quality and standardization and must approve drugs before they are released for public use.
- Drug Enforcement Administration (DEA).
  - Branch of the U.S. Department of Justice that regulates the sale and use of drugs.

What are the requirements for physicians who prescribe, dispense, and administer controlled substances?

- Register with the Drug Enforcement Administration through a division office.
- Keep records concerning the administering or dispensing of a controlled drug on file for two years.
- Note on a patient's chart when controlled substances are administered or dispensed.

- Make a written inventory of drug supplies every two years, and keep such records an additional two years.

- Keep drugs in a locked cabinet or safe, and report any thefts immediately to the nearest DEA office and the local police.

What are schedules under which controlled substances are listed?

- Schedule I—No proven medical use; usually used only for research.

- Schedule II—Potential for abuse high, but accepted medical uses.

- Schedule III—Less potential for abuse; have accepted medical uses.

- Schedule IV—Low potential for abuse compared to other schedules, but may lead to dependency.

- Schedule V—Low potential for abuse, but may lead to dependency.

What is the role of the medical assistant regarding controlled substances in the medical facility?

- Checking to be sure that all controlled substances are kept in a locked cabinet or safe.

- Reminding the physician to keep his or her "black bag" in a safe place.

- Keeping all prescription blanks, especially those used for narcotics, under lock and key.

- Ordering prescription blanks that are serially numbered or otherwise printed to help detect alterations and theft.

- Reporting to the physician any behavior by patients that would suggest an attempt to secure addictive drugs.

- Checking patients' records to verify all prescriptions that may be questioned by a pharmacist.

[ETHICS ISSUES Physicians' Public Duties and Responsibilities]

Two principles are often at odds when health care practitioners must deal with public health issues: the autonomy of each patient and beneficence. As discussed in Chapter 2, *autonomy* refers to the individual's right to make his or her own decisions. *Beneficence* refers to the moral obligation to act in ways that promote the health and welfare of others. As stated in Harman's *Ethical Challenges in the Management of Health Information*, "Beneficence and the closely allied principle of nonmaleficence ['first do no harm'] are among the primary justifications supporting public policies that interfere with the autonomy of individuals."

Ethics ISSUE 1: "Herd immunity" is one of the primary considerations for mandatory vaccinations in the United States. That is, when a large segment of the population is inoculated against certain infectious diseases, individuals—both vaccinated and unvaccinated—benefit, as well as the community as a whole. A true mandate for vaccinating all school-children in the United States has not been enacted since World War I. Today, every state except Mississippi and West Virginia has exceptions that allow parents to exempt their children from state vaccination requirements on the basis of religious or other personal beliefs. Recent epidemics of childhood diseases, such as measles, mumps, and pertussis, in the United States indicate that objections to mandatory vaccinations have increased.

Discussion Questions

1. In your opinion, does a parent's failure to vaccinate his or her child constitute a lack of social responsibility? Explain your answer.

2. Should one's concern for others supersede objections to vaccination on personal or religious grounds? Explain your answer.

3. Should your role as a health care practitioner include encouraging parents to have their children vaccinated? Explain your answer.

Ethics ISSUE 2: A young woman is diagnosed with a sexually transmitted infection and is subsequently reported to the public health department. A public health nurse visits her, but she refuses to name her sexual contacts.

Discussion Questions

1. Should the woman be compelled by law to name her sexual contacts? Why or why not? Does the best interest of the woman's sexual contacts and their contacts supersede the woman's right to privacy? Explain your answer.

2. What values are involved in Ethics Issue 2?

3. What is the first duty of health care practitioners caring for the woman in Ethics Issue 2?

Ethics ISSUE 3: Laws that require the reporting of cases of suspected abuse of children and elderly persons often create a dilemma for health care practitioners. The parties involved, both the suspected offenders and the victims, will often plead that the matter be kept confidential and not be disclosed or reported for investigation by public authorities.

Discussion Questions

1. Assume you are a member of the health care team that has repeatedly treated a woman for injuries that appear to have been inflicted by another. How might you phrase an opening question to learn whether or not she is the victim of abuse?

2. If the woman protests that she is simply "accident prone," how might you phrase your response? Would you drop the matter at this point or continue to question the woman?

_____

_____

3. What could you do to protect the woman if she does not admit abuse, but you are reasonably sure that she is being abused?

_____

_____

Go to **www.mhhe.com/judson6e** to practice your case review skills. Then read on for more information.

[KEY TERMS]

administer	dispense	National Vaccine Injury Compensation Program (VICP)
Amendments to the Older Americans Act	Drug Enforcement Administration (DEA)	prescribe
autopsy	federalism	Smallpox Emergency Personnel Protection Act (SEPPA)
Child Abuse Prevention and Treatment Act	Food and Drug Administration (FDA)	Unborn Victims of Violence Act
Controlled Substances Act	forensics	vital statistics
coroner	medical examiner	
	National Childhood Vaccine Injury Act	

[CHAPTER 9 REVIEW]

Applying Knowledge

Circle the correct answer for each of the following questions.

LO 9.1

1. A physician is required to report all of the following, except
   a. Births
   b. Deaths
   c. Abuse
   d. Stroke

LO 9.2

2. Which of the following is *not* recommended for completing birth and death certificates?
   a. Make entries in ink or typewritten form.
   b. Use rubber stamps for all signatures.

c. Do not skip any blanks.

d. Check entries for correct spelling.

3. Which of the following is *not* included on a death certificate?
   a. Cause of death
   b. Name of attending physician, if any
   c. Time of death
   d. Name of decedent's next of kin

4. Physicians may *not* sign a death certificate in which of the following situations?
   a. Death is suspicious.
   b. Physician was treating the patient.
   c. Death occurred in the home.
   d. Death occurred in the hospital.

5. Which of the following best defines a coroner?
   a. A public official who must be a physician
   b. A public official who is elected by popular ballot
   c. A public official who is appointed by the governor
   d. A public official who investigates and holds inquests over those who die from unknown or violent causes

6. A coroner or medical examiner signs a death certificate if
   a. The death is possibly due to criminal causes or is otherwise suspicious
   b. The death was not attended by a physician within a specified length of time
   c. The death is due to causes undetermined by the physician
   d. All of the above

LO 9.3

7. State public health laws derive indirectly from
   a. A federal law called U.S. Public Health Law
   b. The Tenth Amendment to the U.S. Constitution
   c. City ordinances
   d. None of the above

8. Which of the following best defines the term *federalism*?
   a. Cooperation among federal, state, and local governments
   b. Federal law is accepted as law of the land
   c. State law overrides federal law
   d. Municipal law overrides state law

9. Which of the following falls within the supervision of a state's public health department?
   a. Licensing of public health nurses
   b. Admitting cases of infectious disease to hospitals
   c. Mandatory vaccinating of schoolchildren
   d. Prescribing treatment for STIs

LO 9.4

10. Which of the following should be reported to the health department?
    a. Otitis media
    b. Strep throat
    c. Influenza
    d. Human immunodeficiency virus (HIV)

11. Which of the following will most likely require notification of the appropriate health agencies?
    a. Auto accident
    b. Staph infection
    c. Strep throat
    d. Phenylketonuria

12. Which of the following diseases should be reported to the state health department?
    a. *Escherichia coli* infection of the urinary tract
    b. Candida vaginitis
    c. Staphylococcal pharyngitis
    d. Tuberculous pneumonia

13. Which no-fault federal law compensates for childhood vaccine injury?
    a. Tenth Amendment to the U.S. Constitution
    b. National Childhood Vaccine Injury Act of 1986
    c. Smallpox Emergency Personnel Protection Act of 2003
    d. None of the above

14. Which of the following vaccination information is *not* documented in a patient's medical record?
    a. The date the vaccine was administered
    b. The vaccine manufacturer
    c. The vaccine lot number
    d. The date the vaccine was ordered

15. Which of the following injuries are reportable to the health department?
    a. A restaurant worker falls off a ladder while changing a lightbulb.
    b. A woman tells her physician that her broken ribs occurred when her husband beat her.
    c. A child is severely injured in an automobile accident.
    d. None of the above.

LO 9.5

16. Which of the following is *not* the responsibility of the medical assistant working in a facility where physicians prescribe and administer controlled substances?
    a. Checking to be sure that all controlled substances are kept in a locked cabinet or safe
    b. Reminding the physician to keep his or her "black bag" in a safe place
    c. Ordering prescription blanks that are serially numbered or otherwise printed to help detect alterations and theft
    d. Checking with the patient's pharmacist to be sure prescriptions have been filled

17. Prescriptions for which of the following categories of drugs may *not* be renewed?
    a. Schedule I
    b. Schedule II
    c. Schedule IV
    d. Schedule V

18. Drugs in this category have no accepted medical use and are used for research purposes only.
    a. Schedule V
    b. Schedule II
    c. Schedule I
    d. Schedule III

19. Who must be notified if controlled substances are stolen from a medical facility?
    a. All patients who currently have prescriptions for the stolen drug
    b. The state medical board
    c. The nearest DEA office and the local police
    d. The nearest FDA office

20. A medical facility must keep records concerning the administering or dispensing of a controlled drug on file for
    a. 6 years
    b. 9 years
    c. 10 years
    d. 2 years

21. Which of the following is *not* a requirement for physicians who prescribe, dispense, and administer controlled substances?
   a. Register with the Drug Enforcement Administration through a division office.
   b. Note on a patient's chart when controlled substances are administered or dispensed.
   c. Make a written inventory of drug supplies every two years, and keep such records an additional two years.
   d. Renew permits for prescribing and dispensing controlled substances every six months.

Match each definition with the correct term by writing the letter in the space provided.

_____ 22. Tests and approves drugs for public use.

_____ 23. Also known as the Comprehensive Drug Abuse Prevention and Control Act of 1970.

_____ 24. As a branch of the Department of Justice, regulates the sale and use of drugs.

_____ 25. Require reports of communicable diseases and certain injuries, as mandated by state laws.

_____ 26. Mandates reporting of child abuse.

_____ 27. Created a no-fault compensation program for health care practitioners and/or emergency responders injured by the smallpox vaccine.

_____ 28. The federal law that makes killing or injuring a fetus a crime separate from killing or injuring the pregnant mother, in cases where the federal government has jurisdiction.

a. Unborn Victims of Violence Act

b. Drug Enforcement Administration (DEA)

c. Smallpox Emergency Personnel Protection Act of 2003 (SEPPA)

d. Food and Drug Administration (FDA)

e. Amendments to the Older Americans Act

f. Controlled Substances Act

g. Child Abuse Prevention and Treatment Act of 1974

h. Public health statutes

CASE STUDIES

Use your critical thinking skills to answer the questions that follow each case study.

LO 9.4

One of a physician's patients, a well-respected citizen in a small community, saw the doctor with a complaint of blood in his urine (hematuria). The physician asked the patient if he'd had any new sexual partners recently, and the patient admitted that he had. The physician explained to the patient that his urine specimen had been positive for the STI chlamydia. The physician urged the patient to discuss his medical condition with the patient's wife, who was also the physician's patient, but the man is reluctant.

29. If the patient refuses to confide in the wife, what should the physician do?

_____

_____

30. What are the legal issues in this case? What are the ethical issues?

_____

_____

LO 9.5

Barbara, a medical assistant, noticed that her aunt, who suffered chronic pain from a neck injury, carried two bottles of Percodan in her purse. "Two doctors write prescriptions for me," Barbara's aunt confided, "but neither knows about the other. That's the only way I can get enough medication to control my pain."

31. In Barbara's place, would you report your aunt's deception to the physicians named on her prescriptions? Explain your answer

_____

_____

32. What would you tell your aunt?

_____

_____

33. How can physicians guard against such abuses by patients?

_____

_____

[INTERNET ACTIVITIES LO 9.1, LO 9.3, and LO 9.4]

Complete the activities and answer the questions that follow.

34. Visit the Web site for federal statistics at **www.fedstats.gov**. For what year are the most recent statistics available? How many births and deaths occurred in your state for that year?

_____

_____

35. Search the site for "leading causes of death," and list the top three.

_____

_____

36. Visit the Web site for the National Vaccine Injury Compensation Program (VICP) at **www.hrsa.gov/vaccinecompensation/**. Who is eligible to file a claim?

_____

_____

37. Find the Web site for your state's department of health. Which communicable diseases must be reported in your state? To whom must you report communicable diseases? What is the process involved? At this Web site, can you tell which diseases are prevalent in your state? How?

RESOURCES

Harman, Laurinda B., and Laurie A. Rinehart-Thompson, eds. *Ethical Challenges in the Management of Health Information,* 2nd ed. Sudbury, MA: Jones & Bartlett, 2006.

National Office of Vital Statistics. *Vital Statistics* (United States 2010).

www.hrsa.gov/vaccinecompensation/.

Sanchez, Raf, and David Rose. "Dr. Andrew Wakefield Struck off Medical Register." *The Sunday Times (UK)*, May 25, 2010.

2006 amendments to the Older Americans Act: **www.aoa.gov/aoaroot/ aoa_programs/oaa/resources/faqs.aspx.**

Andrew Wakefield: **www.timesonline.co.uk/tol/news/uk/article 7134893.ece.**

Centers for Disease Control and Prevention, Data & Statistics: **www.cdc. gov/DataStatistics/**.

Centers for Disease Control and Prevention, Health, United States, 2009: **www.cdc.gov/nchs/data/hus/hus09.pdf#highlights.**

Egg recall: Neuman, William. "Egg Farms Violated Safety Rules." *The New York Times*, August 30, 2010.

Federal site discussing vaccination (National Vaccine Program Office): **www.hhs.gov/nvpo/law.htm.**

State immunization laws: **www.immunize.org/laws/.**

State laws on HPV vaccinations: **www.ncsl.org/default.aspx?tabid=14381.**

Vaccine ethics: **www.vaccineethics.org/.**

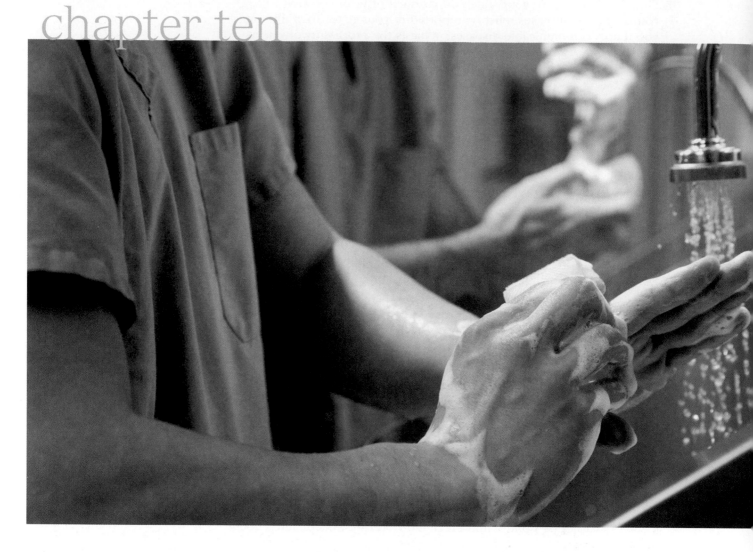

WORKPLACE LEGALITIES

Learning Outcomes

After studying this chapter, you should be able to:

LO 10.1 Identify how the workplace is affected by federal laws regarding hiring and firing, discrimination, and other workplace regulations.

LO 10.2 Identify four areas for which standards are mandated by the Occupational Safety and Health Administration (OSHA) for work done in a clinical setting.

LO 10.3 Discuss the role of health care practitioners in following OSHA standards for infection control in the medical office.

LO 10.4 Define the role of the Clinical Laboratory Improvement Act (CLIA) of 1988 in quality laboratory testing.

LO 10.5 State the purpose of workers' compensation laws and unemployment insurance.

LO 10.6 Determine the appropriate legal process for hiring employees and maintaining the required paperwork while the person is employed.

Cases in This Chapter

Employee Wins Wrongful Discharge Case in Missouri, 302

Fired Employee Sues and Wins, 303

A History-Making Sexual Harassment Case, 303

Employee Alleges Pay Discrimination, 306

from the perspective of . . .

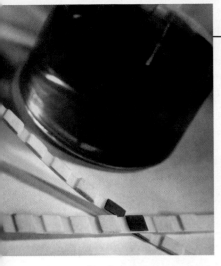

MARILYN is a supervisory medical technologist in the laboratory of a small clinic in the Midwest. Since the clinic does not employ phlebotomists to do blood draws, Marilyn performs this task, as well as all the analytical duties of a medical technologist. When asked the most frequent cause of analytical errors, she says preanalytical personnel practices, rather than equipment malfunction, are most often at fault. "For example, one day a technologist found that the instrument we use for analyzing urine dipsticks was consistently reporting positive for leukocytes on every patient. She asked me if the instrument needed to be checked, and I couldn't find anything wrong with it, so I watched her do a couple of analyses. The manual for the instrument emphasizes cleaning the work table daily after each use, and the technologist admitted that this hadn't been done. In fact, the work table hadn't been adequately cleaned for several days."

The technologist cleaned the work table before the next urine sample was tested, and no leukocytes were reported. "Apparently there was cross contamination from some previous urines with positive leukocyte readings. After that, the technologist made sure to clean the work table thoroughly and often. In the lab, we need to be especially careful about using the instruments according to manual instructions, and about preventing cross contamination of specimens."

From Marilyn's perspective as a laboratory supervisor, sloppy or inattentive work habits can cause inaccurate test results, which can alter a patient's course of medical treatment and cause unnecessary stress and sometimes legal action. Therefore, she generally observes the work habits of employees she supervises before assuming equipment malfunction.

From the technologist's perspective, she realized that urinalyses results were probably incorrect, and asked her supervisor for help. She was eager to correct any errors in preanalytical technique, and took steps to ensure her test results were accurate.

From the perspective of the patients who provided specimens for analysis, and the physicians who ordered the tests, employees who are vigilant and eager to improve job performance are the first line of defense against errors in medical diagnosis and treatment.

> In your opinion, how might the technologist have prevented the problem with urinalyses test results from occurring in the first place?
>
> Why is it important for health care practitioners to constantly check work habits and equipment—perhaps more so than in other occupations?

How the Law Affects the Workplace

LO 10.1

Identify how the workplace is affected by federal laws regarding hiring and firing, discrimination, and other workplace regulations.

This chapter provides an overview of workplace law, but it does not cover every employment statute and situation. For more detail, consult U.S. and state codes and/or an attorney specializing in employment law.

Many federal and state laws govern the workplace. Federal laws may apply only to those businesses with a certain number of employees (such as 15, 20, or 50) who work for a minimum number of weeks during the year. State laws may apply to those areas not covered by federal law, or they may extend or overlap existing federal law.

employment-at-will
A concept of employment whereby either the employer or the employee can end the employment at any time, for any reason.

Traditionally, employment followed the principle of **employment-at-will.** This meant that employees could be refused employment and could be disciplined or fired for any or no reason. In fact, either the employer or the employee could end the employment at any time. Now employment-at-will is affected not only by federal and state statutes, executive orders, and case law, but also by contracts between a worker and an employer, collective bargaining agreements between companies and unions, and civil service rules for government workers.

COURT CASE

Employee Wins Wrongful Discharge Case in Missouri

When a nursing home employee reported allegations of abuse to the Missouri Division of Aging, she was terminated and subsequently brought a wrongful discharge claim. The court found that the Missouri statute concerning reporting such activity created a clear public policy to report such suspicions, and she could not be terminated for having done so. In so finding, the court cited case law from other jurisdictions where employees had reported misconduct of the employer "either to their superiors or to the proper authority pursuant to statutes or ordinances."

Source: *Clark v. Beverly Enterprises-Missouri, Inc.,* 872 S.W.2d 522, 526 (Mo. App. W.D. 1994).

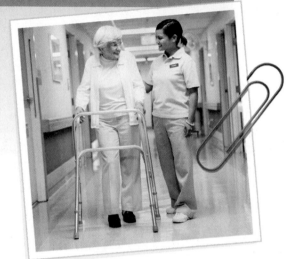

wrongful discharge
A concept established by precedent that says an employer risks litigation if he or she does not have just cause for firing an employee.

just cause An employer's legal reason for firing an employee.

public policy The common law concept of wrongful discharge when an employee has acted for the "common good."

discrimination Prejudiced or prejudicial outlook, action, or treatment.

Hiring and Firing

Employees generally cannot sue their employers simply because they have been fired, but an employer cannot fire an employee for an illegal reason. When no law exists that prohibits a specific reason for firing an employee, the discharged worker may have cause for litigation under precedent for **wrongful discharge.** Generally, in such cases the employer must have documentation that shows **just cause** (a legal reason) for dismissing the employee. Promises made to the employee orally, in a written contract, or in a company handbook may be used as evidence should a suit involving wrongful discharge be filed against his or her employer.

State courts vary in their willingness to accept the common law concept of wrongful discharge, but most recognize **public policy** or "common good" reasons for lawsuits brought by fired employees, such as refusing to commit an illegal act, whistleblowing, performing a legal duty, or exercising a private right.

Discrimination

Discrimination in the workplace—treating employees differently in hiring, firing, work assignments, or other aspects of employment because of personal traits or practices—is illegal. Federal laws prohibit employers from

COURT CASE

Fired Employee Sues and Wins

A discharged radiology technologist brought suit for breach of employment contract. Her complaint alleged that termination of employment-at-will was in retaliation for her refusal to perform catheterizations which were illegal for her to perform since she was not trained to do the procedure.

After the technician's dismissal, the New Jersey Board of Medical Examiners concluded that if she performed such an act she would violate the state's medical practice act. The New Jersey Board of Nursing issued a cease-and-desist order to the defendants to stop ordering unqualified personnel to perform catheterizations.

The court ruled that public policy was an issue, since the public has a "foremost interest" in the administration of medical care. The technician won her suit.

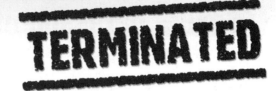

Source: O'Sullivan v. Mallon, 390 Atl.2d 149 (1987).

LANDMARK COURT CASE

A History-Making Sexual Harassment Case

A bank employee worked for Meritor Savings for more than four years. During that time she claimed that her supervisor continued to make sexual propositions. She finally complied, fearing for her job. She also claimed that her supervisor publicly fondled her and forcibly raped her. When she was fired after an indefinite sick leave, she sued for sexual harassment.

A trial court ruled for the bank, finding no *quid pro quo* discrimination, but the employee appealed, and the appellate court found in her favor. The bank appealed, but the U.S. Supreme Court upheld the appellate court's decision in the plaintiff's favor. In a precedent-setting pronouncement, the Court said, "A plaintiff may establish a violation of Title VII by proving that discrimination based on sex has created a hostile or abusive work environment." The court remanded the case to the district court for further proceedings.

Source: Meritor Savings Bank, FSB v. Vinson, 106 S.C. 2399, 91 L.Ed.2d 49, 447 U.S. 57 (U.S. Sup. Ct., 1986).

firing or otherwise discriminating against employees for any of the following reasons:

- Belonging to a particular race or religion, being male or female, or having a particular age or disability.
- Joining a union or engaging in political activity.
- Preventing the collection of retirement benefits.
- Reporting company safety violations.
- Exercising the right to free speech.
- Refusing to take drug or lie detector tests (with some exceptions).

Most states have passed laws that add to the federal list of prohibited discriminatory employment practices. Title VII of the Civil Rights Act makes sexual discrimination illegal, and sexual harassment is considered a form of sexual discrimination. In 1980 the Equal Employment Opportunity

Figure 10-1

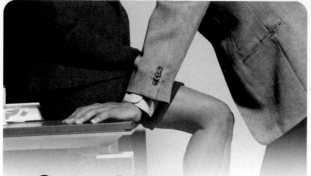

"Sexual harassment in the workplace violates the law."

Commission (EEOC) defined sexual harassment as follows:

Unwelcome sexual advances, requests for sexual favors, and other verbal or physical conduct of a sexual nature constitute sexual harassment when (1) submission to such conduct is made either explicitly or implicitly a term or condition of an individual's employment; (2) submission to or rejection of such conduct by an individual is used as a basis for employment decisions affecting such individual; or (3) such conduct has the purpose or effect of unreasonably interfering with an individual's work performance or creating an intimidating, hostile, or offensive working environment.

Parts 1 and 2 of this definition prohibit what is known as *quid pro quo* (from Latin, meaning "something for something") sexual harassment. Part 3 prohibits conduct that interferes with an employee's work performance or creates a hostile working environment.

Court decisions have affirmed that sexual harassment of employees, either male or female, is cause for legal action. Employers may be found liable even though an employee actually committed the offense. For example, if the offending employee is a supervisor, the employer is usually automatically held liable. If a nonsupervisory employee sexually harasses another worker, the employer is held liable only if he or she knew or should have known about the offense and did nothing to stop it (see Figure 10-1).

check your **progress**

1. Define *employment-at-will*.

2. Define *wrongful discharge*.

3. Define *just cause*.

4. Define *public policy*.

5. Who is liable if sexual harassment in the workplace occurs?

6. Sexual harassment may involve any of the following types of interaction: _____.

7. A federal law called _____ prohibits sexual harassment in the workplace.

8. The demand for sexual favors in exchange for employment benefits is called _____.

9. Sexual harassment can include unwanted physical advances, explicit sexual propositions, and

_____.

Federal Labor and Employment Laws

The following federal laws cover discrimination in hiring and firing, workers' wages and hours, worker safety, and other workplace issues.

Employment Discrimination Laws These laws address discrimination in hiring and firing:

> **Wagner Act of 1935.** This act makes it illegal to discriminate in hiring or firing because of union membership or organizational activities.

Title VII of the Civil Rights Act of 1964. This act applies to businesses with 15 or more employees working at least 20 weeks of the year. The law prevents employers from discriminating in hiring or firing on the basis of race, color, religion, sex, or national origin. Some states have laws that also prohibit discrimination based on marital status, parenthood, mental health, mental retardation, sexual orientation, personal appearance, or political affiliation.

Title VII also specifically prevents federal judges from using **affirmative action** plans—programs intended to remedy the effects of past discrimination—just to correct an imbalance between the percentage of minority persons working for a specific employer and the percentage of qualified minority members in the workplace. Federal judges can order affirmative action plans only when they decide an employer has intentionally discriminated against a minority group.

affirmative action
Programs that use goals and quotas to provide preferential treatment for minority persons determined to have been underutilized in the past.

Title VII created the U.S. Equal Employment Opportunity Commission (EEOC). The EEOC enforces Title VII provisions, the Age Discrimination in Employment Act, the Equal Pay Act, and Section 501 of the Rehabilitation Act. EEOC field offices handle charges or complaints of employment discrimination.

Age Discrimination in Employment Act (ADEA) of 1967. This act applies to businesses with 20 or more employees working at least 20 weeks of the year. It prohibits discrimination in hiring or firing based on age, for persons aged 40 or older.

Rehabilitation Act of 1973. This act applies to employers with federal contracts of $2,500 or more. It prohibits discrimination in employment practices based on physical disabilities or mental health. It also requires federal contractors to implement affirmative action plans in hiring and promoting employees with disabilities.

1976 Pregnancy Discrimination Act. This is an amendment to Title VII of the Civil Rights Act that makes it illegal to fire an employee based on pregnancy, childbirth, or related medical conditions.

Titles I and V of the Americans with Disabilities Act of 1990. This act applies to all employers with 15 or more employees working at least 20 weeks during the year. Titles I and III of the act ban discrimination against persons with disabilities in the workplace, mandate equal access for workers who are disabled to certain public facilities, and require all commercial firms to make existing facilities and grounds more accessible to persons with disabilities.

Civil Rights Act of 1991. This act provided two new important benefits for employees who prove discrimination: (1) Employees may collect punitive damages; (2) employees may collect damages for emotional distress associated with incidents of discrimination.

Genetic Information Nondiscrimination Act of 2008 (GINA). The act prohibits discrimination in health insurance and employment based on genetic information. It is discussed in more detail in Chapter 11.

Lilly Ledbetter Fair Pay Act of 2009. This law responded to the Supreme Court's decision in *Ledbetter v. Goodyear Tire and Rubber Company* (see the court case, "Employee Alleges Pay Discrimination"). It revised sections of the Civil Rights Act of 1964, the Age Discrimination in Employment Act of 1967, the Americans with Disabilities Act of 1990, and the Rehabilitation Act of 1973. The revisions were concerned primarily with statutes of limitation trigger dates, extending the class of plaintiffs to any individual who is "affected by" unlawful discrimination, and recovery of back pay.

Wage and Hour Laws The following laws address wages and hours of work:

1935 Social Security Act. Funded by the Federal Insurance Contribution Act (FICA), the act now encompasses "old age" and survivors insurance (OASI), public disability insurance, unemployment insurance (through the Federal Unemployment Tax Act), and the hospital insurance program (Medicare).

1938 Fair Labor Standards Act. This act prohibits child labor and the firing of employees for exercising their rights under the act's wage and hour standards. It also provides for overtime pay and a minimum wage. New FairPay regulations under the act went into effect on August 23, 2004. The new rules guarantee overtime protection to workers earning less than $23,660 annually and continue exemptions of the overtime rule for certain "learned professional employees." Some nurses may receive overtime pay, depending on how they are paid—hourly or by salary—and licensed practical nurses "and other similar health care employees" are guaranteed overtime pay under the FairPay regulations.

Equal Pay Act of 1963. As an amendment to the Fair Labor Standards Act, this act requires equal pay for men and women doing equal work.

Employee Retirement Income Security Act (ERISA) of 1974. This act regulates private pension funds and employer benefit programs. As part of its provisions, employers cannot prevent employees from collecting retirement benefits from plans covered by the act.

COURT CASE

Employee Alleges Pay Discrimination

Lilly Ledbetter retired from Goodyear Tire and Rubber Company in 1998 after working for 19 years as a night supervisor in the Gadsden, Alabama, plant—a job most often performed by men. Ledbetter discovered six years before her retirement that for most of her career she had earned 20 percent less than her male counterparts, and she filed a charge with the EEOC alleging pay discrimination. Title VII of the Civil Rights Act of 1964 specified that charges of unlawful employment practice must be filed within 180 days of the practice (some states allow filing within 300 days of the practice), but despite this statute of limitations requirement, a lower court declared Goodyear guilty of pay discrimination under Title VII. The case reached the U.S. Supreme Court, where Ledbetter argued that each paycheck she received was an unlawful employment practice and should reset the clock regarding the statute of limitations for filing a claim. The Supreme Court threw out the case on grounds that the statute of limitations, as mandated in Title VII, had run out. This triggered Congress to pass legislation dealing with the statute of limitations issue, and President Barack Obama signed the bill into law on January 29, 2009, eight days after his inauguration.

Source: Ledbetter v. Goodyear Tire and Rubber Company, 550 U.S. 618, 127 S. Ct. 2162 (2007).

While Lilly Ledbetter ultimately lost her case against Goodyear, her lawsuit triggered legislation that would help other employees with similar discrimination claims against their employers.

Workplace Safety Laws One important law addresses health and safety in the workplace:

> **Occupational Safety and Health Act of 1970.** This act ensures the safety of workers and prohibits firing an employee for reporting workplace safety hazards or violations.

Other Terms of Employment Labor and employment laws may also address employees' family emergencies and other family situations.

> **Family Medical Leave Act (FMLA) of 1991.** This act applies to employers with 50 or more employees. It mandates allowing employees to take unpaid leave time for maternity, for adoption, or for caring for ill family members.

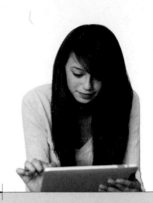

check your **progress**

10. What federal act makes it illegal for employers to discriminate against employees or potential employees on the basis of race, color, religion, sex, or national origin?

11. Which act protects the rights of pregnant employees?

12. Social Security benefits are disbursed under the authority of which act?

13. Which federal act would apply if a job applicant was denied employment because she admitted a family history of Huntington's disease?

14. Which law affected trigger dates for the statute of limitations on alleged acts of discrimination in the workplace?

Employee Safety and Welfare

Certain federal and state laws provide specifically for employee safety and welfare. Major areas covered include workplace safety, including medical hazards, job-related injuries and illnesses, and unemployment or reemployment.

Occupational Safety and Health Administration (OSHA)

In the 1960s job-related disabilities and injuries caused more lost workdays in U.S. companies than did strikes. As a result of increasing concern over such statistics, in 1970 Congress passed the Occupational Safety and Health Act. The act established the **Occupational Safety and Health Administration (OSHA),** charged with writing and enforcing compulsory standards for health and safety in the workplace.

The act covers all employers and employees, with few exceptions. Standards cover four areas of employment—general industry, maritime, construction, and agriculture—and include regulations for the physical workplace, machinery and equipment, materials, power sources, processing, protective clothing, first aid, and workplace administration.

All employers must know those standards that apply to their business. The *Federal Register,* a U.S. government publication that contains all administrative laws, is the primary source of information for OSHA standards.

Under the authority of the U.S. secretary of labor, OSHA inspectors may conduct workplace inspections unannounced; issue citations to employers for violations of the act; and, in some cases, levy fines. The millions of workplaces covered by the Occupation Safety and Health Act cannot

LO 10.2

Identify four areas for which standards are mandated by the Occupational Safety and Health Administration (OSHA) for work done in a clinical setting.

> **Occupational Safety and Health Administration (OSHA)** Established by the Occupational Safety and Health Act of 1970, the organization that is charged with writing and enforcing compulsory standards for health and safety in the workplace.

be inspected at one time; therefore priorities have been established for inspecting the worst situations first. The priority of workplace inspections is as follows:

1. Imminent danger situations receive top priority. An imminent danger is any condition where there is reasonable certainty that a danger exists that can be expected to cause death or serious physical harm immediately or before the danger can be eliminated through normal enforcement procedures.

   If an OSHA inspector finds an imminent danger situation, he or she will ask the employer to voluntarily remedy the situation so that employees are no longer exposed to the dangerous situation. If the employer fails to do this, an OSHA compliance officer may apply to the federal district court for an injunction to stop work until unsafe conditions are corrected.

2. Second priority goes to the investigation of fatalities and accidents resulting in a death or hospitalization of three or more employees. The employer must report such catastrophes to OSHA within 8 hours. OSHA investigates to determine the cause of these accidents and whether existing OSHA standards were violated.

3. Third priority goes to formal employee complaints of unsafe or unhealthful working conditions and to referrals from any source about a workplace hazard. The act gives each employee the right to request an OSHA inspection when the employee believes he or she is in imminent danger from a hazard or when he or she thinks that there is a violation of an OSHA standard that threatens physical harm. OSHA will maintain confidentiality if requested, and will inform the employee of any action taken.

4. Fourth in priority are programmed inspections aimed at specific high-hazard industries, workplaces, occupations, or health substances, or other industries identified in OSHA's current inspection procedures. OSHA selects industries for inspection on the basis of factors such as the injury incidence rates, previous citation history, employee exposure to toxic substances, or random selection.

5. Last on the list of priorities for OSHA inspections are follow-up inspections. A follow-up inspection determines if the employer has corrected previously cited violations. If an employer has failed to abate a violation, the OSHA compliance officer informs the employer that he or she is subject to "Failure to Abate" alleged violations. This involves proposed additional daily penalties until the employer corrects the violation.

Fines are imposed as penalties for violations. Employers and employees may appeal under some circumstances.

Under OSHA standards, both employers and employees have certain rights and responsibilities. Employers must provide a hazard-free workplace and comply with all applicable OSHA standards. Employers must also inform all employees about OSHA safety and health requirements, keep certain records, and compile and post an annual summary of work-related injuries and illnesses. It is the employer's responsibility to ensure that employees wear safety equipment when necessary, to provide safety training, and to discipline employees for violation of safety rules. The law prohibits employers from retaliating in any way against employees who file complaints under the act.

For their part, employees must comply with all applicable OSHA standards, report hazardous conditions, follow all safety and health rules established by the employer, and use protective equipment when necessary. Many states have employee **right-to-know laws,** which allow employees

right-to-know laws State laws that allow employees access to information about toxic or hazardous substances, employer duties, employee rights, and other workplace health and safety issues.

Hazard Communication Standard (HCS) An OSHA standard intended to increase health care practitioners' awareness of risks, improve work practices and appropriate use of personal protective equipment, and reduce injuries and illnesses in the workplace.

access to information about toxic or hazardous substances, employer duties, employee rights, and other health and safety issues.

Federal OSHA authority extends to all private sector employers with one or more employees, as well as to federal civilian employees. In addition, many states administer their own occupational safety and health programs through plans approved under section 18(b) of the federal OSHA act.

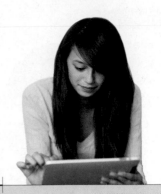

check your **progress**

15. OSHA provides for _____ in the workplace.

16. The primary source of information for OSHA standards is _____.

17. What state laws allow employees access to information about toxic or hazardous substances?

18. As an employee in a health care facility, what are your general responsibilities under OSHA standards?

Infection Control in the Medical Office

OSHA Health Standards and CDC Guidelines

OSHA standards for medical settings and health care workers often are influenced by and/or closely associated with guidelines issued by the Centers for Disease Control and Prevention (CDC). Following are a few of the OSHA standards and CDC guidelines that most often affect health care practitioners working in medical settings.

Medical Hazard Regulations The **Hazard Communication Standard (HCS)** is an OSHA standard that is intended to increase health care practitioners' awareness of risk, improve work practices and appropriate use of personal protective equipment, and reduce injuries and illnesses (see Figures 10-2 and 10-3).

Under the HCS, medical offices must have a written hazard communication program. A list of all office hazards must be compiled, posted on bulletin boards, and placed in a hazard communication manual. The list must include hazardous chemicals, hazardous equipment, and hazardous wastes. Hazards often found in the medical office include disinfectant sprays and lab reagents, electrical and mechanical equipment, and blood and body fluids.

Employers must obtain a Material Safety Data Sheet (MSDS) for each hazardous chemical in use in the office. These sheets should be kept on file, and new ones should be placed in a binder where employees can readily review them. Manufacturers must supply MSDSs when requested. Each hazardous

LO 10.3
Discuss the role of health care practitioners in following OSHA standards for infection control in the medical office.

▶ **Figure 10-2**

"OSHA and CDC regulations govern safety
in medical laboratories. Medical laboratory personnel wearing biohazard suits."

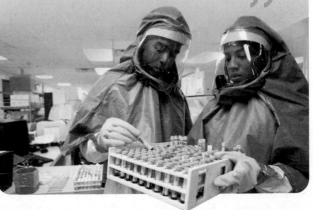

Figure 10-3

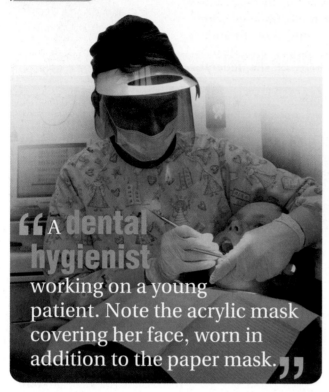

"A dental hygienist working on a young patient. Note the acrylic mask covering her face, worn in addition to the paper mask.**"**

product in use must have a hazard label which is a condensed version of the MSDS (see Figure 10-4).

Employees must determine what hazardous chemicals are used, initial and date new MSDSs as they are read, and initial and date records of safety training. Health care practitioners should see that a hazard communication manual is kept up to date and is accessible to all coworkers. Under the **General Duty Clause** of the HCS, any equipment that may pose a health risk is included as a hazard. This clause covers all areas for which OSHA has not developed specific standards and holds the employer ultimately responsible for the safety of employees: "Each employer shall furnish a place of employment which is free from recognized hazards that are causing or are likely to cause death or serious physical harm to his/her employees."

Chemical Hygiene Plan The Standard for Occupational Exposures to Hazardous Chemicals in Laboratories, or the **Chemical Hygiene Plan,** further clarifies the proper handling of hazardous chemicals in medical laboratories.

Occupational Exposure to Bloodborne Pathogen Standard The **Occupational Exposure to Bloodborne Pathogen Standard** is an OSHA regulation passed in 1991. The standard is designed to protect workers in health care and related occupations from the risk of exposure to bloodborne *pathogens* (disease-causing organisms) such as the human immunodeficiency virus (HIV) and the hepatitis B virus (HBV). The standard requires posting of safety guidelines, exposure incident reporting, and formulation of a written exposure control plan that outlines the protective measures an employer will take to eliminate or minimize employee exposure to blood and other body fluids. The plan must be available to OSHA inspectors and to employees.

As mandated by the Needlestick Safety and Prevention Act, passed by Congress in 2000, the Occupational Exposure to Bloodborne Pathogen Standard, 29 CFR 1910.1030, was revised in 2001 to include new provisions requiring employers to maintain a sharps injury log and to involve non-managerial employees in selecting safer medical devices.

General Duty Clause
A section of the Hazard Communication Standard stating that any equipment that may pose a health risk must be specified as a hazard.

Chemical Hygiene Plan
The Standard for Occupational Exposures to Hazardous Chemicals in Laboratories, which clarifies the handling of hazardous chemicals in medical laboratories.

Figure 10-4

" Usually one practice employee is responsible for filing all **material safety data sheets,** and for making sure that other employees review them. Since MSDSs can be several pages long, a binder is often the choice for displaying them. **"**

By authority of the Bloodborne Pathogen Standard, OSHA can levy fines for violations leading to employee exposure to bloodborne pathogens, based on guidelines issued by the CDC. The CDC's Guidelines for Universal Precautions for Hospitals can apply to any laboratory and include the following:

- Do not contaminate the outside of containers when collecting specimens. All specimen containers should have secure lids.

- Wear gloves when processing patients' specimens, including blood, body fluids containing blood, and other fluids. Masks and goggles should be worn if splashing or aerosolization may occur. Change gloves and wash hands after handling each specimen.

- Use biological safety cabinets for blending and vigorous mixing whenever there is a potential for droplets.

- Do not pipette fluids by mouth. Use mechanical pipetting devices.

- Use extreme caution when handling needles. Do not bend, recap, or remove needles from disposable syringes. Place entire needle assembly in a clearly marked puncture-resistant, leak-proof container.

- Decontaminate work surfaces with a chemical germicide after spills and daily when work is completed. (A clean work surface proved essential in the laboratory scenario at the beginning of this chapter.)

- Clearly and permanently label tissue or serum specimens to be stored as potentially hazardous.

- Never eat, drink, smoke, or apply cosmetics or lip balm in the laboratory.

- Remove protective clothing, and wash hands before leaving the laboratory. (In compliance with this guideline, technologists in Marilyn's medical clinic wear gloves, eye shields, and laboratory coats over street clothes when performing certain duties.)

> **Occupational Exposure to Bloodborne Pathogen Standard** An OSHA regulation designed to protect health care workers from the risk of exposure to bloodborne pathogens.

Medical Waste Tracking Act By authority of the **Medical Waste Tracking Act,** OSHA may inspect hazardous medical wastes and will cite medical facilities for unsafe or unhealthy practices regarding these wastes. Hazardous medical wastes include but are not limited to blood products, body fluids, tissues, cultures, vaccines (live and weakened), sharps, table paper (with body fluids on them), gloves, speculums, cotton swabs, and inoculating loops.

A puncture-proof, leak-proof, approved sharps container must be provided for the disposal of sharp objects. Chemicals should be discarded in a glass or metal container. Flushable chemicals can be washed down the drain with large quantities of water. Other hazardous medical wastes must be contained in plastic, leak-proof biohazard bags. Incineration is often used to dispose of medical wastes. Reputable, licensed waste handlers should be used to handle this material.

> **Medical Waste Tracking Act** The federal law that authorizes OSHA to inspect hazardous medical wastes and to cite offices for unsafe or unhealthy practices regarding these wastes.

Training and Accident Report Documentation Under OSHA standards, each employer must have a written training program detailing how employees will be provided with information and training regarding hazards in the workplace. Training should include information about hazards in the work area, the location of the list of hazards and MSDSs, explanations of MSDSs and the hazardous chemical labeling system, and any measures that employees can take to protect themselves against these hazards. Training logs should be kept, and employees who complete training should sign and date the log.

Accidents occurring in the office must be reported. Reports should include

- Employer's name, address, and phone number.

- Employee's name, address, and phone number.

- Specific information about the accident—when, where, what, and how it occurred.

- Nature of the injury.

- Follow-up information, such as medical treatment or hospitalization.

Each employer who is subject to OSHA record-keeping requirements must maintain a log of all occupational injuries and illnesses. Logs must be kept for five years following the end of the calendar year to which they relate and must be available for inspection by representatives of the U.S. Department of Labor, the U.S. Department of Health and Human Services, and state officials.

OSHA standards for health care settings may be obtained from U.S. Department of Labor, Occupational Safety and Health Administration, Directorate of Health Standards Programs, 200 Constitution Ave. NW, Washington, DC 20210, from state or regional OSHA offices, and from the OSHA Web site at **www.osha.gov**.

Centers for Disease Control and Prevention (CDC) Guidelines

CDC guidelines have always recommended that health care practitioners wear gloves, eye masks, gowns, and other protective equipment when performing such tasks as capillary puncture, phlebotomy, pelvic exams, minor suturing, and throat culture. Health care workers should also wear protective equipment when performing tasks that do not involve direct contact with blood, body fluids, or tissue, in case accidental exposure occurs. These tasks include urinalysis, blood testing, examination of fecal occult blood, injections, positioning for X-rays, performing ultrasound and ECG tests, and examination of sweat, tears, and nasal secretions.

Most recently, the CDC publishes a comprehensive online guide for all health care workers entitled *Guideline for Isolation Precautions: Preventing Transmission of Infectious Agents in Healthcare Settings*, available at **www.cdc.gov/hicpac/pdf/isolation/Isolation2007.pdf.** The document "is intended for use by infection control staff, healthcare epidemiologists, healthcare administrators, nurses, other healthcare providers, and persons responsible for developing, implementing, and evaluating infection control programs for healthcare settings across the continuum of care." It contains references to other guidelines and Web sites for more detailed information and for recommendations concerning specialized infection control problems, such as preventing surgical site infections, recommendations for the prevention, treatment, and control of tuberculosis, prevention of intervascular catheter infections, hand hygiene, and so on.

LO 10.4

Define the role of the Clinical Laboratory Improvement Act (CLIA) of 1988 in quality laboratory testing.

Clinical Laboratory Improvement Act (CLIA) Also called Clinical Laboratory Improvement Amendments. Federal statute passed in 1988 that established minimum quality standards for all laboratory testing.

Clinical Laboratory Improvement Act (CLIA)

The **Clinical Laboratory Improvement Act (CLIA)** of 1988, also called the Clinical Laboratory Improvement Amendments, replaced 1967 laboratory testing legislation that established standards for Medicare and Medicaid. The act established minimum quality standards for all laboratory testing and has been extensively amended since it was first written. The regulations define a laboratory as any facility that performs laboratory testing on specimens derived from humans for diagnosing, preventing, or treating disease or for assessing health. The law requires that laboratories obtain certification, pay applicable fees, and follow regulations concerning testing, personnel, inspections, test management, quality control, and quality assurance.

The Division of Laboratory Services, within the Survey and Certification Group, under the Center for Medicaid and State Operations (CMSO) has the responsibility for implementing the CLIA program. The Federal Drug Administration has responsibility for some CLIA functions. More information about Clinical Laboratory Improvement Act/Amendments is available online at **www.cms.gov/clia/**.

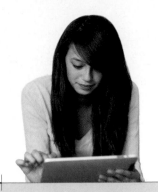

check your **progress**

19. For the facility described in this chapter's opening scenario, which OSHA standards, and/or CDC guidelines discussed earlier would apply?

20. What protective gear does the CDC recommend for laboratory employees?

21. What specific health care procedures/facilities does the Clinical Laboratory Improvement Act cover?

22. Are there penalties for violating any of the OSHA standards concerned with safety in the workplace? Explain your answer.

Workers' Compensation and Unemployment Insurance

Workers' Compensation

Federal and state **workers' compensation** laws establish procedures for compensating workers who are injured on the job. The employer pays the cost of the insurance premium for the employee. These laws allow the injured worker to file a claim for compensation with the state or the federal government instead of suing. However, the laws require workers to accept workers' compensation as the exclusive remedy for on-the-job injuries. Federal laws cover the following employees: workers in Washington, DC; coal miners; maritime workers; and federal employees. State laws cover those workers not protected under federal statutes.

Workers who are injured on the job or who contract an occupational disease may apply for five types of state compensation benefits:

- Medical treatment, including hospital, medical and surgical services, medications, and prosthetic devices.

- Temporary disability indemnity, in the form of weekly cash payments made directly to the injured or ill employee.

- Permanent disability indemnity, which can be a lump sum award or a weekly or monthly cash payment.

- Death benefits for survivors, which consist of cash payments to dependents of employees killed on the job.

- Rehabilitation benefits, which are paid for medical or vocational rehabilitation.

Employees who are injured on the job or become ill due to work-related causes must immediately report the injury or illness to a supervisor. An injury report and claim for compensation are then filed with the appropriate state workers' compensation agency. Forms from the attending or designated workers' compensation physician who examines and treats the

LO 10.5
State the purpose of workers' compensation laws and unemployment insurance.

workers' compensation
A form of insurance established by federal and state statutes that provides reimbursement for workers who are injured on the job.

employee must also be filed with the appropriate agency as proof of the employee's injury or illness.

A medical office employee may be responsible for filing the physician's report with the state workers' compensation agency. Requirements concerning waiting periods and other filing specifics vary with each state. When a claim is filed, all questions must be answered in full and as thoroughly as possible.

Unemployment Insurance

Unemployment insurance (sometimes called reemployment insurance) funds are managed jointly by state and federal governments. Under the Federal Unemployment Tax Act (FUTA), employers contribute to a fund that is paid out to eligible unemployed workers. Each state also provides unemployment insurance, and credit is given employers against the FUTA tax for amounts paid to the state unemployment fund. The total cost is borne by the employer in all but a few states.

Out-of-work employees should contact a state unemployment office to determine whether they qualify for unemployment benefits. Former employees are denied unemployment compensation for three main reasons: (1) They quit their jobs without cause, (2) they were fired for misconduct, or (3) they are unemployed because of a labor dispute. Independent contractors and self-employed individuals usually do not qualify for unemployment compensation.

Individuals may file for unemployment benefits at state unemployment offices. A claimant needs

- A Social Security card.
- W-2 statements for the past one to two years.
- Other wage records for the past 18 months.
- Employers' names and addresses for the past 18-month employment period.
- A statement of the reasons for leaving the job.
- The employer's unemployment insurance account number, if available.

LO 10.6

Determine the appropriate legal process for hiring employees and maintaining the required paperwork while the person is employed.

Hiring and the New Employee

When interviewing for a position or when asked to interview a job applicant, the health care practitioner must know legal boundaries.

Interviews

Because of federal and state laws against discrimination in hiring, inquiries cannot be made concerning an applicant's

- Race or color.
- Religion or creed.
- Gender.
- Family.
- Marital status.
- Method of birth control.
- Age, birth date, or birthplace.
- Disability.
- Arrest record (with some exceptions in many states).
- Residency duration.

- National origin. (However, the Immigration Reform and Control Act of 1986 requires new employees to complete an I-9 form, intended to prevent the employment of illegal aliens.)
- General military experience or discharge.
- Membership in organizations.

Questions concerning one's Social Security number, qualifications (including license or certificate), and job experience are proper, and they should be answered as thoroughly and truthfully as possible. As part of the hiring process, applicants may be asked to take a physical examination.

During a job interview, applicants may refuse to answer a question that is clearly improper or not job-related, but this could cost them the job. The question "May I ask how this relates to the position?" is generally more acceptable than a blunt, "That question is illegal, and I don't have to answer it." Furthermore, the mere asking of an improper preemployment interview question does not in itself give an applicant grounds for a legal challenge if he or she is not hired.

The following guidelines can help those employees who are responsible for conducting preemployment interviews:

- Make a list of questions that relate specifically to the job description of the position to be filled, and stick to them.
- Do not rush the interview, nor let it drag on beyond reasonable time limits.
- General questions that may prove helpful include these: What are your qualifications for this position? Why are you leaving your present position? Why do you want this job? What salary do you expect? When can you begin work? What are your professional strengths? What are your professional goals?
- Remain objective and listen well.
- End the interview on a positive note. Indicate when a decision will be made, and follow through on your promise to inform the applicant of your decision, one way or the other.

Bonding

In some medical offices and other workplace locations where employees are responsible for collecting fees and handling financial matters, prospective employees may be asked whether they are bondable. An employer can purchase a **surety bond** for a specific amount from an insurance carrier. If a bonded employee should embezzle or otherwise abscond with funds, the employer can collect from the insurance carrier up to the amount of the bond. However, the employer must have filed a complaint against the alleged dishonest employee in order to collect on the bond. If the insurance company pays the bond, it will then seek to recover the amount from the offending employee.

surety bond A type of insurance that allows employers, if covered, to collect up to the specified amount of the bond if an employee embezzles or otherwise absconds with business funds.

Employment Paperwork

Once employed, the new worker will be asked to provide certain information so that the employer may comply with federal and state regulations. Complete records for every employee must include

- Social Security number.
- Number of exemptions claimed.
- Gross salary.
- Deductions for Social Security; Medicare; and federal, state, and city taxes.
- Withholding for state disability insurance, state unemployment tax, and health care plans, if applicable.

The law requires employers to withhold specified amounts from employees' pay and to keep records of and send these sums to the proper income tax center. The amount to be withheld is based on the employee's total salary, the number of exemptions he or she claims, marital status, and the length of the pay period involved.

Health care practitioners who are self-employed do not have to deduct withholding, but they must make quarterly city, state, and federal income tax payments. Self-employed individuals must also pay Social Security taxes (FICA), via a self-employment tax percentage that is higher than the rate paid by individuals who are not self-employed. The difference lies in the fact that a self-employed individual is making both the employer and the employee contribution.

Employers must provide each employee with a Form W-2, Wage and Tax Statement, by January 31 of each year. The W-2 shows the following information:

- Employer's tax identification number.

- Employee's Social Security number.

- Total earnings (wages and other compensation) paid by the employer.

- Amounts deducted for income tax and Social Security.

- Amount of advance earned income credit payment, if any.

Most employers want the workplace to be as pleasant and safe for employees as it can possibly be. However, it is still the employee's responsibility to know the employment legalities most likely to affect him or her and to work within this legal framework to help ensure a satisfying and productive employer–employee relationship.

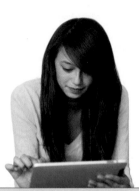

check your **progress**

23. Distinguish between workers' compensation and unemployment insurance.

24. Is it permissible for an employer to ask a job applicant to take a physical exam? Why might such a requirement exist?

25. Place a check mark beside those questions that are considered to be illegal if asked in a preemployment interview.

_____ Why are you leaving your present position?

_____ Do you belong to a church?

_____ What do you hope to achieve over the next five years?

_____ How many children do you have, and how old are they?

_____ Who will watch your children while you work?

_____ Why do you want to work for us?

_____ How many years' experience do you have as a medical assistant/dental assistant/physician assistant/nursing assistant?

_____ Are you married?

_____ Is your husband/wife employed, and if so where?

_____ What nationality are you?

CHAPTER SUMMARY

LO 10.1 What issues affected by federal law have traditionally affected employees in the workplace?

- Employment-at-will.
- Wrongful discharge.
- Just cause.
- Public policy.

What categories do federal and state laws generally address, regarding employees in the workplace?

- Discrimination.
  - Sexual harassment.
  - Physical disability.
  - Pregnancy.
  - Age.
  - Genetic discrimination.
- Wages and work hours.
  - Equal pay.
  - Retirement income security.
- Safety and welfare.

LO 10.2 and LO 10.3 What is the role of the health care practitioner following OSHA standards for work done in the clinical setting and for infection control in the medical office?

- Right-to-know.
- Hazard Communication Standard.
- Chemical Hygiene Plan.
- Occupational Exposure to Bloodborne Pathogen Standard.
- Medical Waste Tracking Act.

LO 10.4 What is the role of the Clinical Laboratory Improvement Act (CLIA) in quality laboratory testing?

LO 10.5 What is the purpose of worker's compensation and unemployment insurance.

- Five types of benefits.
  - Claimant requirements.

LO 10. 6 What should health care practitioners know about hiring and paperwork for new employees?

- Prohibited questions to ask job applicants.
- Guidelines for conducting interviews.
  - Required paperwork.
  - Surety bond.

Ethics ISSUE 1: All ethical guidelines for health care practitioners remind them to be aware that, even though sexually suggestive behavior may not have crossed the line legally, any form of sexual harassment or exploitation between medical supervisors and trainees, employers and employees, coworkers, or medical practitioners and patients is unethical.

Discussion Questions

1. You are a surgical technologist in a large hospital. Whenever you work with a certain surgeon, she tells off-color jokes to you and your coworkers and makes suggestive comments to workers of the opposite sex. One coworker tells you that he might quit his job because he is married, and the surgeon's behavior makes him so uncomfortable that he dreads coming to work. Is the surgeon's behavior illegal or simply in bad taste? Explain your answer.

_____

_____

2. Do you or your coworkers in the previous situation have grounds for a sexual harassment complaint? Explain your answer.

_____

_____

3. If you have determined that you do have a complaint, how would you proceed?

_____

_____

Ethics ISSUE 2: The *Code of Medical Ethics* for the American Medical Association states: "Sexual contact that occurs concurrent with the patient-physician relationship constitutes sexual misconduct. . . . At a minimum, a physician's ethical duties include terminating the patient-physician relationship before initiating a dating, romantic, or sexual relationship with a patient" (AMA *Code of Medical Ethics*, E-8.14).

Patients are often accompanied by third parties who play an important part in the health care practitioner–patient relationship. The health care practitioner interacts and communicates with these individuals and often is in a position to offer them information, advice, and emotional support. The more deeply involved the individual is in the clinical encounter and in medical decision making, the more troubling sexual or romantic contact with the health care practitioner would be. Key third parties include, but are not limited to, spouses or partners, parents, guardians, and proxies.

Discussion Questions

1. As a medical assistant, you have been present when a young, single father brings his infant in for checkups. The child is seriously ill, and the father begins consulting you about his emotional anguish. You are also single and sense an attraction. When the young man asks you out, should you accept? Explain your answer.

_____

_____

2. Do you believe ethical standards governing such relationships are stricter for health care practitioners than for other professions, such as law professors and students? In your view, is this as it should be? Explain your answer.

_____

_____

Ethics ISSUE 3: Health care practitioners have legal and ethical responsibilities to follow laws and procedures that protect their safety and patient safety.

Discussion Question

1. Assume you are the medical technologist in the chapter's opening scenario, and you observe that every urine specimen analyzed during a hectic morning has a high leukocyte count. You realize this is unusual, but you don't want to fall behind, and you do not report the anomaly to your supervisor. Have you acted ethically? Explain your answer.

_____

_____

Go to **www.mhhe.com/judson6e** to practice your case review skills. Then read on for more information.

KEY TERMS

affirmative action	just cause	public policy
Chemical Hygiene Plan	Medical Waste Tracking Act	right-to-know laws
Clinical Laboratory Improvement Act (CLIA)	Occupational Exposure to Bloodborne Pathogen Standard	surety bond
discrimination		workers' compensation
employment-at-will	Occupational Safety and Health Administration (OSHA)	wrongful discharge
General Duty Clause		
Hazard Communication Standard (HCS)		

CHAPTER 10 REVIEW

Applying Knowledge

Circle the correct answer for each of the following questions.

LO 10.1

1. Under the concept of employment-at-will, who has the right to terminate employment?
   a. The government
   b. Both the employer and the employee
   c. The business owner
   d. The employee's legal representative

2. When might an employee who is fired sue his or her former employer for wrongful discharge?
   a. Never
   b. Only one year after the discharge
   c. At any time if the employee was discharged for an illegal reason
   d. Six months after the discharge

3. Which of the following reasons for discharge is *not* illegal under antidiscrimination laws?
   a. The employee is too old.
   b. The employee joined a union.
   c. The employee has been unable to master the requirements of the job.
   d. The employee is too religious.

4. Which of the following common law concepts protects an employee who reports his employer's illegal chemical dumping activities?
   a. Employment-at-will
   b. Public policy
   c. Wages and hour law
   d. Antisexual harassment law

5. Which of the following federal laws protects employees from potential discrimination?
   a. Civil Rights Act of 1967
   b. Affirmative action
   c. Social Security Act
   d. ERISA

6. Which of the following federal laws protects employees from sexual harassment in the workplace?
   a. Equal Pay Act
   b. ERISA
   c. Civil Rights Act of 1967
   d. Social Security Act

7. Which of the following is *not* a form of sexual harassment in the workplace?
   a. A supervisor promises an employee a pay raise in exchange for sexual favors.
   b. A male employee makes unwelcome sexual advances to a male coworker.
   c. A female employee makes unwelcome sexual advances to a male coworker.
   d. A female supervisor hires a male assistant.

8. Which federal office can be contacted to report charges or complaints of employment discrimination?
   a. Wages and Hours Office
   b. Social Security Office
   c. Equal Employment Opportunity Office
   d. Internal Revenue Office

9. Which of the following employment issues do federal laws generally address?
   a. Employment discrimination
   b. Wages and hours
   c. Safety and welfare
   d. All of the above

10. A form of sexual harassment that means "something for something" is called
    a. Right-to-know
    b. *Quid pro quo*
    c. ERISA
    d. *Res judicata*

11. Which of the following types of evidence may an employee produce to substantiate a wrongful discharge claim?
    a. Oral promises to the employee
    b. A written contract
    c. Company handbook
    d. All of the above

12. What federal publication is the primary source for locating OSHA standards?
    a. Publication of Labor Statistics
    b. CDC list of OSHA regulations
    c. *Federal Register*
    d. Workers' Compensation Guide

LO 10.2

13. Which of the following does not govern work done in a clinical setting?
    a. Hazard Communication Standard
    b. Occupational Exposure to Bloodborne Pathogen Standard
    c. Needlestick Safety and Prevention Act
    d. Social Security Act

14. Which of the following is an OSHA regulation that applies to hazardous equipment in the workplace?
    a. Occupational Exposure to Bloodborne Pathogen Standard
    b. General Duty Clause
    c. Chemical Hygiene Plan
    d. None of the above

15. Which of the following is *not* true of OSHA's Hazard Communication Standard?
    a. Requires medical offices to have a written hazard communication program
    b. Requires employers to obtain and post a Material Safety Data Sheet for each hazardous chemical in use in the workplace
    c. Requires at least one safety session per month on use of hazardous chemicals
    d. Requires a hazard communications manual be kept up to date and accessible to all employees

LO 10.3 and LO 10.4

16. Infection control in the medical office requires employees to
    a. Wear protective equipment when handling hazardous materials
    b. Post Material Safety Data Sheets for hazardous chemicals in use
    c. Initial and date records of safety training
    d. All of the above

17. The Clinical Laboratory Improvement Act (CLIA)
    a. Established minimum quality standards for all laboratory testing
    b. Has been extensively amended since it was first written
    c. Requires laboratories to obtain certification
    d. All of the above

18. Which of the following does *not* help control infections in the medical office?
    a. Wearing protective equipment when appropriate
    b. Disposing of sharps appropriately
    c. Cleaning/disinfecting work areas
    d. All of the above help control infections

LO 10.5

19. Which laws allow an injured employee to file a claim with the state or federal government?
    a. Workers' Compensation
    b. Needlestick Safety and Prevention Act
    c. General Duty Clause
    d. Clinical Laboratory Improvement Act

20. Which of the following is generally *not* a reason for an ex-employee to be denied an unemployment claim?
    a. Quit job without cause
    b. Fired for misconduct
    c. Quit due to sexual harassment
    d. Quit when spouse was transferred

21. Which of the following are generally *not* eligible for unemployment benefits?
    a. Women who quit to give birth
    b. Men who quit to care for young children
    c. Independent contractors and the self-employed
    d. Seasonal employees, such as construction workers

LO 10.6

22. Which of the following questions is illegal to ask a job applicant?
    a. Why did you leave your previous employment?
    b. Why do you want to work here?
    c. What are your five-year employment goals?
    d. Do you have children?

23. Which of the following types of employee information is *not* routinely collected and maintained by employers?
    a. Salary/hours worked
    b. Number of exemptions
    c. Married or divorced
    d. Social Security number

24. A W-2 form typically does *not* include
    a. Change in employee's marital status
    b. Employer's tax identification number
    c. Total wages paid
    d. Employee's Social Security number

25. A type of insurance that allows employers to collect if employees embezzle or otherwise steal business funds is called
    a. Disability insurance
    b. Workers' compensation
    c. Unemployment insurance
    d. Surety bond

Match each definition with the correct term by writing the letter in the space provided.

_____ 26. Established the EEOC.

_____ 27. Makes it illegal to discriminate because of pregnancy, childbirth, or related medical conditions.

_____ 28. Protects employees aged 40 or older.

_____ 29. Protects employees who engage in union or other organizational activities.

_____ 30. Regulates private pension funds and employer benefit programs.

_____ 31. Requires equal pay for equal work.

_____ 32. Ensures a safe work environment.

_____ 33. Regulates child labor, and provides for minimum wages and overtime pay.

_____ 34. Provides for Medicare, unemployment insurance, disability, and OASI, through FICA funding.

_____ 35. Protects individuals who are disabled or mentally ill.

_____ 36. Provides minimum federal standards for quality laboratory testing.

a. Wagner Act

b. Social Security Act

c. Fair Labor Standards Act

d. Equal Pay Act

e. Civil Rights Act of 1964

f. Age Discrimination in Employment Act

g. Occupational Safety and Health Act

h. Rehabilitation Act

i. Employee Retirement Income Security Act

j. Pregnancy Discrimination Act

k. Clinical Laboratory Improvement Act/Amendments

CASE STUDIES

Use your critical thinking skills to answer the questions that follow each case study.

LO 10.1

You have recently graduated from a two-year medical assistant program, have earned certification, and want to apply for the following advertised positions: (1) a CMA in a pediatric clinic and (2) a CMA/receptionist for a physician in private practice. Write letters of application for each position and a résumé to be included with the cover letters. Consider the following questions:

37. What information will you give about your educational, employment, and personal background?

38. If interviewed for the position, how will you follow up?

LO 10.2

While many people think of the health care industry as "clean," medical providers continue to accidentally contract diseases from incidents in the workplace. For example, Sheila, an emergency room nurse with 15 years' experience, had just finished drawing blood from a patient when she disposed of the needle in the sharps container and felt a prick through her glove from a used needle that had hung up in the drop-down sharps lid. Several months later, Sheila learned that she had not only been infected with the human immunodeficiency virus (HIV), but also the hepatitis C virus (HCV). Other diseases health care practitioners often contract through needle sticks include methicillin-resistant *Staphylococcus aureus* (MRSA), hepatitis B, malaria, syphilis, herpes, and many less common diseases.

39. In your opinion, were there precautions that Sheila could have taken in the emergency room where she worked to prevent her accidental infection? Explain your answer.

40. What other common hazards do health care practitioners face in a medical office or other medical setting? How would you deal with each?

INTERNET ACTIVITIES LO 10.1, LO 10.2, and LO 10.3

Complete the activities and answer the questions that follow.

41. Visit the Web site for the Equal Employment Opportunity Commission (EEOC) at **www.eeoc.gov/index.html**. Choose two headlined articles and briefly summarize their importance to health care workers.

42. Visit the Web site for OSHA's bloodborne pathogen site at **www.osha.gov/SLTC/bloodbornepathogens/**. What are five of the most frequently asked questions about the Bloodborne Pathogen Standard that interest you? Include the answers to the questions.

43. Visit the Web site for the Mayo Clinic's recommendations on effective hand washing at **www.mayoclinic.com/health/hand-washing/HQ00407**. List the steps for the recommended procedure, and explain how the guidelines can prevent the spread of infection in a health care setting.

RESOURCES

Kubasek, Nancy, et al. *Dynamic Business Law*. New York: McGraw-Hill, 2009.

Liuzzo, Anthony L. *Essentials of Business Law*. New York: McGraw-Hill, 2010: employment-at-will, p. 445; workers' compensation, pp. 456–458; Occupational Safety and Health Act, Civil Rights Act of 1964, Age Discrimination in Employment Act, etc., pp. 458–462.

Genetic Information Nondiscrimination Act (GINA) of 2008: **www.genome.gov/24519851**.

Ledbetter case: **http://thomas.loc.gov/home/thomas.html**.

Ledbetter v. Goodyear Tire & Rubber Co., 550 U.S. 618 (2007).

Lilly Ledbetter: **www.kuow.org/program.php?id=19571**.

OSHA Web site: **www.osha.gov/**.

THE BEGINNING OF LIFE AND CHILDHOOD

Learning Outcomes

After studying this chapter, you should be able to:

LO 11.1 Define *genetics* and *heredity*.

LO 11.2 List several situations in which genetic testing might be appropriate, and explain how it might lead to genetic discrimination.

LO 11.3 Define *genetic engineering*, and explain why cloning and stem cell research are controversial issues.

LO 11.4 Discuss three possible remedies for couples experiencing infertility problems.

LO 11.5 List and discuss those laws affecting health care that pertain especially to children's rights.

Cases in This Chapter

Baby M—First Surrogacy Case, 339

Gestational Surrogacy Contract Held Valid, 340

Minor Appeals for Judicial Bypass to Obtain an Abortion, 344

Judge Rules That Minor May Consent to Her Own Medical Treatment, 345

Minor Says No to Surgery, 345

MEMORY

STEVE, a 32-year-old auto mechanic, lives in a large midwestern city with Gloria, his fiancé. While growing up, he has watched as his paternal grandfather, his maternal grandmother, his father's two brothers, and his mother's sister all develop Alzheimer's disease, the most frequent cause of dementia in older adults. In each case, the disease began with what appeared to be occasional memory loss—forgetting names, appointments, purses, and car keys—then progressed rather rapidly to forgetting how to perform routine tasks, such as making coffee, preparing a shopping list, or following a recipe. "I was riding with my granddad in his car one day when he signaled to make a left-hand turn across traffic and suddenly seemed confused about what to do next," Steve recalls. "I told him to step on the gas and get us across, and he made the turn, but after that he quit driving."

Eventually Steve's grandfather was placed in a skilled nursing facility, as were other members of his family who developed Alzheimer's disease as they aged.

"Now, I'm thinking of being genetically tested to see if I've inherited genes for Alzheimer's," Steve reveals. (The genetic test for Alzheimer's disease looks for variations of the apolipoprotein E—APOE—gene.) "I'm not sure I really want to know, but it seems likely that I could develop the disease, and if I knew I could set aside some funds—maybe take out long-term care insurance—now, looking toward the day when I won't be able to care for myself."

From Steve's perspective, the knowledge that he could be genetically predisposed to developing a devastating disease is frightening, but on the other hand, such knowledge would give him time to prepare for the day when, if the disease develops, funds would be available for his care.

From Gloria's perspective, Steve's genetic test results, if negative for the variations of the APOE gene that predict the development of late-onset Alzheimer's, could allow her to view the future with less trepidation. Positive results, on the other hand, might allow her to prepare herself emotionally and financially for whatever Steve's future holds.

From a genetic counselor's perspective, Steve might benefit, in terms of peace of mind, from examining the pros and cons of predictive genetic testing.

In Steve's position, would you want to be tested?

In Gloria's position, would you want your fiancé to be tested?

Should a positive result to Steve's test influence the couple's decision about having children?

In all of the previous questions, what factors influenced your answers?

Genetics and Heredity

Genetics was often in the news from the mid-1990s into the 21st century, as scientists published the results of experiments in genetics research. **Genetics,** as you probably remember from earlier science courses, is the science that accounts for natural differences and resemblances among organisms related by descent. The science of **heredity,** or the process by which organisms pass genetic traits on to their offspring, is part of the wider scope of the term *genetics*.

As a result of genetics research, improved science education, and extensive media coverage of genetics procedures and issues, health care practitioners and members of the general public have become familiar with

LO 11.1

Define *genetics* and *heredity*.

genetics The science that accounts for natural differences and resemblances among organisms related by descent.

heredity The process by which organisms pass genetic traits on to their offspring.

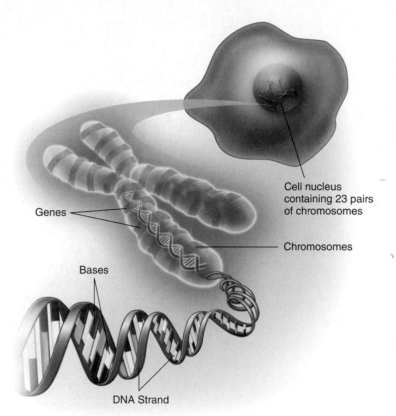

> **Figure 11-1** DNA is the combination of proteins called nucleotides that make up each human chromosome.

Genes

Cell nucleus containing 23 pairs of chromosomes

Chromosomes

Bases

DNA Strand

DNA (deoxyribonucleic acid) The combination of proteins, called nucleotides, that is arranged to make up an organism's chromosomes.

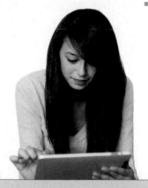

the term **DNA (deoxyribonucleic acid).** DNA is the combination of proteins called nucleotides that are arranged to make up each human **chromosome** (see Figure 11-1).

Forty-six chromosomes (23 pairs) are found inside the nucleus of every human cell, except egg and sperm cells, which have 23 chromosomes each. We inherit half of our chromosome complement from our mother and half from our father. These 46 chromosomes carry the genes responsible for all our human characteristics, from eye, skin, and hair color to height, body type, and intelligence. Each **gene** is a tiny segment of DNA that holds the formula for making a specific enzyme or protein.

The genes that make up the human **genome**—all the genetic information necessary to create a human being—are responsible for all the cells, organs, tissues, and traits that make up each individual.

The Human Genome Project

The **Human Genome Project,** funded by the U.S. government, was started in 1990 to analyze the entire human genome. A genome is all the DNA in an organism, including its genes. Scientists around the world who worked on the project set out to map all of the genes within the 23 pairs of human chromosomes. The project was scheduled for completion in 2003 but was finished ahead of time, in mid-2000. One surprising finding was that instead of a suspected 100,000 genes, humans have approximately 20,000 to 25,000 genes.

Goals of the Human Genome Project that have largely been accomplished were to locate and map the location of each gene on all 46 chromosomes and to create a data bank of the information that would be available to all scientists or physicians who could use it. The scientists involved in the project also vowed to continue to examine the ethical, legal, and social issues originating

check your **progress**

Give the term that is defined by each phrase.

1. The science that studies inherited traits.

2. The threadlike structures inside cell nuclei that are composed of DNA and carry an organism's genes.

3. A tiny segment of DNA that holds instructions for making a specific enzyme or protein.

4. All the genes necessary to replicate a human being.

5. A worldwide project to locate and map the location of all human genes.

with human genetics research, and to train other scientists to use the technologies developed to improve human health (see Figure 11-2).

▶ Figure 11-2

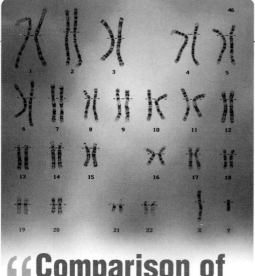

Genetic Testing

Our increasing knowledge about DNA has led to tests that have widespread applications. Specially trained technicians perform DNA tests. The tests are conducted on samples of solid tissues such as hair roots, skin, or bone, and from body fluids such as blood, semen, or saliva.

Uses of genetic testing include

1. *Predictive testing.* This testing is used to see if genes are present that could lead to hereditary diseases or other harmful genetic conditions. Individuals who come from families where certain inherited diseases have appeared may opt for predictive genetic testing to confirm or rule out the presence of a disease-causing gene. For example, Huntington's disease (also known as Huntington's chorea) runs in families, but symptoms typically do not develop until individuals reach middle age. Since the disease is incurable, debilitating, and fatal, affecting the brain and the nervous system, adults with relatives who have developed the disease may opt to be tested to plan for any eventuality. (Steve, in the chapter's opening scenario, was considering predictive genetic testing to determine if his genome included variations of the APOE gene associated with the development of Alzheimer's disease.)

2. *Carrier testing.* Used to determine if individuals carry harmful genes that could be passed on to offspring.

3. *Prenatal testing.* This testing is used to see, through a process called **amniocentesis,** if harmful genes are present in a fetus. During amniocentesis, the physician withdraws a sample of amniotic fluid (the fluid surrounding the developing fetus inside the mother's womb) from the uterus of a pregnant woman. The fluid is then tested for genetic or other conditions that may lead to abnormal development of the fetus. Down syndrome is one inherited condition that is often detected through amniocentesis.

4. *Preimplantation testing.* Tests for harmful genes in embryos after artificial insemination but before implantation. Usually offered to couples who have a reasonable chance of passing on harmful genes.

5. *Forensic testing.* Forensic testing is used in law enforcement to eliminate or designate suspects in a crime, identify homicide victims, or to otherwise analyse DNA samples for law enforcement purposes.

6. *Tracing linage.* This testing is used in determining parentage or other relationships within families.

7. *Newborn screening tests.* Usually performed routinely to check for treatable, harmful genetic conditions or diseases, such as PKU (see Table 11-1).

8. *Diagnostic testing.* If symptoms have appeared, doctors can order tests for patients to confirm or rule out certain genetic diseases.

"Comparison of chromosomes to check for disease."

LO 11.2

List several situations in which genetic testing might be appropriate, and explain how it might lead to genetic discrimination.

chromosome A microscopic structure found within the nucleus of all living cells that carries genes responsible for the organism's characteristics.

gene A tiny segment of DNA found on a chromosome within a cell's nucleus. Each gene holds the formula for making a specific enzyme or protein.

genome All the DNA in an organism, including its genes.

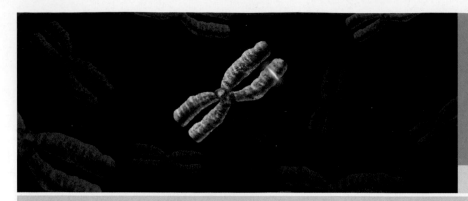

GENETIC DISEASES

Table 11-1

As of mid-2010, genetic tests were available for approximately 1,700 genetic disorders, although some genetic tests are more reliable than others. Some inherited diseases for which reliable genetic tests are available include:

Aarskog syndrome—linked to the X chromosome and found mostly in males, affects height, muscle and skeletal formation, and appearance of the face.

Aicardi syndrome—found mostly in females because it involves a gene on the X chromosome; the corpus callosum, which connects right and left sides of the brain, is absent. Causes spasms in infants.

Alzheimer's disease—the most frequent cause of dementia in older adults that eventually leads to organ breakdown and death.

Cancer—especially some types of breast, ovarian, and colon cancer.

Cystic fibrosis—affects the mucus glands of the lungs, liver, pancreas, and intestines, causing progressive disability due to multisystem failure. There is no cure and many individuals with the disease die young, often in their twenties and thirties.

Down syndrome—causes mental retardation and other physical problems.

Duchenne muscular dystrophy—causes rapidly worsening muscle weakness; usually appears before age six.

Elliptocytosis—red blood cells are abnormally shaped causing fatigue, shortness of breath, an enlarged spleen in adults, and jaundice in infants.

Fragile X syndrome—a rare condition causing mental retardation.

Gaucher's disease—affects fat metabolism.

Hemochromatosis—an iron storage disorder and the most commonly occurring inherited disease.

Huntington's disease, also called Huntington's chorea—an adult-onset, untreatable, ultimately fatal disease of the brain and nervous system.

Mucopolysaccharidosis (MPS)—a metabolic disorder causing skeletal deformities and usually mental retardation.

Neurofibromatosis—causes tumors that grow along the body's nerves and under the skin.

Phenylketonuria (PKU)—a metabolic disorder for which all newborns are tested. It results in mental retardation if left untreated.

Sickle cell anemia—a malformation of the red blood cells most often diagnosed in African Americans.

Spinocerebellar ataxia—a rare disorder that eventually destroys the brain's cerebellum.

Tay-Sachs disease—a lipid metabolism disorder that affects some people of Jewish descent. Children with the disease seldom survive childhood.

Genetic Diseases

Permanent changes in DNA, or **mutations,** often cause genetic diseases. Mutations can involve one gene, as in sickle cell anemia, hemophilia, cystic fibrosis, Aicardi syndrome, and Huntington's disease, or they can involve more than one gene. When more than one gene is involved, environmental factors, such as the changes caused by aging, smoking, exposure to environmental toxins, or other factors may trigger the onset of a genetic disease, as in cases of Alzheimer's disease, diabetes, obesity, and some forms of cancer. Another type of genetic disease can arise from abnormalities in the structure or number of whole chromosomes. Down syndrome, for example, results from an extra copy of chromosome 21.

These mutations occur in nuclear DNA, but diseases can also result from mutations in mitochondrial DNA (mtDNA), which multicelled organisms inherit mostly from mothers. (Mitochondria exist outside cell nuclei, but within cell membranes, and are responsible for cell metabolism and respiration.) Mutations in mtDNA may contribute to the loss of neurons in Alzheimer's and Parkinson's disease, and have been associated with diabetes, autism, and a variety of metabolic disorders. Health care practitioners should refer any patient who wants to undergo genetic testing to a **genetic counselor.** Genetic counselors can explain test results and help patients deal with difficult questions concerning those results.

As genetic testing has become more widely available and more reliable, use of test results has become an important issue. For example, if a couple learns through amniocentesis that the fetus the mother is carrying will be born with Down syndrome (Figure 11-3), should they consider aborting the fetus? Should the young man who learns he has the gene for Huntington's disease opt not to marry, to avoid taking the chance of passing the gene on to offspring? And will the woman in her twenties who learns she has one of two genes known to predispose her to breast cancer live her life any differently than she would have had she not been tested?

Genetic testing has also raised the issue of privacy. For instance, should employers and health and life insurance companies have access to genetic test results? How can individuals be certain that information about their genetic makeup is not shared with unknown sources?

Clearly, advances in genetics and genetic testing have led to difficult ethical, social, and medical questions for patients and their families and for health care practitioners.

Genetic Discrimination

With the increased ability to identify genetic differences comes increasing concern for the proper use of such information. The term **genetic discrimination** describes the differential treatment of individuals based on their actual or presumed genetic differences.

Harvard Medical School's Lisa N. Geller and her colleagues conducted a comprehensive and still often-quoted study of genetic discrimination throughout the 1990s. The landmark study found that a number of institutions were reported to have engaged in genetic discrimination, including health and life insurance companies, health care providers, blood banks, adoption agencies, the military, and schools. Geller's study included individuals at risk for or related to people with hemochromatosis, phenylketonuria (PKU), mucopolysaccharidosis (MPS), and Huntington's disease.

Four hundred and fifty-five respondents out of 917 who returned questionnaires for Geller's study said they had experienced genetic discrimination. In one case, a health maintenance organization had covered the medical expenses of a child since birth but refused to pay for occupational

Human Genome Project A scientific project funded by the U.S. government, begun in 1990 and successfully completed in 2000, for the purpose of mapping all of a human's genes. This Web site is an excellent resource: **www.ornl.gov/ sci/techresources/Human_ Genome/home.shtml.**

amniocentesis A test whereby the physician withdraws a sample of amniotic fluid (the fluid surrounding the developing fetus inside the mother's womb) from the uterus of a pregnant woman. The fluid is then tested for genetic or other conditions that may lead to abnormal development of the fetus.

mutation A permanent change in DNA.

genetic counselor An expert in human genetics who is qualified to counsel individuals who may have inherited genes for certain diseases or conditions.

genetic discrimination Differential treatment of individuals based on their actual or presumed genetic differences.

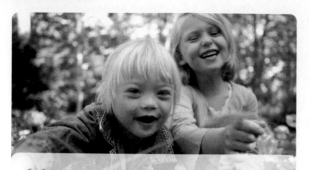

Figure 11-3

" Parents of children with **Down syndrome** often describe their offspring as 'affectionate, kind, and full of fun.' Individuals with Down syndrome have an extra copy of chromosome 21. "

therapy after she was diagnosed with mucopolysaccharidosis, claiming that the condition was preexisting.

In another case, a 24-year-old woman was denied life insurance due to her family history of Huntington's disease and the fact that she had not been tested for the presence of the gene. If she agreed to be tested and was found not to carry the gene, the insurance company would issue her a policy.

Geller also reported that in several cases, medical professionals reportedly pressured patients at risk for having children with serious genetic conditions to undergo prenatal diagnostic testing or to decide against having children.

Partially due to Geller's extensive study, there are now laws in place to prevent genetic discrimination. Many states have laws against genetic discrimination in employment, and the federal Genetic Information Nondiscrimination Act (GINA) of 2008 prohibits discrimination in health insurance and employment based on genetic information. The act defines genetic information as data about an individual's genetic tests and about genetic tests among that individual's family. Provisions within the law also apply to family members' medical histories. The law forbids genetic discrimination in any aspect of employment, and also prohibits harassment in the workplace based on an employee's genetic condition or history. The health insurance aspect of the law prohibits insurance companies from discriminating against clients and their families because of genetic testing results or other information, but in an article for *Science and Engineering Ethics*, Joseph S. Alper and John Beckwith point out that unless legislation addresses the problem of how to distinguish between genetic tests and nongenetic medical tests, it can be severely flawed:

> [W]e argue that much of this legislation is severely flawed because of the difficulty in distinguishing genetic from nongenetic tests. . . . In addition, barring the use by insurance companies of a genetic test but not a nongenetic test (conceivably for the same multifactorial disease) raises issues of fairness in health insurance. These arguments suggest that ultimately the problems arising from genetic discrimination cannot be solved by narrowly focused legislation but only by a modification of the entire health care system.

In addition to state laws against genetic discrimination and GINA at the federal level, the Health Insurance Portability and Accountability Act (HIPAA) passed in 1996 prevents health insurers from denying coverage based on genetic information. HIPAA, however, applies only to individuals moving between group health insurance plans (see Chapter 8, which discusses HIPAA in detail).

The Americans with Disabilities Act (ADA) of 1990, discussed in Chapter 10, also offers some protection against genetic discrimination in the workplace. It protects those who have a genetic condition or disease, or are regarded as having a disability, against discrimination. Under a 1995 ruling by the Equal Employment Opportunities Commission, the ADA applies to anyone who is discriminated against on the basis of genetic information relating to illness, disease, condition, or other disorders. Furthermore, under the ADA, a person with a disability cannot be denied insurance or be subject to different terms or conditions of insurance based on disability alone, if the disability does not pose increased risks.

Since Steve, in the chapter's opening scenario, has considered long-term care insurance, now, while he is healthy, what might happen to his application for insurance if the results of his genetic tests were available to insurance companies?

Genetic Engineering

Our increased body of knowledge about DNA, chromosome structure, and the basis of heredity has allowed scientists to manipulate DNA within the cells of plants, animals, and other organisms to ensure that certain advantageous traits will appear and be passed on, or that certain harmful trails are eliminated. This is called **genetic engineering.** Because the chemical composition of DNA is nearly identical throughout the plant and animal kingdoms, genes can often be interchanged among plants and animals to transfer desirable characteristics to different species. Through this process, for example, genes from a species of Arctic flounder have been added to strawberry plants to make them better able to withstand cold temperatures. Genetic engineering has also created corn and soybean crops that are resistant to insect-borne diseases, "golden" rice with increased beta-carotene content, and bacteria that can devour oil spilled into oceans.

However beneficial a genetic engineering result may sound, controversy is almost guaranteed as a new project is announced. Objections may be raised on the religious or moral grounds that humans simply should not tamper with the time-honored progression of life as dictated by nature. Or opponents may fear that the process will harm the environment by releasing genetically engineered super-species that may crowd out naturally occurring species and lead to the eventual disappearance of many original organisms. Critics may also fear that the undisclosed addition of genes to plants or animals ingested by humans can have unforeseen effects. For instance, some fear that genes from peanut plants added to a product might cause harmful reactions in unsuspecting consumers who are allergic to peanuts.

Clearly, if genetic engineering is to truly benefit society, scientists and governments must consider the objections and fears of concerned individuals and proceed with research in a manner that takes these concerns into account.

Cloning

One type of genetic engineering that is extremely controversial is cloning. The word **clone** comes from the Latin root meaning "to cut from." A clone is an organism grown from a single cell of the parent, and so it is genetically identical to the parent. In other words, the genes and chromosomes found in each cell's nucleus are the same in clone and parent. Identical twins are clones. So are all the cells in our bodies except for eggs and sperm: Somatic (body) cells divide to produce clones or exact replicas of themselves. Therefore, cells within the liver and other organs, within walls of blood vessels and arteries, within the skin, and so on are exactly like the cells that divided to produce them.

The term **cloning** was thrust into the public consciousness with the birth of Dolly, a Finn Dorset sheep, in July 1996 (Figure 11-4). Dolly was the product of scientists at the Roslin Institute near Edinburgh, Scotland, and was the only lamb born of 277 attempts. Her birth was controversial because she was the world's first mammal cloned from an adult parent cell. That is, Dolly was not the product of union of egg and sperm, but was created from a single cell scraped from the inside of her six-year-old mother's udder. Scientists used a process called nuclear transfer to clone Dolly from the udder cell.

LO 11.3

Define *genetic engineering,* and explain why cloning and stem cell research are controversial issues.

genetic engineering Manipulation of DNA within the cells of plants, animals, and other organisms through synthesis, alteration, or repair to ensure that certain harmful traits will be eliminated in offspring and that desirable traits will appear and be passed on.

clone An organism produced asexually, usually from a single cell of the parent.

cloning The process by which organisms are created asexually, usually from a single cell of the parent organism.

Dolly, the first mammal to be cloned from an adult cell, died relatively young in 2003 at age six and a half from progressive lung disease.

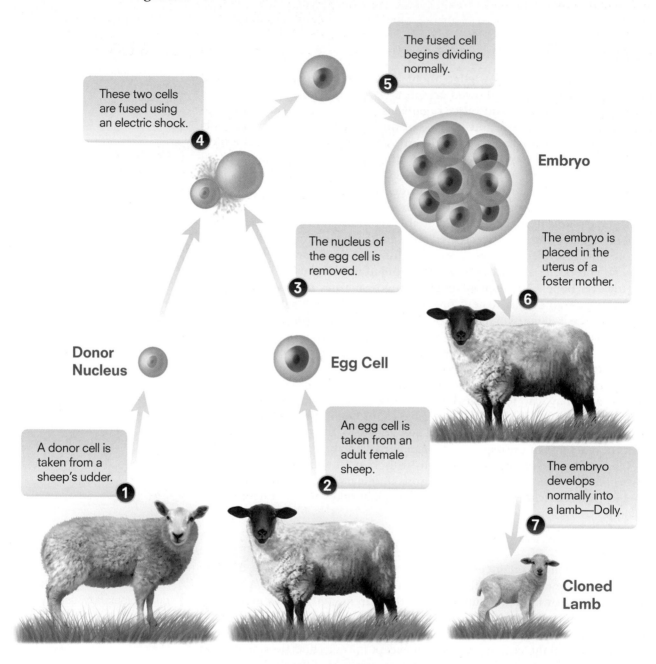

The fused cell begins dividing normally. **5**

These two cells are fused using an electric shock. **4**

The nucleus of the egg cell is removed. **3**

Embryo

The embryo is placed in the uterus of a foster mother. **6**

Donor Nucleus

Egg Cell

A donor cell is taken from a sheep's udder. **1**

An egg cell is taken from an adult female sheep. **2**

The embryo develops normally into a lamb—Dolly. **7**

Cloned Lamb

Dolly lived until February 2003, when she was put down to prevent further suffering from a progressive lung disease. She had also developed arthritis, leading to speculation that she aged more quickly than normal. Since normal sheep live to 11 or 12 years, Dolly's death at 6½ years fueled intensive debate about the health and longevity of cloned animals.

Scientists have continued to clone cattle, goats, mice, monkeys, pigs, and sheep. One objective of the cloning of farm and laboratory animals is to breed genetically identical animals that can produce substances useful in medicine, such as insulin and growth hormone. Another objective in cloning farm animals is the consistent production of prime, low-fat meat.

Some cloned animals have lived normal life spans while others, like Dolly, have died young, suffering from conditions usually associated with aging.

A third objective of animal cloning is to clone animal tissues and organs for human medical use. Because pigs are similar to humans in organ size and other biological aspects, an objective in cloning them is to grow a potential source of organs and tissue for transplanting into human patients. Transplanting animal tissues and organs into humans is called **xenotransplantation.** Research in this area is continuing, but at least two major difficulties make the process problematic. Animal cells produce a sugar that human cells do not, causing a severe immune rejection reaction in humans when animal tissues are transplanted. In addition, scientists have found that human cells can be infected with some viruses that exist in animals.

> **xenotransplantation** Transplantation of animal tissues and organs into humans.

Many animal rights proponents object on ethical grounds to using animals in this way. They argue that animals should be allowed to exist in nature without being subjected to experiments for the benefit of humankind. Furthermore, other groups object to introducing animal cells into humans on ethical grounds and on grounds that the animal tissue can harm people.

Objections against animal cloning are sometimes also based on grounds that such experiments could lead to the cloning of human beings—for several reasons a frightening prospect:

1. To date, animal cloning does not always yield viable offspring, with only 1 or 2 healthy animals resulting from approximately every 100 experiments.

2. Not only do most attempts to clone mammals fail; about 30 percent of clones born alive are affected with "large-offspring syndrome" and other debilitating conditions. Large-offspring syndrome occurs primarily in cloned lambs and calves which are the result of embryo manipulation. The process often creates oversized offspring due to deactivation of insulinlike growth factor 2 receptors which would normally block the growth of cells at a certain point. When the receptor is deactivated, the embryos grow too large. Other symptoms can include enlarged hearts, immature lungs, and damaged kidneys.

3. Scientists do not yet understand the processes involved in reproductive cloning well enough to ensure success, and a large failure rate in human clones is unacceptable.

4. Like Dolly the sheep, many cloned animals have died prematurely from infections and other complications. The same problems would be expected to occur in human cloning.

5. Scientists do not know how cloning could impact mental development. While factors such as intellect and mood may not be important for a cloned cow or mouse, they are crucial for the development of healthy humans.

With so many unknowns concerning reproductive cloning, many scientists and physicians believe the attempt to clone humans at this time is potentially dangerous and ethically irresponsible (see Figure 11-5).

Congress has made several attempts to pass legislation banning human cloning research in the United States, but to date no such laws have been passed. Most states have laws banning the cloning of humans.

Human Stem Cell Research

Early-stage human embryos, called *blastocysts,* consist of about 20 cells and are considered valuable for research because they are composed of **stem cells.** These early embryonic cells have the potential to become any type of body cell. Interest in this type of research—the *therapeutic* use of stem cells—remains intense because stem cells have shown promise for treating patients with a wide variety of medical problems. For example, stem cells that develop into neuronal tissue could be used to treat patients with Parkinson's and Alzheimer's diseases, as well as patients with strokes, spinal cord injuries, and other neurological disorders. Stem cells that become

> **stem cells** Cells that have the potential to become any type of body cell.

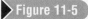
Figure 11-5

"Is **Human Cloning** in our **Future?**"

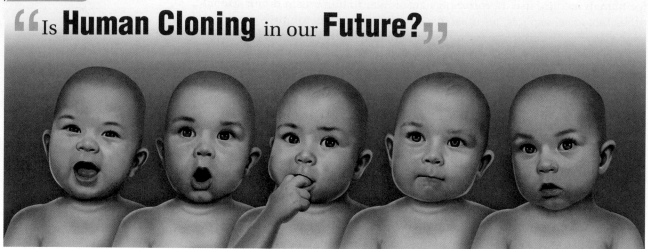

pancreatic islet cells might help those with diabetes. Skin tissue grown from stem cells could replace burned tissue, and cultivated cardiac tissue might help damaged arteries and hearts.

Most embryos used in stem cell research in the United States are the frozen products of in vitro fertilization that were not used to produce a pregnancy and are destined to eventually be destroyed. In 2001, President George W. Bush ordered that federal financing could be allowed only for stem cell research using cells grown from human embryos destroyed before August 9, 2001. By 2004, in contrast, England, Australia, Israel, and Portugal actively supported stem cell research without such restrictions.

In March 2009, President Barack Obama issued an executive order that reversed George W. Bush's order, stating he would "vigorously support scientists who pursue this research." Obama's order would allow the National Institutes of Health (NIH) to fund scientists working on embryonic stem cell research. In August 2010, however, a federal judge blocked U.S. government funding of embryonic stem cell research, on grounds that federal law prohibits the use of taxpayer money to fund such research. U.S. District Judge Royce C. Lamberth cited the Dickey-Wicker Amendment of 1996, which prohibits federal funding for "research in which a human embryo or embryos are destroyed, discarded, or knowingly subjected to risk of injury or death greater than that allowed for research on fetuses in utero." The ruling appeared to bar further government legal action, assuming the Dickey-Wicker Amendment remains in force, but in April 2011, the U.S. Court of Appeals for the District of Columbia lifted the 2010 injunction and gave the go-ahead for federal funding of embryonic stem cell research.

Opponents to human embryonic stem cell research of any kind argue that regardless of how the embryos were created, they are human beings with inherent rights to ethical and legal protection. Others argue that since the embryos are not growing within a uterus, they are not subject to the same protection as fetuses, and since most would be destroyed anyway, the good that could come from such research far outweighs any downside. To date, the U.S. government can fund embryonic stem cell research. Some state governments such as California, Connecticut, Illinois, Maryland, Massachusetts, New Jersey, New York, and Wisconsin have funded embryonic stem cell research, but many states prohibit funding all or certain aspects of the research.

Because of the controversy over using human embryonic cells in research, scientists are searching for other sources of stem cells. They have discovered that some adult human body tissues, such as bone marrow and fat, also contain cells that can function as stem cells. Adult stem cells are **multipotent,** however, which means that they can become only a limited number of types of tissues and cells in the body. For example, adult blood-forming stem cells (found in bone marrow) have been used successfully to treat only blood-based diseases such as leukemia and lymphoma. Embryonic stem cells have greater potential to treat a wider variety of diseases because they are **pluripotent**—they can become almost all types of tissues and cells in the body. A breakthrough development in 2010 offered the possibility that within a year, peripheral blood drawn from adult donors could be used to culture pluripotent stem cells.

Stem cells are found in small quantities in adult tissues and in umbilical cord blood, but scientists have found they do not have the same capacity to produce diverse tissues or to multiply as do embryonic stem cells. If a patient receives an adult stem cell transplant from a donor, the patient's body might reject it—a problem that researchers anticipate could be overcome with therapeutic cloning. Furthermore, adult stem cells may have more genetic abnormalities, which occur naturally during the aging process and with exposure to harmful agents.

Some scientists are exploring the possibility that adult stem cells are more flexible than previously thought, but many questions remain about the potential of adult stem cells, and much more research is required to answer them.

Amniotic stem cells are another possibility as a source for researchers. Amniotic stem cells are found in the fluid that surrounds a fetus. Scientists recently showed that they can be induced to create more cell types than was previously thought. However, the research is not intended as a replacement for embryonic stem cell research.

Some individuals within the scientific community agree that both adult and embryonic stem cell research show great potential to revolutionize the practice of medicine and that both types of research should be pursued.

> **multipotent stem cells**
> Stem cells that can become a limited number of types of tissues and cells in the body.

> **pluripotent stem cells**
> Stem cells that can become almost all types of tissues and cells in the body.

Gene Therapy

Gene therapy is rapidly becoming an effective tool for correcting and preventing certain diseases. In fact, therapy for genetic disease is often very similar to therapy for other types of disorders, as in the following cases:

- Special diets can eliminate compounds that are toxic to patients. This applies to such diseases as phenylketonuria and homocystinuria.

- Vitamins or other agents can improve a biochemical pathway and thus reduce toxic levels of a compound. For example, folic acid reduces homocysteine levels in a person who carries the 5,10-methylene-tetrahydrofolate reductase polymorphism gene.

> **gene therapy** Treating harmful genetic diseases or traits by eliminating or modifying the harmful gene.

Gene therapy may involve replacing a deficiency or blocking an overactive pathway. For instance, a fetus can sometimes be treated by treating the mother (e.g., corticosteroids for congenital virilizing adrenal hypoplasia) or by using in utero (inside the uterus) cellular therapy (e.g., bone marrow transplantation). Similarly, a newborn with a genetic disease may be a candidate for treatment with bone marrow or organ transplantation.

Genetic therapy may also involve the insertion of normal copies of a gene into the cells of persons with a specific genetic disease (this is called somatic gene therapy). Such somatic gene therapy has been undertaken for severe genetic disorders such as adenosine deaminase deficiency, an immunodeficiency that usually results in death during the first few months of life.

Germ-line gene therapy involves the correction of an abnormality in the genes of sperm or egg but is presently considered an inappropriate way to deal with genetic diseases because of ethical issues, cost, lack of research in humans, lack of knowledge about whether or not changes would be

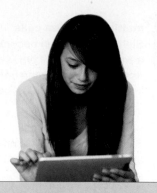

maintained in the growing embryo, and the relative ease of treating the pertinent conditions somatically when needed.

Gene therapy could also involve turning off genes before their harmful properties can be expressed. For example, if the gene for Huntington's disease could be turned off before carriers reached adulthood, theoretically the disease could not develop.

check your **progress**

6. List five possible uses for genetic testing.

7. The process of manipulating the DNA of organisms to produce desired results is called
   _____.

8. Define *genetic discrimination*.

9. Define *cloning*.

10. Distinguish between multipotent and pluripotent stem cells.

11. What are the foremost objections to embryonic stem cell research?

12. Name and briefly define five methods of gene therapy.

LO 11.4

Discuss three possible remedies for couples experiencing infertility problems.

infertility The failure to conceive for a period of 12 months or longer due to a deviation from or interruption of the normal structure or function of any reproductive part, organ, or system.

in vitro fertilization (IVF) Fertilization that takes place outside a woman's body, literally "in glass," as in a test tube.

artificial insemination The mechanical injection of viable semen into the vagina.

homologous artificial insemination The process in which a husband's sperm is mechanically injected into his wife's vagina to fertilize her eggs.

Conception and the Beginning of Life

Fortunately, most couples who decide to have a child are able to conceive naturally, and most pregnancies proceed without problems. However, it is estimated that about 10 to 15 percent of reproductive-age couples in the United States will have difficulty conceiving. Of this percentage, either husband or wife will experience **infertility**—that is, the failure to conceive for a period of 12 months or longer due to a deviation from or interruption of the normal structure or function of any reproductive part, organ, or system.

Infertility

When couples have reproductive difficulties and consult physicians who specialize in infertility problems, diagnoses are made and appropriate treatment recommended. Several options for infertile couples exist, depending on the type of fertility problem:

- **In vitro fertilization (IVF).** In this process, eggs and sperm are brought together outside the body in a test tube or petri dish. When fertilization takes place, the resulting embryo can then be frozen in liquid nitrogen for future use or implanted in the female uterus for pregnancy to occur.

- **Artificial insemination.** This process involves the mechanical injection of viable semen into the vagina. If the husband's sperm cells are used to fertilize the wife's eggs, the process is called **homologous artificial insemination.** If the husband's sperm cells are not viable, a donor's sperm may be used to fertilize the wife's eggs. This is called **heterologous artificial insemination.**

- **Surrogacy.** If a woman cannot carry an embryo to term, the couple may elect to contract with a surrogate mother.

Surrogacy

A **surrogate mother** is a woman who agrees to carry a child to term for a couple, often for a fee. If the surrogate is not genetically related to the embryo, the type of surrogacy is called *gestational* surrogacy. If the surrogate contributes eggs to produce the embryo or is related to either husband or wife, the type of surrogacy is called *traditional* surrogacy. (In one much-publicized case in the United States, a woman carried her own grandchild to term for her married daughter who was born without a uterus.) Traditional surrogacy differs from gestational surrogacy in that a traditional surrogate is genetically related to the fetus she carries.

Infertility treatments can cost several thousand dollars, with no guarantee of success. Most insurance plans do not cover expenses for infertility treatments or for contracting with a surrogate mother to bear a child. The law has been slow to catch up with technology, but many states have passed legislation regulating infertility clinics and surrogacy. Health care practitioners dealing with infertility should check state laws for current regulations.

Surrogacy is a relatively new concept in reproductive technology; thus, there is not a large volume of case law. The two cases, "Baby M—First Surrogacy Case" and "Gestational Surrogacy Contract Held Valid," however, have contributed to establishing precedent for legal decisions.

> **surrogate mother** A woman who becomes pregnant, usually by artificial insemination or surgical implantation of a fertilized egg, and bears a child for another woman.

> **heterologous artificial insemination** The process in which donor sperm is mechanically injected into a woman's vagina to fertilize her eggs.

LANDMARK COURT CASE

Baby M—First Surrogacy Case

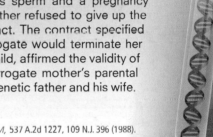

In 1985, a woman signed a contract agreeing to serve as a surrogate for a couple who could not conceive. She was then medically inseminated with the husband's sperm and a pregnancy resulted. When the child was born in March 1986, the surrogate mother refused to give up the infant. The genetic father sued for violation of the surrogacy contract. The contract specified that the genetic father and his wife held custody and that the surrogate would terminate her parental rights. The trial court, considering the best interests of the child, affirmed the validity of the contract. In March 1987, an appellate court terminated the surrogate mother's parental rights and gave full custody of the then one-year-old Baby M to her genetic father and his wife. The genetic father's wife legally adopted the baby.

Source: In re Baby M, 537 A.2d 1227, 109 N.J. 396 (1988).

Adoption

Adoption is also an option for those couples who want to raise children. All 50 states have laws regulating adoption. Certain areas of federal law may also affect some aspects of the parent–child relationship established by adoption. For example, the Adoption Assistance and Child Welfare Act of 1980, the Child Abuse Prevention and Treatment and Adoption Reform Act, and the Indian Child Welfare Act all contain provisions that pertain to adoptive parents and their children.

Typically, any adult who shows the desire to be a fit parent may adopt a child. Depending on state law, both married and unmarried couples may adopt, and single people may adopt through a process called single-parent adoption. Some states list special requirements for adoptive parents, such as requiring an adoptive parent to be a specified number of years older than the child. There may also be state requirements concerning residency, or the marital state of the prospective parent. Any adult who wishes to adopt will need to check state law before proceeding, and if potential adoptive parents use an adoption agency, they will also have to meet any agency requirements.

Some single individuals or couples may have a more difficult time qualifying as adoptive parents than others. For example, single men, gay singles, and homosexual couples may not specifically be prevented from adopting

Gestational Surrogacy Contract Held Valid

A married couple was unable to have a child because the wife had undergone a hysterectomy. The wife's ovaries had not been removed, however, and could still produce eggs, so the couple opted for gestational surrogacy. They entered into a surrogacy contract with a woman who agreed to relinquish her parental rights after the child was born in exchange for a $10,000 fee and a paid life insurance policy. The wife's eggs were fertilized in vitro with the husband's sperm, and the resulting embryo was implanted into the surrogate's uterus. While she was still pregnant, the surrogate demanded immediate payment and threatened not to relinquish the child when it was born. The couple who had contracted with the surrogate filed a lawsuit seeking a legal determination that the surrogate had no parental rights to the baby. The surrogate countersued and the court consolidated the two cases.

A trial court found for the married couple. It determined that the couple was the child's "natural parents" and held that the surrogate had no parental rights to the child. An appellate court and the state supreme court upheld this decision.

Source: Johnson v. Calvert, 5 Cal. 4th 84, 851 P.2d 776 (1993).

by state law, but they may have a more difficult time meeting state and agency requirements than married couples would. All states strive to find placements that meet the best interest of the child, so in some cases potential adoptive parents may be asked additional questions about lifestyle and why they want to adopt. (See "Best Interest of the Child Concept" on page 341 for a more thorough explanation of "best interest of the child.")

Generally, couples can adopt a child of a different race. Adoptions of Native American children, however, are governed by the Indian Child Welfare Act, and the act's provisions outline specific rules and procedures that must be followed if the adoption of a Native American child is to be approved.

There are several different types of adoptions, depending on services used and whether or not a blood or marital relationship exists between adoptive parents and children:

- Agency adoptions occur when state-licensed and/or state-regulated public or private adoption agencies place children with adoptive parents. Charities or religious or social service organizations often operate private agencies. Adoption agencies usually place those children who have been orphaned or whose parents have lost or relinquished parental rights through abuse, abandonment, or inability to support.

- Independent or private adoptions are arranged without the involvement of adoption agencies. Potential adoptive parents may hear of a mother who wants to give up her child, or they may advertise in newspapers or on the Internet to find such a mother. At some point in the process, an attorney must be involved to ensure the legality of the adoption. A few states prohibit independent adoptions. In those states where independent adoptions are allowed, they are usually strictly regulated.

- Identified adoptions are those in which adopting parents locate a birth mother, or vice versa, and then ask an agency to take over the adoption process. Prospective parents who find a birth mother willing to give up her child can bypass the long waiting lists that most agencies maintain for adoptions and can perhaps be better assured that the adoption will proceed in an orderly and legal fashion.

- International adoptions occur when couples adopt children who are citizens of foreign countries. In these procedures, adoptive parents must not only meet requirements of the foreign country where the child resides; they must also meet all U.S. state requirements and U.S. Immigration and Naturalization Service rules for international adoptions.

- Relative adoptions are those in which the child is related to the adoptive parent by blood or marriage. Stepparent and grandparent/grandchildren adoptions fall within this category.

Rights of Children

Common law has established the rights of parents to make health care decisions for minor children. In some circumstances, under the doctrine of *parens patriae,* literally "father of the people," the state may act as the parental authority. This doctrine is the legal principle that grants the state the broad authority to act in the child's *best interest,* sometimes overriding parental decisions, and allowing the state to remove abused or neglected children from the custody of offending parents.

Best Interest of the Child Concept

When alternatives are available for child placement or for determining medical treatment for minor children, the common standard is the "best interest of the child." In other words, which alternative will best safeguard the child's growth, development, and health? This standard is used in child placement situations. It is also used when legal authorities must work with health care practitioners to determine the least harmful and most appropriate treatment for an ailing child.

Rights of the Newborn

Legally, the legal rights of newborns are the same as those of any other American citizen of any age. For newborns who are severely disabled, however, existing law provides for several treatment options. Under the federal Child Abuse Amendments (U.S. Code, Title 42, Section 5106g), if the parents agree, physicians may legally withhold treatment, including food and water, from infants who

- Are chronically and irreversibly comatose.
- Will most certainly die and for whom treatment is considered futile.
- Would suffer inhumanely if treatment were provided.

Treatment of newborns who are severely disabled raises many ethical questions. Should the federal government intrude into physicians' and parents' decisions with imposed regulations? Is it ever in an infant's "best interest" to die, or should medical treatment be administered regardless of the probable outcome? Is quality of life an issue that can ethically be considered? Who should decide among treatment options for newborns who are disabled if the parents are unwilling or unable to make such decisions?

Abandoned Infants

Throughout the 1990s, newborn babies abandoned and left to die in dumpsters, public bathrooms, and other locations led to legislation allowing a parent to abandon a newborn at a safe location without legal prosecution or with reduced legal prosecution. By 2010, all 50 states had enacted some form of **safe haven law,** allowing abandonment at certain locations. State laws vary greatly:

- In some states, the baby can be handed to a doctor or police officer, or left at a fire station or hospital.
- Some states allow either reduction or elimination of prosecution.

parens patriae A legal doctrine that gives the state the authority to act in a child's best interest.

safe haven laws State laws that allow mothers to abandon newborns to designated safe facilities without penalty.

- In some states the parent can remain anonymous, while in others he or she must reveal identity and give a medical history. In some states, medical histories can also be dropped off anonymously.

- Some states place a limit on the age of a baby that can be abandoned. This is to encourage a parent to abandon the baby early, so it can receive adequate nutrition and medical care, rather than hiding the baby and letting it become malnourished or otherwise unhealthy.

- Nebraska is one state that did not specify that its safe haven law, passed in July 2008, applied to infants only, and within a short time 16 children, including teenagers, had been abandoned to the care of the state. Nebraska legislators convened an emergency session to change the word "child" in the state's safe haven law to "infant." (Ironically, in 2010 some states were pushing to up the age for abandonment to four or five, in light of several cases where mothers had murdered their small children.)

See **www.childwelfare.gov/systemwide/laws_policies/statutes/ safehavenall.pdf** for state-specific information about safe haven laws.

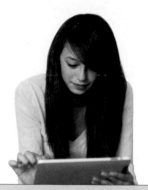

Reports by the National Conference of State Legislatures and the national Evan B. Donaldson Adoption Institute in 2003 indicated that the problem of abandonment of newborns has not been resolved and that, in fact, the laws have caused some undesirable results:

- The "no hassle" provisions discourage mothers from using established adoption and child welfare policies, while encouraging irresponsible and destructive behavior.

- The laws seem to some to be government statements that it's OK to abandon a baby.

- The abandoned children have little hope of learning family medical histories.

- The laws allow one parent to abandon a child, thus stripping the other parent of all rights.

The issue of abandonment also raises many ethical questions for society and for health care practitioners. Is the "safe haven" concept ethical—since prosecution is usually waived for parental abandonment under safe haven laws—or is it a form of child abuse and neglect? Should abandoned infants be eventually returned to the parent(s) who abandoned them, or should such parents be forced to relinquish parental rights? What public health measures might help prevent such events from occurring?

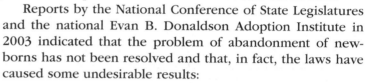

check your **progress**

13. Define *infertility*.

14. List and define three medical procedures that might be available to infertile couples.

15. Adoptions are regulated primarily by _____.

16. Name four types of adoptions.

17. Under existing child abuse amendments, physicians may, with the consent of parents, withhold treatment for those infants who _____.

18. What are safe haven laws designed to prevent?

19. What are the disadvantages of safe haven laws?

Teenagers

While common law has dictated that parents have a right to decide what medical care their young children receive, laws for older children differ from those for newborns. For example, states recognize that some older minors have the capacity to consent to their own medical care. For instance, teenagers considered mature or emancipated minors may give consent for medical treatment.

Mature minors are individuals in their mid- to late teens who are considered mature enough to comprehend a physician's recommendations and give informed consent. Most states allow mature minors to seek medical treatment without the consent of a parent or guardian in certain critical areas, such as mental health, drug and/or alcohol addiction, treatment for sexually transmitted diseases, pregnancy, and contraceptive services.

Emancipated minors legally live outside their parents' or guardians' control. A judge may issue an emancipation order at the request of parents or a minor child after certain important factors have been considered:

- Does the minor live at home with parents or other supervising adults, or is he or she living independently? If living at home, does he or she pay for room and board?

- Does the minor have a job, and does he or she spend his or her earnings without parental supervision?

- Does the minor pay his or her own debts?

- Is the minor claimed as a dependent on the parents' tax return?

The court may declare minors emancipated if one or more of the following criteria are met:

- They are self-supporting.

- They are married, provided the marriage is legal. In most states, persons must be at least 16 to marry and those under the age of 18 must have parental consent. Emancipation is not forfeited if the minor divorces or is separated or widowed.

- They are serving in the armed forces.

Emancipated minors do not usually gain all the rights of adults. Some limits, such as the legal age for purchasing alcohol or tobacco products, voting age, mandatory school attendance age (unless married), and other legal age restrictions, still apply.

Minors have the same constitutional rights as adults, including the right to privacy. This is especially relevant for the increasing numbers of adolescents in the United States who are sexually active. Many hesitate to seek birth control or family planning counseling if they must inform or seek consent from their parents.

No state explicitly requires parental involvement for a minor to obtain any of the services listed above. In some states, however, laws leave the decision about whether or not to inform parents that minor sons and daughters have received or are seeking contraceptives, prenatal care, or STI services to the discretion of the treating physician, based on the best interest of the minor.

In addition to the ability to consent to these specific services, laws in some states give minors the right to consent to general medical and surgical care under some circumstances, such as being a parent themselves, being pregnant, or reaching a certain age.

Several states also allow minors who are parents to consent to medical care for their children. In many states, mothers who are minors may also legally place their children for adoption without the consent or knowledge of the mothers' parents.

mature minors Individuals in their mid- to late teens who, for health care purposes, are considered mature enough to comprehend a physician's recommendations and give informed consent.

emancipated minors Individuals in their mid- to late teens who legally live outside parents' or guardians' control.

In many states, minors seeking an abortion must involve at least one parent in the decision. This means that teenagers who do not tell their parents about a pregnancy must either travel out of state or obtain approval from a judge—a process known as *judicial bypass*—to obtain an abortion. Currently, the trend is toward state and federal legislation making it increasingly difficult for minors to obtain an abortion without parental involvement.

COURT CASE

Minor Appeals for Judicial Bypass to Obtain an Abortion

Texas state law says that minors seeking abortions must notify their parents. Exceptions may be made for a minor who can show that

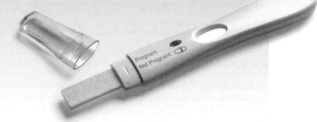

1. She is mature and sufficiently well-informed to make the decision to obtain an abortion without notifying a parent.

2. Notifying a parent would not be in her best interest.

3. Notifying a parent may lead to physical, sexual, or emotional abuse of the minor.

A minor petitioned a Texas court for authorization to consent to an abortion without notifying her parents. An appeals court denied the minor's petition, and she appealed to the Texas Supreme Court. The supreme court overturned the appellate court's decision and authorized the minor to consent to an abortion without notifying a parent. The court determined that the evidence the petitioner presented conclusively established that she was mature and sufficiently well-informed to consent to an abortion without parental notification.

Source: In Re Jane Doe, 19 S.W.3d 346; 2000 Tex., 43 Tex. Sup. J. 910.

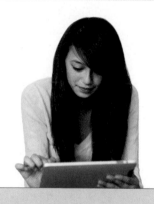

For exact legal restrictions regarding minors, health care practitioners should check statutes in the states where they practice.

In certain cases, the legal right of a minor to decline medical treatment has been upheld.

As we progress into the 21st century, health care practitioners will be constantly challenged to stay current with developments in genetics and reproductive science.

check your **progress**

20. Define the term *mature minor*.

21. Name three criteria that may be considered to determine if a minor is to be declared *emancipated*.

22. What effect do the previous designations *mature minor* and *emancipated minor* have on a minor's health care decisions?

23. In what treatment areas are minors most likely to make their own health care decisions?

Judge Rules That Minor May Consent to Her Own Medical Treatment

Nancy, a 17-year-old Kansas girl, gave permission for a doctor to transplant some skin from her wrist to her finger. Her mother later sued on Nancy's behalf, on the grounds that Nancy was a minor.

Nancy's mother had been hospitalized for major surgery. After the operation, Nancy accompanied her mother to her hospital room. A nurse asked Nancy to wait in the hallway. She didn't notice that Nancy's hand was resting on the wall near the door jamb, with her right ring finger in the space between the door and the jamb. As the nurse closed the door, Nancy cried out in pain. The door had closed on her finger, severing the tip.

Nancy was taken to the emergency room, where a doctor decided to graft a small piece of skin from Nancy's wrist over the raw tip of her finger. Nancy's mother was still recovering from her surgery, and it would be hours before she could give consent for her daughter's treatment. Nancy's parents were divorced, and her father lived in another city. To spare Nancy a long, uncomfortable wait, the emergency room physician called the girl's family physician and received his agreement that he should treat Nancy.

When Nancy's mother recovered, she sued the hospital, claiming that the nurse had been negligent in causing her daughter's injury and that the doctor had not obtained proper consent to treat her minor daughter.

The nurse was not found negligent. Regarding the question of consent, the Kansas Supreme Court ruled that Nancy "was of sufficient age and maturity to know and understand the nature and consequences of the 'pinch graft' utilized in the repair of her finger."

Source: Younts v. St. Francis Hosp. and School of Nursing, 205 Kan. 292, 469 P.2d 330, 338 (1970)

Minor Says No to Surgery

Believing they were acting in the best interests of a minor, a county health department in New York State tried to obtain the court's permission to seek surgery for a 14-year-old boy who had a cleft palate and upper lip.

The boy's father would not consent to surgery for his son because he believed that forces in the universe would heal all ailments. Influenced by his father, the boy refused the offer of surgery for his condition.

The court ruled that the boy could not be forced to have surgery. He could turn down the procedure, because his cooperation would be needed for the speech therapy that would follow. A majority of the judges saw less harm in letting him wait until he was an adult and could make the choice for himself than in pursuing surgery.

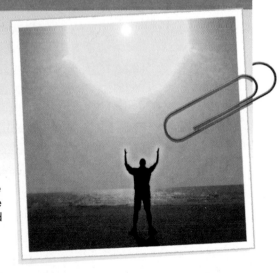

Source: In the Matter of S., 309 N.Y. 80, 127 N.E. 2d 820 (1955).

CHAPTER SUMMARY

LO 11.1 How does the term *genetics* differ from the term *heredity*?

- Genetics is the science that accounts for natural differences and resemblances among organisms related by descent.
- Heredity is the process by which organisms pass on genetic traits to their offspring.

What terms, integral to the study of genetics, are defined in this chapter?

- DNA—deoxyribonucleic acid: The combination of proteins, called nucleotides, that is arranged to make up an organism's chromosomes.
- Chromosome: A microscopic structure found within the nucleus of all living cells that carries genes responsible for the organism's characteristics.
- Gene: A tiny segment of DNA that holds the formula for making a specific enzyme or protein.
- Genome: All the DNA in an organism, including its genes.

What is the Human Genome Project?

- A scientific project funded by the U.S. government, begun in 1990 and successfully completed in 2000, for the purpose of mapping all of a human's genes.

LO 11.2 What is genetic testing?

- Testing one's DNA to discover one's genetic makeup.

What are the different types of genetic testing explained in this chapter?

- Predictive
- Carrier
- Prenatal
  - Amniocentesis—testing a sample of amniotic fluid for genetic or other conditions in a developing fetus—is a common prenatal test.
- Preimplantation
- Forensic
- Tracing linage
- Newborn screening
- Diagnostic

What is a mutation?

- A permanent change in DNA.

What does a genetic counselor do?

- Genetic counselors are qualified to counsel individuals before and after genetic testing.

What is genetic discrimination?

- Genetic discrimination is different treatment of individuals based on actual or presumed genetic differences.

What federal laws are in place to protect Americans against genetic discrimination in health insurance and employment?

- Genetic Information Nondiscrimination Act (GINA) of 2008.
- Health Insurance Portability and Accountability Act (HIPAA).
- Americans with Disabilities Act (ADA).

LO 11.3 What is genetic engineering?

- Genetic engineering is the manipulation of DNA within an organism's cells through synthesis, alteration, or repair to ensure that certain harmful traits will be eliminated in offspring and that desirable traits will appear and be passed on.

What is a clone?

- An organism produced asexually, usually from a single cell of the parent.

What is xenotransplantation?

- Transplantation of animal tissues and organs into humans.

What are stem cells?

- Cells that can become another type of body cell.
  - Multipotent: Adult cells that can become a limited number of types of tissues and cells.
  - Pluripotent: Embryonic cells that can become almost all types of tissues and cells.

What is gene therapy?

- Treatment of harmful genetic diseases or traits by eliminating or modifying the harmful gene.

LO 11.4 What is infertility?

- The failure to conceive for a period of 12 months or longer due to a deviation from or interruption of the normal structure or function of any reproductive part, organ, or system.

What alternatives are available for infertile couples who want to become parents?

- In vitro fertilization (IVF).
- Artificial insemination.
  - Homologous: husband's sperm/wife's eggs.
  - Heterologous: donor sperm/wife's eggs.
- Surrogacy.
- Adoption.

LO 11.5 Under what doctrine may the state act as a child's parental authority?

- *Parens patriae.*
  - Best Interest of the child concept.

When may physicians, with the parents' consent, legally withhold treatment and nourishment from a newborn who is severely disabled?

- If the child is chronically and irreversibly comatose.
- If the child will most certainly die, and treatment is considered futile.
- If the child would suffer inhumanely if treatment were provided.

What are safe haven laws?

- Laws that allow mothers to abandon newborns to designated safe facilities without penalty.

How do mature minors differ from emancipated minors?

- Mature minors: Individuals in mid- to late teens who legally live outside parental or guardian control.
- Emancipated minors: Individuals in mid- to late teens who legally live outside parental or guardian control, usually through judicial decree, as long as minor

  - Is self-supporting.
  - Is legally married.
  - Is serving in the armed forces.

[ETHICS ISSUES The Beginning of Life and Childhood]

Ethics ISSUE 1: Reproductive science has progressed so rapidly that laws have not kept pace. For example, in 1996 a couple lost their adult single daughter, Julie, to leukemia. Before her death, Julie had paid a fertility clinic to harvest and freeze several of her eggs. When Julie died, her parents inherited the frozen eggs, along with Julie's furniture and other material possessions. Julie's parents then paid a surrogate mother to carry one of Julie's implanted eggs, fertilized by a sperm donor. Julie's parents did not plan to raise their grandchild themselves.

"This field [of reproductive medicine] is screaming for oversight, regulation and control," Arthur Caplan, director of the Center for Bioethics at the University of Pennsylvania, told *The Washington Post* in 1998 when asked about the previous scenario. "If you are going to make babies in new and novel ways, you have to be sure it's in the interest of the baby."

Discussion Questions

1. Although no laws prevented the parents in the previous situation from paying a surrogate mother to carry one of their deceased daughter's fertilized eggs, in your opinion did they act ethically? Why or why not? What values are involved in your answer?

_____

_____

_____

2. In your opinion, how should the child's parents have been determined in the previous scenario? (The surrogate mother miscarried.)

_____

_____

Ethics ISSUE 2: Your neighbor's daughter, who is 16, has made an appointment to see a physician in the clinic where you work as a medical assistant. You have assisted the physician with the examination of the girl, and he has determined that she is pregnant.

Discussion Questions

1. The patient's mother telephones you at home, demanding to know why her daughter saw the physician. What do you tell her?

_____

_____

2. When the patient learns she is pregnant, she tearfully requests information about an abortion. What are you and the girl's physician allowed to tell her—both legally and ethically? Based on your personal values, what would you tell the girl?

_____

_____

Ethics ISSUE 3: Predictive genetic testing is offered to asymptomatic adults even when there is no effective treatment. Testing of young people in similar circumstances is controversial, and guidelines recommend against it. Most young people seeking genetic testing want to know (or their parents want to know) if they have a genetic predisposition to develop Huntington's disease.

Discussion Questions

1. In your opinion should immature young people—say under the age of 14—be genetically tested for adult-onset diseases that have no effective treatment or cure? Explain your answer.

_____

_____

2. Should mature young people who express a genuine desire to know be genetically tested for Huntington's disease or any other adult-onset disease for which there is no effective treatment? Explain your answer.

_____

_____

Go to **www.mhhe.com/judson6e** to practice your case review skills. Then read on for more information.

KEY TERMS

amniocentesis	genetic discrimination	in vitro fertilization (IVF)
artificial insemination	genetic engineering	mature minors
chromosome	genetics	multipotent stem cells
clone	genome	mutation
cloning	heredity	*parens patriae*
DNA (deoxyribonucleic acid)	heterologous artificial insemination	pluripotent stem cells
emancipated minors	homologous artificial insemination	safe haven laws
gene		stem cells
gene therapy	Human Genome Project	surrogate mother
genetic counselor	infertility	xenotransplantation

CHAPTER 11 REVIEW

Applying Knowledge

Circle the correct answer for each of the following questions.

LO 11.1

1. Which of the following best describes the term *genetics*?
   a. The science of heredity
   b. The science that accounts for natural differences and resemblances among organisms related by descent
   c. The process by which organisms pass genetic traits on to their offspring
   d. The science of studying genes

2. The complex arrangement of proteins that comprises genes and chromosomes is called
   a. Deoxyribonucleic acid
   b. DPA
   c. Amino acids
   d. Hydrochloric acid

3. *Heredity* is best defined as
   a. One's family tree
   b. The science of genetics
   c. The process by which organisms pass on genetic traits to their offspring
   d. The science of studying genes

4. A *genome* is
   a. A type of gene
   b. A type of chromosome
   c. All the DNA in an organism, including its genes
   d. A family's genetic history.

5. The Human Genome Project
   a. Mapped all the genes on a human's chromosomes
   b. Was funded by the U.S. government
   c. Was so successful it was completed early
   d. All of the above

LO 11.2

6. Susan's father developed Huntington's disease when she was 28. She is healthy, but wants to be tested to see if she has the gene to develop the disease. What type of genetic testing will she have?
   a. Predictive genetic testing
   b. Diagnostic genetic testing
   c. Carrier genetic testing
   d. Preimplantation genetic testing

7. A permanent change in DNA is called a
   a. Gene
   b. Chromosome
   c. Mutation
   d. Genome

8. A test performed to determine if harmful genes are present in a fetus is called
   a. Diagnostic genetic testing
   b. Amniocentesis
   c. Carrier genetic testing
   d. Preimplantation genetic testing

9. In which of the following situations might DNA testing be indicated?
   a. A man involved in a paternity suit
   b. Parents who suspect they brought the wrong baby home from the hospital
   c. A woman who is a suspect in a murder
   d. All of the above

10. *Genetic discrimination* is best described as
   a. A government-sponsored project
   b. A form of favoritism in employment
   c. Differential treatment of individuals based on their actual or presumed genetic differences
   d. None of the above

LO 11.3

11. Dolly the sheep was created through a genetic engineering process called
   a. Heredity
   b. Stem cell transfer
   c. DNA testing
   d. Cloning

12. One serious concern with the genetic engineering process referred to in question 11, after Dolly's death, was
   a. Lung disease, which was a result
   b. Premature aging
   c. That the process was unsuccessful
   d. That more Dollys would be produced

13. Genetic engineering is often accomplished through the use of specialized cells referred to as
   a. Leukocytes
   b. Nuclear cells
   c. Autosomal cells
   d. Stem cells

14. Specialized cells described as *pluripotent* are capable of
    a. Dividing very quickly
    b. Decaying very quickly
    c. Becoming nearly any type of body cell
    d. Becoming only one type of body cell

15. *Multipotent* cells are capable of
    a. Dividing just once
    b. Becoming a limited number of types of body cells
    c. Becoming any type of body cell
    d. Decaying very quickly

LO 11.4

16. *Artificial insemination* may be an acceptable remedy for
    a. Pregnancy
    b. Infertility
    c. Surrogacy
    d. Cloning

17. Which of the following best defines *in vitro fertilization*?
    a. The union of egg and sperm
    b. The fusion of egg and cell nucleus
    c. Fertilization taking place outside a woman's body
    d. Cloning

18. Which of the following best defines *surrogacy*?
    a. A woman bears a child for another woman.
    b. A woman is artificially inseminated.
    c. Fertilization takes place outside a woman's body.
    d. None of the above.

LO 11.5

19. Which term means the government serves as parent to a child?
    a. Surrogacy
    b. In vitro fertilization
    c. *Parens patriae*
    d. Adoption

20. What is the common standard when the government must enter into decision making for minor children?
    a. Civil Rights Law
    b. Adoption law
    c. Surrogacy
    d. Best interest of the child

21. In which of the following situations is it legal and ethical for physicians to withhold life support for a newborn?
    a. Child is chronically and irreversibly comatose.
    b. Child has no reasonable hope of survival.
    c. Treatment would be painful and inhumane.
    d. All of the above.

22. Federal regulations concerning newborns who are severely disabled take their authority from which federal regulation?
    a. Safe haven law
    b. federal child abuse amendments
    c. Civil Rights Act
    d. None of the above

23. State laws that allow mothers to abandon newborns to designated safe facilities without penalty are called
    a. Best interest of the child laws
    b. Safe haven laws

    c.   Newborn treatment laws

    d.   Civil rights laws

24. In most states, which of the following age groups can receive some types of medical care without parental permission?

    a.   Mature minors

    b.   Minors over age 14

    c.   Minors under age 18

    d.   None of the above

25. Minors may be declared emancipated only if they

    a.   Go to court and request emancipation

    b.   Receive parental permission to request emancipation

    c.   Are self-supporting

    d.   None of the above

26. Once declared emancipated, a minor can lose that status if he or she

    a.   Was married but divorces

    b.   Was in the military but is discharged

    c.   Was self-supporting but loses a job

    d.   None of the above causes loss of emancipated minor status

27. A physician or other health care practitioner who treats a minor in a nonemergency situation, without parental consent, risks being charged with

    a.   Kidnapping

    b.   Assault and/or battery

    c.   Violating the Civil Rights Act

    d.   No charges can ever be made

[CASE STUDIES]

Use your critical thinking skills to answer the questions that follow each case study.

LO 11.1

Since the 1980s it has been legal in the United States to patent genes. That fact was brought home to Lisbeth Ceriani, a Massachusetts woman who developed an aggressive form of cancer in both breasts at age 42. She wanted to be tested for mutations in the BRCA gene, to find out if she was also at high risk for ovarian cancer. "I didn't want to just go ahead and have my ovaries removed if I didn't necessarily have to," Ceriani told a reporter for *USA Today*.

Unfortunately, Ceriani discovered that the company that manufactures the tests, Myriad Genetics of Salt Lake City, owns the patent on the gene. Myriad Genetics refused to contract with Ceriani's insurance provider, a Massachusetts form of Medicaid, because reimbursement fees were too low. Ceriani waited a year and a half to be tested, until Myriad Genetics donated 200 tests to Massachusetts.

The test showed that Ceriani had the gene mutation, and she then had her ovaries removed.

Ownership of the patents for both BRCA1 and BRCA2—the mutations for a common type of breast cancer—meant that researchers and others who wanted to look at or use the gene for research had to pay Myriad Genetics, the patent holder. Ceriani joined an ACLU lawsuit to overturn Myriad's patent, and in March 2010, U.S. District Court Judge Robert Sweet in New York State invalidated part of seven patents granted to Myriad on the two breast cancer genes. The ruling was expected to reach the U.S. Supreme Court on appeal, but if left in place, could change the 30-year practice of gene patenting.

28. In your opinion, should genes be considered private property? Why or why not?

29. Should individuals receive payment if they turn over ownership of genes to researchers? Why or why not?

30. Should scientists or drug companies be allowed to patent genes as they do other discoveries and inventions? Why or why not?

31. The ACLU said in the previous lawsuit that the proper time for a patent is not when a company or researcher isolates a gene, but when a marketable product, such as a drug or a test, is developed based on that gene. Do you agree or disagree?

LO 11.4

As reproductive technology advanced, headlines announcing "Couple Battles over Frozen Embryos" became more and more commonplace. For example, in the 1980s a man went to court and succeeded in preventing his ex-wife from using their frozen embryos to become pregnant. He maintained that after he and his wife had divorced, he no longer wanted to become a parent, and should not be forced to do so against his will.

In 1998, a divorced woman in New Jersey won a legal battle with her ex-husband over custody of seven frozen embryos the couple had created in vitro while still married. The wife wanted to have the embryos destroyed, while the ex-husband argued his right to adopt his own embryos to be implanted in a future partner or donated to an infertile couple.

32. In your opinion, should frozen embryos be considered property to be awarded during a divorce? Why or why not?

33. Should a man who loses custody of frozen embryos in a lawsuit be responsible for child support if his ex-wife is implanted with the embryos and becomes pregnant at a later date? Explain your answer.

34. Should the husband or wife who wins custody of frozen embryos be allowed to destroy them, against the wishes of the ex-husband or ex-wife? Why or why not?

[INTERNET ACTIVITIES LO 11.1, LO 11.4, and LO 11.5]

Complete the activities and answer the questions that follow.

35. Visit the Web site for the Human Genome Project at **www.ornl.gov/ sci/techresources/Human_Genome/home.shtml**. What are three of the medical applications expected to result from the project or presently in use as a result of the project?

36. Visit the fact sheet page for the American Society for Reproductive Medicine at **www.asrm.org/detail.aspx?id=2322**. How does the page define *infertility*? Briefly summarize additional information presented.

37. Visit the Planned Parenthood Federation of America's Web site for teens at **www.plannedparenthood.org/teen-talk/**. Briefly summarize the topics available there. In your opinion, does the site promote

valid health care issues? Why or why not? The site is controversial. Comment on why you think this is so.

[RESOURCES]

Geller, Lisa N., Joseph S. Alper, Paul R. Billings, Carol I. Barash, Jonathan Beckwith, et al. *Science and Engineering Ethics* 2, no. 1 (1996), 71–88.

Weise, Elizabeth Weise. "Is It Unfair to Patent Genes?" *USA Today*, April 13, 2010, p. 10B.

Zimmer, Carl. "Voices: What's Next in Science?" *The New York Times*, online ed., November 9, 2010, **www.nytimes.com/interactive/2010/11/09/ science/20111109_next_feature.html?nl=todaysheadlines&emc=ab1**.

Alzheimer's disease gene: **http://ghr.nlm.nih.gov/gene/APOE**.

Cases of genetic discrimination: **www.genome.gov/12513976**.

Cloning humans: **www.ornl.gov/sci/techresources/Human_Genome/ elsi/cloning.shtml#humans**.

Disadvantages to safe haven laws: **www.ncsl.org/IssuesResearch/ HumanServices/UpdateSafeHavensforAbandonedInfants/ tabid/16434/Default.aspx#Policymakers**.

Distinguishing genetic from nongenetic medical tests, Joseph S. Alper and Jon Beckwith: **www.springerlink.com/content/lu7v417x88884185/**.

Dolly dies: **www.newscientist.com/article/dn3393-dolly-the-sheep-dies-young.html**.

Dolly "277 attempts": **www.animalresearch.info/en/medical/timeline/ Dolly**.

Evan B. Donaldson Adoption Institute Web site: **www.adoptioninstitute. org/whowe/lastreport coverpage.html**

Geller study: **www.springerlink.com/content/739823h426q50x51/**.

Genetic testing: **http://ghr.nlm.nih.gov/handbook/testing/uses** and **www.genome.gov/19516567#al-2I**.

Genetic testing/diseases: **www.nlm.nih.gov/medlineplus/genetictesting. html**.

Genetics articles: **www.mayoclinic.com/health/genetic-testing/ MY00370/TAB=expertblog**.

Judge blocks stem cell funding by NIH: **www.washingtonpost.com/ wp-dyn/content/article/2010/08/23/AR2010082303448.html**.

How many genetic diseases + types of genetic diseases: **www.genetic-diseases.net/http://www.aicardisyndrome.org/site/**.

Obama stem cell research: **www.cbsnews.com/stories/2009/03/09/ politics/100days/domesticissues/main4853385.shtml**.

Tests for 1,700 diseases: **www.cdc.gov/genomics/gtesting/**.

Uses of genetic testing (University of Washington): **www.genetests.org/**.

chapter twelve

DEATH AND DYING

Learning Outcomes

After studying this chapter, you should be able to:

LO 12.1 Discuss how attitudes toward death have changed over time.

LO 12.2 Discuss accepted criteria for determining death.

LO 12.3 Determine the health care professional's role in caring for the dying.

LO 12.4 Discuss benefits to end-of-life health care derived from the right to die movement.

LO 12.5 Identify the major features of organ donation in the United States.

LO 12.6 Discuss the various stages of grief.

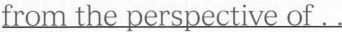

from the perspective of . . .

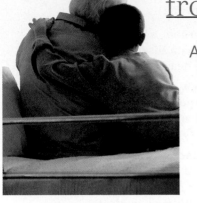

ANGELA HAS BEEN A REGISTERED NURSE FOR 18 YEARS. Just as some hospital nurses are drawn to surgery, the emergency room, or the intensive care unit, Angela prefers hospice and palliative care. "Broadly speaking," Angela explains, "medicine is about repairing, extending, and medicating, while end-of-life care is more about the patient as an individual, about basic human needs. In addition, it isn't just the patient you are caring for; you are caring for the entire family group—everybody needs you.

"We live in a time when death has been removed from family and home for the most part," Angela continues, "and people generally have less understanding of the process than a hundred years ago. . . . The family most often feels helpless and confused. The hospice nurse is able to help not just the patient, but the family, too, through a sad and often frightening time."

Sometimes family members are hesitant about approaching a dying loved one. For example, Angela remembers a situation where the mother of two siblings in their thirties was dying. "When I arrived they were practically plastered against the walls of the room, clearly unsure of what they should be doing." Angela encouraged the two family members to come to their mother's bedside and comfort her. "The son pulled a chair to the side of the bed and held his mother's hand. The daughter climbed onto the bed and cradled her mother. . . . I like to think that because I urged them to take a more active part in her passing that they found comfort after their mother was gone."

Angela also recalls a patient in his eighties whose 32 family members joined him in his hospice room. "It was almost a living wake. They talked for hours about his life and the experiences they had each shared with him. They laughed and they cried and it was wonderful. This sharing in their loved one's death was a beautiful experience for those left behind, and I hope it helped him in some way as well."

From Angela's perspective as a hospice nurse, the end of a life is a time when family members can come together to comfort their dying loved one and each other. She sees her job as a facilitator for this natural process.

From the perspective of the individual who is dying, the nearness of family members is comforting, as well as the presence of a nurse who is not uncomfortable with end-of-life issues.

From the perspective of surviving family members, Angela has heard many times that her attitude—don't be afraid to comfort your loved one—gave them the courage to participate in the process, and comforted them after the death occurred.

In your opinion, what personal characteristics make Angela an effective hospice nurse?

Could you care for dying patients in a situation such as Angela's? Why or why not?

Attitudes toward Death and Dying

LO 12.1

Discuss how attitudes toward death have changed over time.

Prior to the twentieth century, death was an intimate experience for most families. Antibiotics and chemotherapies had not yet been discovered; genetically engineered drugs, organ transplantation, and life-support machines were still science fiction; and infectious diseases periodically decimated populations. Nearly every husband and wife, mother and father, brother and sister had lost a loved one. Loved ones customarily died at home, surrounded by family members who bade them goodbye and then mourned their passing with funeral rituals and rites, including the following:

- Black has long been worn by undertakers, mourners, and pallbearers to show grief. In ancient times it was also used as a disguise to protect against malevolent spirits that might be lurking nearby.

- An early custom for mourners was to go barefoot and to wear sackcloth and ashes. This was said to discourage the dead from becoming envious as they might be if mourners appeared at funerals wearing new clothes and shoes.

- Pagan tribes began the custom of covering the face of the deceased with a sheet, since they believed that the spirit of the deceased escaped through the mouth. They often held the mouth and nose of a sick person shut, hoping to retain the spirit and thus delay death.

- In earlier times, traffic was halted for a funeral procession because any delay in transporting a soul might turn it into a restless ghost, reluctant to pass over into the next world.

- Wakes held today come from the ancient custom of keeping watch over the deceased, hoping that life would return. In England the dead were always carried out of the house feet first; otherwise, their spirits might look back into the house and beckon family members to come with them.

- Pagan beliefs concerning funeral wreaths held that the circle formed by the wreath would keep the dead person's spirit within bounds.

- The firing of a rifle volley over the deceased is similar to the tribal practice of throwing spears into the air to ward off spirits hovering over the deceased.

- In the past, holy water was sprinkled on the body to protect it from demons.

> **Figure 12-1**

"Individuals around the United States contributed to the **AIDS memorial quilt,** shown here in Washington, DC."

By the late twentieth century, individuals were more likely to die in the hospital, at least in the Western world. Once admitted to hospitals, the dying were isolated from family members and surrounded by machines designed to prolong life as long as possible. Consequently, modern technology has effectively hidden death from view, but in so doing it has also made the end of life a fearful prospect.

Attitudes toward death and dying vary with individuals, of course, but as each of us ages, we will likely begin to think of our own mortality and perhaps to wonder how the end will come. Will I die alone, in an impersonal, clinical hospital environment? Will my health care providers be so committed to preserving life that they delay my dying to an irrational degree? Will I suffer in pain? Will I feel a sense of tasks left unfinished and goals left unrealized, or will I experience a peaceful letting go?

Because the fears associated with death and dying are universal, health care practitioners should evaluate their own attitudes to effectively and compassionately respond to dying patients and their families (Figure 12-1).

Determination of Death

Modern medical technology and life-support equipment may keep a person's body "alive"—the heart may beat and blood may circulate—long after the brain ceases to function. This makes it difficult in some cases to determine the moment when death actually occurs. For this reason, in 1981 a **Uniform Determination of Death Act** was proposed by the President's Commission for the Study of Ethical Problems in Medicine and Biomedical Research working in cooperation with the American Bar Association, the American Medical Association, and the National Conference of Commissioners on Uniform State Laws. The National Conference of Commissioners on Uniform State Laws has no legislative authority. Acts the commissioners propose must still be approved by state legislatures, and that is sometimes difficult to accomplish. States have their own criteria for determining when death actually occurs, but most have adopted the act's definition of **brain death** as a means of determining when death actually occurs:

- Circulatory and respiratory functions have irreversibly ceased.
- The entire brain, including the brain stem, has irreversibly ceased to function.

When the brain is injured or shuts down due to lack of oxygen, a patient may appear near death when, in fact, he or she is in a **coma,** which is a condition of deep stupor from which a patient cannot be roused by external stimuli. Patients can and do recover from comas, as opposed to a persistent vegetative state. **Persistent vegetative state (PVS)** exists as a result of severe mental impairment, characterized by irreversible cessation of the higher functions of the brain, most often caused by damage to the cerebral cortex. In PVS, only involuntary bodily functions are present, and there exists no reasonable expectation of regaining significant mental function (Figure 12-2).

Before pronouncing an unresponsive and unconscious patient dead, physicians may perform a series of tests to determine whether death has occurred. Death is indicated if the following signs are present. The patient

- Cannot breathe without assistance.
- Has no coughing or gagging reflex.
- Has no pupil response to light.
- Has no blinking reflex when the cornea is touched.
- Has no grimace reflex when the head is rotated or ears are flushed with ice water.
- Has no response to pain.

Today the declaration of death occurs only when the last signs of brain and respiratory activity are gone. Technically, death results from lack of oxygen. When deprived of oxygen, cells cannot maintain metabolic function and soon begin to deteriorate.

Autopsies

After a patient is declared dead, family members (next of kin) may be asked to consent to an autopsy. An autopsy is a postmortem examination to determine cause of death and/or to obtain physiological evidence when necessary. Autopsies performed in hospitals may confirm or correct clinical diagnoses, thus providing a measure of quality assurance.

LO 12.2

Discuss accepted criteria for determining death.

Uniform Determination of Death Act   A proposal that established uniform guidelines for determining when death has occurred.

brain death   Final cessation of bodily activity, used to determine when death actually occurs; circulatory and respiratory functions have irreversibly ceased, and the entire brain (including the brain stem) has irreversibly ceased to function.

coma   A condition of deep stupor from which the patient cannot be roused by external stimuli.

persistent vegetative state (PVS)   Severe mental impairment characterized by irreversible cessation of the higher functions of the brain, most often caused by damage to the cerebral cortex.

> Figure 12-2

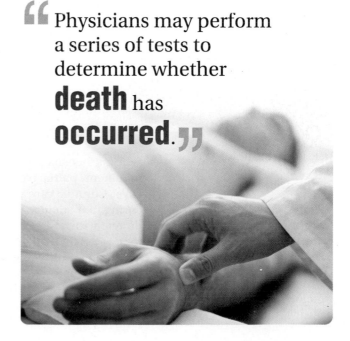

" Physicians may perform a series of tests to determine whether **death** has **occurred**. "

Autopsy results can also highlight those cases in which diagnoses tend to be incorrect, or treatments tend to be ineffective, thereby adding to scientific knowledge and revealing areas that need further study. In cases of suspicious deaths, autopsy results can provide information to help law enforcement authorities, such as cause and time of death. (Legal requirements concerning autopsies are discussed in Chapter 9.)

While autopsies must be performed in cases in which the death is suspicious or due to homicide, the number of autopsies performed in all other deaths each year has steadily declined. One reason that fewer autopsies are performed today is cost—insurance companies and government health care programs usually do not pay for autopsies. (However, when patients die in hospitals, often an autopsy can be performed free of charge.) Some clinicians argue that technological advances have made clinical diagnoses more accurate, so that postmortem diagnoses are less essential. Another reason for the decline in autopsies is that in many smaller hospitals, pathologists are not readily available.

Furthermore, even though autopsies can yield information that may clarify causes of death, reveal genetic disease that runs in families, or reassure survivors that their loved ones could not have been saved, when an autopsy is not mandated by law, family members are often reluctant to give consent. They may feel that their loved one has "suffered enough," that the physician already knows the cause of death, or that the procedure would interfere with viewing of the body during funeral rites. Health care practitioners may believe that these perceptions of autopsies are inaccurate, but they must remain sensitive to the beliefs and emotions of surviving family members.

check your **progress**

1. Briefly explain how attitudes toward death and dying in the United States have changed over the years.

   _____

2. The _____ , while not a law, was proposed as a universal means of determining when death actually occurs.

3. Distinguish between *comatose* and *persistent vegetative state*.

4. Define *brain death*.

5. Name six signs for which physicians may test that indicate death has occurred.

   _____

LO 12.3

Determine the health care professional's role in caring for the dying.

palliative care Treatment of a terminally ill patient's symptoms to make dying more comfortable; also called comfort care.

curative care Treatment directed toward curing a patient's disease.

Caring for Dying Patients

When it becomes evident that a patient's disease is incurable and death is imminent, **palliative care** may serve the dying patient better than **curative care**. Curative care consists of treatments and procedures directed toward curing a patient's disease. Palliative care, also called comfort care, is directed toward providing relief to terminally ill patients through symptom and pain management. The goal is not to cure, but to provide comfort and maintain the highest possible quality of life. Going beyond relief of disease symptoms, palliative care includes relief of emotional distress and other problems, so that a patient's last months and days may be as comfortable as possible.

Palliative care is also emerging as a way to help patients with serious illnesses live a more comfortable and fulfilling life, whether their diseases are terminal or not. For example, through palliative care

- A 90-year-old stroke patient with limited mobility is able to continue living independently in his home.

- An ovarian cancer patient is more comfortable and can actually continue working as she undergoes aggressive chemotherapy treatment.

- A lung cancer patient receives counseling about his disease and help in navigating the complex U.S. health care system.

The Center to Advance Palliative Care, based in New York, provides information to help patients and their families receive care that addresses all of the patient's needs. According to the organization's statistics, some 58 percent of U.S. hospitals provide palliative care—up from just half that number since 2000. (Visit the center's Web site at **www.capc.org** for information about goals and services.)

Traditionally, in educational programs for health care practitioners, courses of study have placed more emphasis on curative care than on palliative care. Treatments included in curative care include surgery, chemotherapy, radiation therapy, and other treatments and procedures, and may be used more aggressively as a patient's disease progresses. Since most physicians are taught to fight disease with every product and technique at their command, it is sometimes difficult for them to recognize or admit that curative care has failed or is no longer effective in treating a patient's disease. Through use of palliative care, health care providers can help relieve a dying patient's pain and emotional distress and ease the journey toward life's end (Figure 12-3).

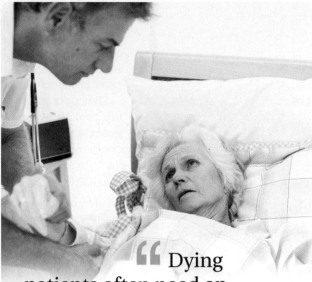

▶ Figure 12-3

"Dying patients often need an **understanding listener** and this may be a health care practitioner."

Hospice Care

Terminally ill patients are often referred to facilities or agencies that provide **hospice** care. A hospice in medieval times was a way station for travelers. The first modern hospice facilities were established in England in the 1960s as places where patients could go to die in comfort.

In the United States, hospice care may be provided in facilities built especially for that purpose, in hospitals and nursing homes, or at home. (Angela, in the chapter's opening scenario, practices in a hospital. The floor she supervises is designated a hospice.) Hospice care focuses on relieving pain, controlling symptoms, and meeting emotional needs and personal values of the terminally ill, instead of targeting the underlying disease process. The hospice philosophy also recognizes that family members and other caregivers deserve care and support, continuing after the death of the patient. Hospice programs ease dying; they do not support active euthanasia (a Greek term meaning 'good death') or assisted suicide.

Bereavement services are also available through hospice care to help patients discuss such issues as preparing a will and planning a funeral, and to help surviving family members cope with grief and loss after the patient dies. Hospice programs generally provide bereavement services through discussion groups, follow-up visits from hospice personnel, and sometimes referral to appropriate mental health professionals.

hospice A facility or program (often carried out in a patient's home) in which teams of health care practitioners and volunteers provide a continuing environment that focuses on the physical, emotional, and psychological needs of the dying patient.

Most in-home hospice programs are independently run in a fashion similar to visiting nurse or home health care agencies. Patients receive coordinated care at home by multidisciplinary teams composed of physicians, nurses, social workers, home health aides, pharmacists, physical therapists, clergy, volunteers, and family members. Hospice teams meet regularly to work on patients' needs concerning pain and other serious symptoms, depression, family problems, inadequate housing, financial problems, or lack of transportation. The team then expands, amends, or otherwise revises each patient's care plan, as necessary.

For patients to be eligible for hospice care, physicians usually must certify that they are not expected to live beyond six months. Hospice care is generally reimbursed by Medicare, Medicaid, and many private insurance companies and managed care programs.

Educating Health Care Practitioners about End-of-Life Issues

While modern medicine has effectively delayed the moment of death, in many cases it has dealt less conscientiously with compassionate, comfort care for **terminally ill** patients: those who are not expected to live beyond six months, usually because of a chronic illness that has progressed beyond effective treatment or for which there is no cure.

Studies published within the last two decades have shown the need for educating health care practitioners in end-of-life care:

- A 1995 study published in the *Journal of the American Medical Association (JAMA)* found that nearly 4 out of every 10 terminally ill patients spend at least 10 days in intensive care connected to life-sustaining machines. The same study found that half of patients who die in hospitals experience moderate to severe pain.

- In November 1996, the Robert Wood Johnson Foundation published results of the largest study ever conducted on patients near death. The six-year Study to Understand Prognoses and Preferences for Outcomes and Risks of Treatment (SUPPORT) showed that more than 50 percent of people dying in hospitals suffered from uncontrolled pain, and that decisions to medicate were inappropriately timed. The study of 9,100 hospitalized

terminally ill Referring to patients who are expected to die within six months.

check your **progress**

6. Distinguish between *palliative care* and *curative care*.

_____

7. Define *hospice*.

_____

Indicate with a "C" or a "P" whether each of the following actions constitutes a form of curative care or palliative care.

_____ 8. Allowing a patient who is terminally ill with lung and stomach cancer to self-administer morphine patches as needed for pain relief.

_____ 9. Administering radiation treatments after breast cancer surgery.

_____ 10. Surgical severing of certain nerves to relieve suffering for a patient terminally ill with cancer of the spine.

_____ 11. Counseling a terminally ill patient and his or her family concerning funeral arrangements and other end-of-life decisions.

_____ 12. Administering antibiotics to cure an infected tooth.

_____ 13. Cosmetic surgery for a teenaged patient whose face was burned in a fire.

patients also showed that most physicians did not know their patients' end-of-life wishes or did not follow them, and that half of those patients who were conscious during the last three days of life died in pain.

- A survey by the Association of American Medical Colleges in 1998 found that 122 medical schools (96.1 percent) included information about death and dying as part of an existing course, but just 6 schools (4.7 percent) featured the subject as a separate required course. Fifty schools (39.4 percent) offered a course in death and dying as an elective.

- A survey of medical textbooks, published in the February 9, 2001, issue of *JAMA* showed that most "don't deal with the end of life," according to the article's lead author, Michael Rabow of the University of California at San Francisco Medical School. Of the 50 top-selling textbooks that were reviewed, 56.9 percent did not discuss end-of-life care at all. The remaining books either covered the topic minimally (19.1 percent) or did include some helpful information on end-of-life care (24.1 percent).

- A report by the National Research Council and the Institute of Medicine issued in June 2001 states that U.S. physicians and hospitals are not prepared to handle the suffering of dying cancer patients. The report, *Improving Palliative Care for Cancer: Summary and Recommendations,* says that federal research and training efforts have focused largely on treatment and finding cures, while neglecting symptom control measures that could relieve a patient's suffering.

- In 2001, the American Medical Association (AMA), an organization for physicians, first implemented a program called Education for Physicians on End of Life Care (EPEC). The project, now funded by Northwestern University Medical School, is designed to educate all health care practitioners on the essential clinical competencies required to provide quality end-of-life care.

- In 2004, the American Medical Students Association (AMSA) formed a death and dying interest group, in response to medical students' consensus that medical school leaves students inadequately prepared to communicate with terminally ill patients, as well as poorly equipped emotionally to deal with matters of death and dying. The AMSA interest group continues to provide guidance, support, and resources for students who wish to supplement their medical education in the area of death and dying.

- A 2010 study of 12 Washington State hospitals found that programs aimed at improving health care practitioners' ability to communicate with patients and families in ICUs did not improve end-of-life care, according to results published online in the *American Journal of Respiratory and Critical Care Medicine.* For example, wrote J. Randall Curtis, MD, one of the study's authors, "Many patients [in the intensive care unit] die with moderate or severe pain and physicians are often unaware of patients' preferences regarding end-of-life care." In addition, the study found, "Family of ICU patients have a high prevalence of symptoms of anxiety, depression, and post-traumatic stress disorder . . . and report physician and nurse behaviors that increase their burden." Study conclusions supported improving education among doctors, patients, family members, nurses, and social workers to improve end-of-life care and patient/family satisfaction. "This is an area of care that is especially important in our current time," Curtis added.

- A 2010 British study that surveyed 8,500 physicians found that their religious beliefs often affected the quality of end-of-life care administered. The more religious the physician, the more likely he or she is to avoid discussions with very ill patients about comfort care only. Physicians who describe themselves as agnostics or atheists were more open to patient requests for less aggressive end-of-life care.

thanatology The study of death and of the psychological methods of coping with it.

Fortunately, the need to teach end-of-life care to physicians and other health care practitioners has been recognized. Increasingly, schools that train health care providers are offering courses in **thanatology**—the study of death and of the psychological methods of coping with death. In addition, many organizations exist that list their primary mission as advocacy for improved care for the dying and educating health professionals and the public about end-of-life issues. A sampling of such groups includes Americans for Better Care of the Dying (ABCD) (**www.abcd-caring.org**), Compassion & Choices (**www.compassionandchoices.org**), Finding Our Way (FOW) (**www.findingourway.net**), Partnership for Caring (**www.partnershipforcaring.com/**), Growth House (**www.growthhouse.org**), and the American Institute of Life-Threatening Illness and Loss (**www.lifethreat.org**). An Internet search for "death and dying" will provide URLs for many more organizations. Many of these organizations provide living will and medical power of attorney forms, and all provide useful information to the public. Some routinely file *amicus curiae* (friend of the court) briefs in legal cases addressing end-of-life issues. Others are engaged in research, public advocacy, and education activities to improve the care of the dying and their families.

Despite a conscious effort to improve training and attitudes regarding dying patients, end-of-life care remains one of the most emotional issues for health care practitioners.

LO 12.4

Discuss benefits to end-of-life health care derived from the right to die movement.

The Right to Die Movement

Americans have long been concerned that advancing medical technology may allow health care practitioners to delay death beyond the point where any quality of life can be maintained or a cure realized, thus depriving individuals of the right to die as they wish. This concern led to the first living will, created and made available to the public by attorney Luis Kutner, who founded the Euthanasia Society. Kutner's goal was to help dying people exercise their rights to control end-of-life medical care.

The right to die first became a matter for the courts to deliberate in 1976, with the death of Karen Ann Quinlan.

The *Quinlan* case raised important questions in bioethics, euthanasia, and the legal rights of guardians. The case resulted in the development of formal ethics committees in hospitals, long-term care facilities, and hospices. It also called attention to the need for advance health directives.

Another landmark case in the right to die movement involved Nancy Cruzan, a 26-year-old woman who was severely injured in a car crash.

While the previous landmark legal cases furthered certain right to die arguments, other events in the nation's history have also furthered the cause. Here is a timeline:

- 1946—Committee of 1776 Physicians for Legalizing Voluntary Euthanasia is formed in New York State.

- 1967—Attorney Luis Kutner and members of the Euthanasia Society (later called Choice in Dying and then Partnership for Caring, both organizations now defunct) devise the original living will.

- 1973—American Hospital Association creates the Patient's Bill of Rights. (To date, attempts to pass a federal Patient's Bill of Rights have consistently failed.)

- 1976—California's Natural Death Act, the nation's first right to die statute, is signed into law.

- 1977—Laws dealing with the refusal of treatment are passed in Arkansas, Idaho, Nevada, New Mexico, North Carolina, Oregon, and Texas.

LANDMARK COURT CASE

Right to Die Precedent

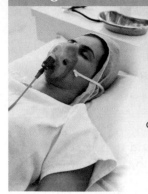

In 1976, the parents of Karen Ann Quinlan, then 22, obtained permission from a New Jersey court to remove their daughter from a respirator. Karen Ann had been in a persistent vegetative state for several months, after allegedly ingesting an unknown combination of alcohol and drugs. Karen Ann's father, as her legal guardian, had asked her physicians to remove the respirator believed to be sustaining her life. The physicians refused, and the Quinlans sued for their daughter's right to die. A lower court held for the physicians, but on appeal, judges allowed Karen Ann's respirator to be disconnected. She continued to live via a feeding tube, but died in June 1985 of pneumonia, at the age of 31.

Source: In re Quinlan, 70 N.J. 10, 49, 355 A.2d 647, 668 (1976).

LANDMARK COURT CASE

Legal Struggle to Remove Feeding Tube

On January 11, 1983, Nancy Beth Cruzan was driving alone when she lost control of her older model car that had no seat belts. Nancy was thrown from the car and landed face down in a water-filled ditch. When emergency medical technicians arrived Nancy had no vital signs, but the EMTs resuscitated her. After about two weeks Nancy had not awakened and her condition was diagnosed as persistent vegetative state, following irreversible brain damage. Physicians inserted a feeding tube for Nancy's long-term care.

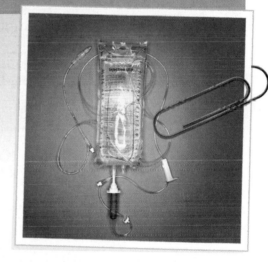

After four years with no improvement, Nancy's parents asked to have the feeding tube removed. The hospital demanded a court order, and a three-year legal battle ensued. The trial court ruled that the feeding tube could be removed, based on testimony given by one of Nancy's friends that she would not want to live on artificial life support. The Missouri State Supreme Court reversed the trial court's ruling, holding that the lower court did not meet the *clear and convincing evidence* standard. The case reached the U.S. Supreme Court, where justices affirmed the Missouri State Supreme Court ruling and recognized that the right to refuse medical treatment is guaranteed by the U.S. Constitution. The case was sent back to the trial court, for the purpose of gathering clear and convincing evidence that Nancy Cruzan would not have wanted to live in a persistent vegetative state. Three of Nancy's friends testified as to her wishes, and the court ruled that this met the clear and convincing evidence standard, and that the feeding tube could be removed. This decision was also appealed, but the appeal failed to change the court's ruling, and Nancy's feeding tube was removed in December 1990. She died 11 days later.

Source: Cruzan v. Director, Missouri Department of Health, 497 U.S. 261 (1990).

- 1984—The District of Columbia and 22 states have statutes that recognize advance directives.
- 1989—The **Uniform Rights of the Terminally Ill Act** serves as a guideline for state legislatures in constructing laws addressing advance directives.
- 1990—Congress passes the Patient Self-Determination Act, the first federal act concerning advance directives.

Uniform Rights of the Terminally Ill Act   A 1989 recommendation of the National Conference of Commissioners on Uniform State Laws that all states construct laws to address advance directives.

- 1992—Pennsylvania becomes the 50th state to enact advance-directive legislation.
- 1997—The U.S. Supreme Court holds that state bans on physician-assisted suicide do not violate the U.S. Constitution. The Court leaves the decision up to each state on whether to ban physician-assisted suicide.
- 1997—Oregon's Death with Dignity Act is passed, making the state the first to permit physician-assisted suicide in certain circumstances.
- 1997—By this date, 35 states have enacted statutes expressly criminalizing assisted suicide; 9 states criminalize assisted suicide through common law.
- 2001—The California Supreme Court clarifies the right to die in a decision that states the right to die does not extend to people who are conscious and in a twilight state, are unable to communicate or care for themselves, and have not left formal written directions for health care.
- 2006—The U.S. Supreme Court upholds Oregon's Right to Die law. As published on ABC's Web site, "Writing for a 6–3 majority, Justice Anthony Kennedy rebuffed efforts by the nation's top law enforcement official, Attorney General Alberto Gonzales, to criminally charge doctors who helped people end their lives. According to Gonzales, federal drug laws did not permit or condone doctor-assisted suicide." The Supreme Court held, however, that the federal government did not have the authority to prosecute a state's physicians.
- 2010—Only Oregon and Washington have passed laws allowing physician-assisted suicide. Thirty-four states explicitly criminalize assisted suicide. Ohio's Supreme Court ruled in 1996 that assisted suicide is not a crime; three states do not have laws criminalizing assisted suicide, but have not passed laws allowing it.

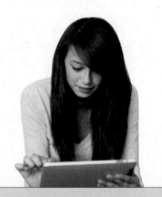

check your **progress**

14. Define *terminally ill*.

_____

15. Define *thanatology*.

_____

16. How were decisions in the *Quinlan, Cruzan,* and *Shiavo* cases significant in the right to die movement?

_____

In the United States, by 2011 two states—Oregon and Washington—had laws that allow physician-assisted suicide (see Table 12-1). Oregon's Death with Dignity Act went into effect in November 1997, and was the first in the United States to permit physician-assisted suicide In 2008, voters in Washington passed a death with dignity law, making that state the second to allow physician-assisted suicide. The law was implemented in 2010.

LANDMARK COURT CASE

Right to Die or the Right to Live?

In 1990, 27-year-old Terri Schindler Schiavo suffered an apparent heart attack at her home in Florida. Emergency medical technicians restored a heartbeat, but Terri remained comatose at first, then later semicomatose. Terri's husband, Michael Schiavo, was appointed her guardian, and she was placed in a long-term care facility, where she was finally diagnosed as being in a persistent vegetative state (PVS).

In 1992, Michael Schiavo sued Terri's physician for malpractice, and was awarded $600,000. Terri was awarded $1.4 million and $250,000 in separate medical malpractice trials.

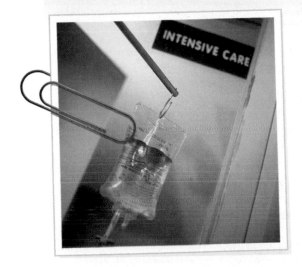

In 1993, Michael Schiavo refused medically recommended rehabilitative therapy for Terri, and her parents intervened. Bob and Mary Schindler, Terri's parents, petitioned the court to remove Michael Schiavo as Terri's guardian. A judge denied the guardianship petition. In 1997, a judge approved Michael Schiavo's petition to remove the tubes delivering Terri's hydration and nutrition. Terri seemed semiconscious, and her parents insisted she might be successfully rehabilitated.

In 1998 the court appointed a guardian *ad litem* to investigate Terri's case. The guardian *ad litem* recommended against removing Terri's feeding tubes and was dismissed for bias. In 2001, the court ordered the feeding tubes removed, despite physicians' testimonials that Terri was not in a PVS and could swallow. Many physicians also testified that Terri was in a PVS. In April of that year, Terri's feeding tubes were removed, but in light of new evidence, a new judge ordered feeding restored.

Court battles continued, with Michael Schiavo petitioning the court to end Terri's life and her parents counterpetitioning to keep Terri alive. Finally, in October 2003, the Florida legislature passed a law—"Terri's Law"—allowing then Governor Jeb Bush to issue an executive order to let Terri continue to receive nutrition and hydration. The law was repealed in September 2004.

In March 2005, Terri's husband, Michael Schiavo, won court approval to have his wife's feeding tube removed. Terri died 13 days later, on March 31, 2005, after having been in an apparent persistent vegetative state for 15 years. An autopsy performed in June 2005 confirmed that Schiavo was in a persistent vegetative state.

Source: Schindler v. Schiavo, Florida Supreme Court, 900 So.2d 554 (2005).

There are many sides to the debate over physician-assisted suicide. Some advocates believe a person has the right to control his or her own life, including choosing to end it. Others see the question from a quality-of-life perspective. That is, when one suffers from an incurable, debilitating, and/or painful disease, he or she should have the right to end the suffering. Another group argues that physician-assisted suicide should be permissible only if a person is nearly brain-dead with no chance of recovery.

Those who argue against physician-assisted suicide also hold a variety of opinions. Some simply say that killing a human being is always wrong. Others cite the Hippocratic oath as evidence that physicians are always bound to protect life and, therefore, should not be asked to assist a suicide. Opponents also claim that the potential for abuse is too great. For example, if physician-assisted suicide is sanctioned, will relatives of wealthy patients advocate for their deaths? Does serious illness alter mental states

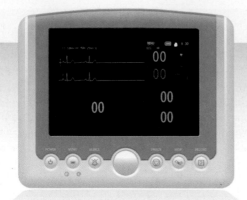

EUTHANASIA AND PHYSICIAN-ASSISTED SUICIDE

Table 12-1

In the United States, debate has raged over whether or not physicians should play a state-sanctioned role in ending a patient's life. *Euthanasia,* which in Greek means "good death," refers to mercy killing of the hopelessly ill. Physicians may be involved in a variety of ways:

Active euthanasia	Is a conscious medical act that results in the death of a dying person.
Passive euthanasia	Is the act of allowing a patient to die naturally, without medical interference.
Voluntary euthanasia	Requires the patient's consent, or that of his or her designated representative, to use medical means to end the patient's life.
Involuntary euthanasia	Is the act of ending a patient's life by medical means without the consent of the patient or his or her representative.
Physician-assisted suicide	Loosely refers to any of these euthanasia situations in which a doctor takes part in a patient's suicide.

Most states have laws against physician-assisted suicide, but many have been challenged in court. All states have some form of right-to-die laws that allow patients to decide whether they want to receive medical treatment when they are no longer competent to make decisions. Physician-assisted suicide is legal in several countries, including Germany and the Netherlands.

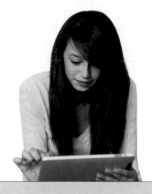

so that these patients cannot be trusted to make such decisions rationally? Will quality-of-life issues take precedence in deciding who should take advantage of statues that regulate physician-assisted suicide?

The debate over physician-assisted suicide will continue for years to come, but until legal issues are settled, health care practitioners are reminded that, legally and ethically, they are bound to consider existing law and the welfare of patients.

check your **progress**

17. Define *euthanasia.*

18. How does passive euthanasia differ from active euthanasia? Is either process legal in the United States?

19. How does voluntary euthanasia differ from involuntary euthanasia? Is either process legal in the United States?

20. In your opinion, are the death with dignity acts in Oregon and Washington ethical? Explain your answer.

Planning Ahead

In today's health care environment, individuals are well advised to be prepared for the time when they or their legal representatives may have to make decisions about medical treatment, including the use of life-sustaining measures. To address this concern, the federal **Patient Self-Determination Act** was passed in 1990 and took effect December 1, 1991. The act requires hospitals and other health care providers to provide written information to patients regarding their rights under state law to make medical decisions and execute advance directives. (Advance directives include the living will; durable power of attorney; and the health care proxy, which is simply a durable power of attorney for medical care.) The act also provides that

- Health care providers will document in the patient's medical record whether he or she has executed an advance directive.
- Providers may not discriminate against an individual based on whether or not he or she has executed an advance directive.
- Providers must comply with state laws respecting advance directives.
- Providers must have a policy for educating staff and the community regarding advance directives.

Congress's action in passing this law was due, in large part, to the *Nancy Cruzan* case, decided by the U.S. Supreme Court in June 1990.

As a result of the Patient Self-Determination Act, patients are encouraged to execute living wills or durable powers of attorney while still able to do so and before life-sustaining measures become necessary for life to continue.

Living Will

A **living will** directly provides instructions to physicians, hospitals, and other health care providers involved in a patient's treatment. It may detail circumstances under which treatment should be discontinued, such as coma, brain death, or a terminal condition. It may also detail which treatments or medications to suspend (for example, invasive surgery, artificial nutrition or hydration, and measures that serve no purpose except to delay death) and which to maintain (for example, kidney dialysis and drugs for pain). In addition, it may list which "heroic measures" (for example, emergency surgery and CPR) should and should not be used. A living will may also indicate preferences regarding organ donation, autopsy, and alternative treatments. Living wills may designate an agent to carry out these wishes if the patient is incapable of making decisions.

All 50 states accept the validity of living wills, although they also specify various requirements that must be met. Standard state forms may be obtained from a number of sources for completion by individuals and their attorneys.

Generic living will forms may also be obtained from various sources, but users should be aware of any state-specific requirements. Copies of completed forms should be given to designated family members or agents and may be filed with medical records upon a patient's admission to the hospital (see Figure 12-4).

Durable Power of Attorney

The **durable power of attorney** is not specifically a medical document, but it may serve that purpose. It confers upon a designee the authority to make a variety of legal decisions on behalf of the grantor. It takes effect when the grantor loses the capacity to make decisions, through either unconsciousness or mental incompetence. The document may place limits on the rights and responsibilities of the designee (usually an attorney or a spouse), and it may give specific instructions regarding the grantor's medical and other preferences. Standard forms are available and are governed by state law.

active euthanasia A conscious medical act that results in the death of a dying person.

passive euthanasia The act of allowing a dying patient to die naturally, without medical interference.

voluntary euthanasia The act of ending a dying patient's life by medical means with his or her permission.

involuntary euthanasia The act of ending a terminal patient's life by medical means without his or her permission.

Patient Self-Determination Act A federal law passed in 1990 that requires hospitals and other health care providers to provide written information to patients regarding their rights under state law to make medical decisions and execute advance directives.

living will An advance directive that specifies an individual's end-of-life wishes.

durable power of attorney An advance directive that confers upon a designee the authority to make a variety of legal decisions on behalf of the grantor, usually including health care decisions.

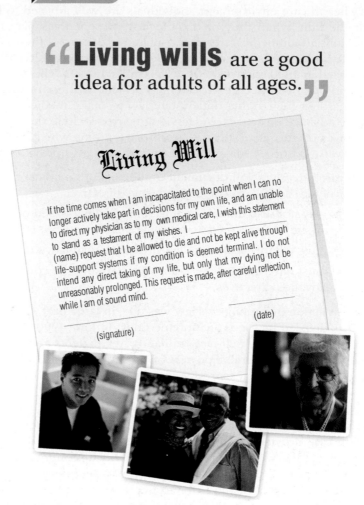

Figure 12-4

❝**Living wills** are a good idea for adults of all ages.❞

Living Will

If the time comes when I am incapacitated to the point when I can no longer actively take part in decisions for my own life, and am unable to direct my physician as to my own medical care, I wish this statement to stand as a testament of my wishes. I _____ (name) request that I be allowed to die and not be kept alive through life-support systems if my condition is deemed terminal. I do not intend any direct taking of my life, but only that my dying not be unreasonably prolonged. This request is made, after careful reflection, while I am of sound mind.

_____ (signature)   _____ (date)

---

health care proxy A durable power of attorney issued for purposes of health care decisions only.

Health Care Proxy

A **health care proxy,** or *health care power of attorney,* is a state-specific, end-of-life document. The health care proxy or health care power of attorney differs from the durable power of attorney in that it pertains just to health care decisions and not to other legal decisions. With it, individuals specify their wishes and designate an agent to make medical decisions for them in the event that they lose the ability to reason or communicate. As with the living will, this document outlines specific types of care and treatment that should be permitted or excluded. It also carefully outlines the specific responsibilities and authority of the proxy. Some states prohibit attending physicians, hospital employees, or other health care providers from serving as proxies, unless related to the patient by blood. Patients should name one or more alternates in case the primary proxy cannot serve when called (see Figure 12-5).

do-not-resuscitate (DNR) order Orders written at the request of patients or their authorized representatives that cardiopulmonary resuscitation not be used to sustain life in a medical crisis.

Do-Not-Resuscitate (DNR) Order

When admitted to a hospital, most patients or their authorized representatives are allowed by state law to specify that they are not to be revived if their heart stops. The request can be made via a standard **do-not-resuscitate (DNR) order** which is then placed with the patient's chart. In some hospitals patients may also wear a bracelet alerting medical personnel to the existence of a DNR order.

Figure 12-5 Health Care Proxy

I, _____, designate and appoint:

Name: _____

Address: _____

Telephone Number: _____

to be my agent for health care decisions and pursuant to the language stated below, on my behalf to:

(1) Consent, refuse consent, or withdraw consent to any care, treatment, service or procedure to maintain, diagnose or treat a physical or mental condition, and to make decisions about organ donation, autopsy and disposition of the body;

(2) Make all necessary arrangements at any hospital, psychiatric hospital or psychiatric treatment facility, hospice, nursing home or similar institution; to employ or discharge health care personnel to include physicians, psychiatrists, psychologists, dentists, nurses, therapists or any other person who is licensed, certified or otherwise authorized or permitted by the laws of this state to administer health care as the agent shall deem necessary for my physical, mental and emotional well-being; and

(3) Request, receive and review any information, verbal or written, regarding my personal affairs or physical or mental health including medical and hospital records and to execute any releases of other documents that may be required in order to obtain such information. In exercising the grant of authority set forth above my agent for health care decisions shall:

The powers of the agent herein shall be limited to the extent set out in writing in this durable power of attorney for health care decisions, and shall not include the power to revoke or invalidate any previously existing declaration made in accordance with the natural death act.

The agent shall be prohibited from authorizing consent for the following items:

The durable power of attorney for health care decisions shall be subject to these additional limitations:

This power of attorney for health care decisions shall become effective immediately and shall not be affected by my subsequent disability or incapacity or upon the occurrence of my disability or incapacity.

Any durable power of attorney for health care decisions I have previously made is hereby revoked. This durable power of attorney for health care decisions shall be revoked in writing, executed and witnessed or acknowledged in the same manner as required herein.

Executed this _____, at _____

_____
(Signature of principal)

State _____ County _____ S.S. No. _____

This instrument was acknowledged before me _____ (date) by _____ (name)

_____
(Signature of notary public)

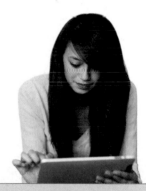

check your **progress**

21. What purpose do advance directives serve?
_____

22. Distinguish between a living will and a durable power of attorney.
_____

23. Distinguish between a health care proxy and a durable power of attorney.
_____

24. How must health care practitioners proceed if a patient has a do-not-resuscitate order in place?
_____

25. Generic living will forms are acceptable, legal documents, with what caveat?
_____

LO 12.5

Identify the major features of organ donation in the United States.

The National Organ Transplant Act

Passed in 1984, the **National Organ Transplant Act** addresses the severe shortage of organs available for transplantation. It provides funds for (1) grants to qualified organ procurement organizations (OPOs) and (2) the establishment of an Organ Procurement and Transplantation Network (OPTN) to assist OPOs in the distribution of unused organs outside their geographical area.

The Organ Procurement and Transplantation Network maintains the only national patient waiting list. It is a unique public/private organization that links all the professionals involved in the organ donation and transplantation system. OPTN goals are to

- Increase the effectiveness and efficiency of organ sharing and equity in the national system of organ allocation.
- Increase the supply of donated organs available for transplantation.

The United Network for Organ Sharing (UNOS), based in Richmond, Virginia, administers the OPTN under contract with the Health Resources and Services Administration of the U.S. Department of Health and Human Services.

Studies conducted by UNOS in 2004 found the increasing need for more donor organs a recurring theme, especially for pancreas, liver, and kidney transplants. Over the decade from 1992 to 2002, the organ transplant waiting list increased by 150 percent, and long wait times for transplant candidates also indicated that supply was not meeting demand.

As of mid-2010, there were 117,531 people waiting for transplants. Of that number, the breakdown by organ type was as follows: kidney, 91,763; liver, 16,718; pancreas, 1,446; kidney and pancreas, 2,275; heart, 3,165; lung, 1,834; heart and lung, 79; intestines, 251.

The number of people waiting for organ transplants is updated hourly at **http://optn.transplant.hrsa.gov/latestData/rptData.asp**. In February 2002, UNOS made a significant change to policy for determining the order for liver transplants, based on studies that showed that U.S. surgeons were transplanting livers into their own patients first, even when those patients were not as sick as others. Changes to the UNOS liver policy addressed the equitable allocation of human livers for transplant based on two formulas that put sickest transplant candidates on the waiting list ahead of others: one for adults, known as the Model for End-Stage Liver Disease (MELD), and one for children, known as the Pediatric End-Stage Liver Disease (PELD) Model. Higher MELD and PELD scores (and thus greater priority for a transplant) are associated with a higher risk of death while awaiting a transplant. In 2004, however, transplant officials said that despite the new UNOS rule, federal regulations governing transplants may need changing so that the sickest patients receive organ transplants ahead of others on the waiting list who are not as sick.

Although there is a national coordinated effort to maintain a list of people in need of an organ transplant, there is no national registry for donors. There are coordinated efforts through organ procurement organizations nationwide to coordinate donor information through OPTN. The Association of Organ Procurement Organizations (**www.aopo.org**) provides a list of organizations at the local level in each state.

The Organ Donation and Recovery Improvement Act, passed in 2004, established programs to increase organ donation through public awareness campaigns and education projects, and provided grants programs for individual states supporting use of hospital-based organ procurement

National Organ Transplant Act Passed in 1984, a statute that provides grants to qualified organ procurement organizations and established an Organ Procurement and Transplantation Network.

coordinators, research and demonstration projects, and reimbursement to living donors for travel-related expenses.

Organ Donor Directives

Patients may also want to make clear to hospital personnel that they wish to donate organs for transplantation or medical research in the event of their death. This can be accomplished in several ways:

- Some states allow licensed drivers to fill out organ donation forms on the back of their licenses.

- Nondrivers or residents of states where driver's licenses do not include this information may carry an organ donor card in their wallets, specifying their desire to donate organs (Figure 12-6).

- Organizations such as the National Kidney Foundation, the United Network for Organ Sharing (UNOS), and the Living Bank provide donor registration materials in response to requests.

- In addition to having an organ donor card, patients should make clear to family members their wishes regarding organ donation in the event of their death.

Uniform Anatomical Gift Act

In 1968 the **Uniform Anatomical Gift Act** was approved by the National Conference of Commissioners on Uniform State Laws for the purpose of allowing individuals to donate their bodies or body parts, after death, for use in transplant surgery, tissue banks, or medical research or education. The act was not officially enacted as law, but states accepted it because it made certain provisions uniform throughout all states. Major provisions include the following:

- Any person 18 years of age or older who is of sound mind may make a gift of his or her body, or certain bodily organs, to be used in medical research or for transplantation or storage in a tissue bank.

- Donations made through a legal will are not to be held up by probate.

- Except in autopsies, the donor's rights override those of others.

- Survivors may speak for the deceased if arrangements were not made prior to his or her death (provided the deceased did not express an objection to donation before his or her death).

- Physicians who rely on donation documents for the acceptance of bodies or organs are immune from civil or criminal prosecution. However, if the physician (or hospital) knows the deceased was opposed to donation or if, in the absence of prior arrangements, survivors express an objection, then the donation should be refused.

- Hospitals, surgeons, physicians, accredited medical or dental schools, colleges and universities, and tissue banks or storage facilities may accept anatomical gifts for research, advancement of medical or dental science, therapy, or transplantation.

- Time of death of the donor must be established by a physician who is not involved in transplanting the donor's designated organs,

> **Figure 12-6** Sample Uniform Donor Card

Uniform Donor Card

I,_____, have spoken to my family about organ and tissue donation. The following people have witnessed my commitment to be a donor. I wish to donate the following:

☐ any needed organs and tissue,
☐ only the following organs and tissue: _____
Donor Signature: _____ Date: _____
Next of Kin: _____
Telephone:(___) _____

Uniform Anatomical Gift Act A recommendation of the National Conference of Commissioners on Uniform State Laws, that all states accepted, allowing individuals to donate their bodies or body parts, after death, for use in transplant surgery, tissue banks, or medical research or education.

and the donor's attending physician cannot be a member of the trans-plant team.

- Donors may revoke the gift, and gifts may be rejected.

Frequently Asked Questions about Organ Donation

Since there are more people waiting for organ transplants than there are organs available, individuals are encouraged to designate their willingness to become donors. One way to increase the numbers of possible organ donors is to make sure that potential donors understand the process. Here are a few of the most commonly asked questions about organ donation, fol-lowed by summarized answers from the experts:

Q: What organs and tissues can be transplanted?

A: Organs that can be transplanted include heart, kidney, pancreas, lung, stomach, and small and large intestines. Other tissues often trans-planted include bone, corneas, skin, heart valves, veins, cartilage, and other connective tissues.

Q: Is the donor or the donor's family responsible for paying for transplantation of donated organs?

A: No. Costs are borne by the recipient or his or her insurance plan, when applicable.

Q: If a prospective, designated donor is injured in an accident, will the attending doctors allow that person to die in order to harvest donated organs?

A: Absolutely not. A willingness to donate organs in no way compromises the medical care provided to accident victims. The organ procurement organization (OPO) is notified that organs are available only after a patient is declared dead, and the transplant team is not notified until surviving family members have consented to donation.

Q: How old or young can a donor be?

A: Donors range from newborns to persons about the age of 70.

Q: If a person donated an organ, would the recipient and/or the recipi-ent's family learn the donor's identity and contact the donor or his or her family?

A: A donor's name is released to recipients only if the recipient asks for the information and the donor's family agrees.

Q: Are organs transplanted only after a prospective donor has died?

A: Not necessarily. Voluntary transplants from living donors to living recipients may also take place. For example, kidneys, lungs, skin, and other tissues are successfully transplanted from compatible living donors to recipients.

Q: May a family member who is an acceptable medical match for a recipient refuse to donate an organ to a relative in need of a transplant?

A: Of course. No laws exist that would compel a person to donate an organ against his or her will, regardless of relationship to the intended recipient.

Q: If I, as a willing organ donor, sign the back of my driver's license indicating that I am a donor, and then die, can my relatives legally "undo" my wishes?

A: No. A signed declaration on the back of a driver's license still is legally effective to authorize donation in every state in the United

States. Moreover, the relevant laws specify that the consent of the donor's relatives is not needed in such circumstances. However, prospective organ donors should also make their wishes known to family members while they are able, because in spite of their having signed a card, if relatives protest the donation, fear of bad publicity regarding organ donation will likely prevent the donation from occurring.

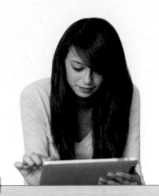

check your **progress**

26. What law made organ donation possible in the United States?

   _____

27. In your opinion, why is there a shortage of transplant organs in the United States?

   _____

28. What suggestions do you have for alleviating the shortage of transplant organs?

   _____

29. What is UNOS, and what is its function?

   _____

30. A widely circulated urban legend tells of a person who has a sexual tryst with a stranger and awakens in a bathtub minus a kidney. Why do you know the story is untrue?

   _____

The Grieving Process

Regardless of our personal philosophy and belief system concerning death and dying, we are all destined to experience the loss of an acquaintance, a friend, or a loved one. At that time, we need to grieve. Unfortunately, in our modern-day culture we are often uncertain of how to deal with grief in our own lives or how to help someone else who is grieving. The following facts and guidelines can help us respond helpfully to others.

What Is Grief?

Grief is the human reaction to loss. Individuals may grieve over a divorce, the loss of a job, or relocation, but grief after the death of a loved one is undoubtedly the most painful. Patients who are diagnosed with a terminal illness also experience profound grief. The grieving process is necessary, in both instances, for healing or resolution to take place.

Stages of Grief

The late Elisabeth Kübler-Ross, MD, recognized for many years as an authority in the field of death and dying, was the first to list and describe the coping mechanisms of people who grieve. Such individuals experience five stages of grief, she maintained, not necessarily in any particular order, before coming to terms with the death of a loved one or the prospect of imminent death.

   Stage 1. This first stage is identified with feelings of denial and isolation. This is the it-can't-be-true stage, in which patients believe the physician's diagnosis must be a mistake, or relatives informed of a loved one's death deny that the person is gone. They may suggest that

LO 12.6

Discuss the various stages of grief

X-rays or results of blood tests were somehow mixed up or that identities of accident victims were somehow mistaken. Denial is usually a temporary state, claims Kübler-Ross, and is soon replaced by partial acceptance. A terminally ill patient seldom continues to deny his or her disease until death comes, and grieving relatives realize all too soon that a loved one has, in fact, died.

Stage 2. When denial can no longer be maintained, the patient or grieving relative progresses to anger, rage, and resentment. "Why me?" is the typical reaction. Patients are angry over the "betrayal" of once-healthy bodies and the loss of control over their lives. Grieving relatives may feel anger toward a God that took the loved one away. Even the terminally ill family member may feel the same anger at God for leaving others behind to bear the pain of loss. Anger is a normal reaction to death and may be expressed in different ways. For example, a bereaved person may yell at others or withdraw in sullen silence.

Stage 3. Grieving individuals next respond with attempts at bargaining and guilt. Just as children continue to ask for a favor after parents have said no, patients may ask for "just enough time to see my daughter married" or "one more week at work before I have to quit." Something in the human psyche seems to believe, if only for a short time, that if we are "good," the "bad" will be taken away or postponed.

A corresponding experience for individuals grieving the loss of a loved one is guilt. The bereaved person may somehow feel responsible for the death, especially if the relationship with the deceased was not good. He or she might be tortured by thoughts of how things might have been different if only the loved one had lived.

Stage 4. The fourth stage involves depression or sadness, which is the most expected reaction to loss. Patients coping with terminal illness may face not only physical pain and debilitation but also loss of financial security and inevitable changes in lifestyle—all of which can cause

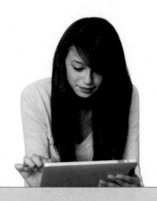

check your **progress**

The following questionnaire is intended to generate discussion. Check each statement that tells how you feel. There are no correct or incorrect answers.

_____ **31.** I feel uncomfortable talking to someone who is dying.

_____ **32.** I do not know what to say to a person who is dying.

_____ **33.** I would not want to tell a patient that he or she has a terminal condition.

_____ **34.** I think I can help a dying patient be more comfortable with his or her impending death.

_____ **35.** I am afraid of becoming too attached to a dying patient, and as a result I will not be able to control my feelings.

_____ **36.** I do not think a person should be told that his or her condition is terminal, because doing so adds to his or her suffering.

_____ **37.** I do not think death should be discussed in the presence of children.

_____ **38.** The thought of being around a dying person makes me uncomfortable.

_____ **39.** I think elderly people are the most fearful of death.

_____ **40.** Being around a dying person reminds me that someday I, too, will die.

Source: Adapted from a book by W. Worden, *Grief Counseling and Grief Therapy* (New York: Springer, 1982).

them to feel that their situation is hopeless. Individuals grieving the loss of a loved one may see no point in going on.

During this state bereaved persons may cry frequently or may be unable to cry at all, expressing their grief in body language—downcast eyes, shuffling steps, and stooped shoulders. Daily routines may be difficult or impossible to maintain. If depression continues for a prolonged period of time, health care providers, family members, or friends should help the bereaved person seek professional counseling.

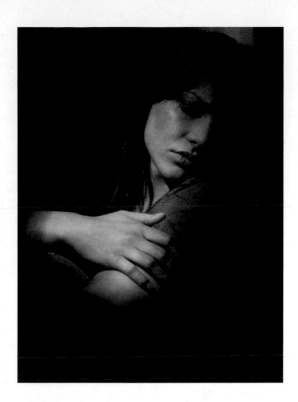

Stage 5. Finally, those experiencing the grieving process reach a stage of acceptance. At this point the person has finally accepted his or her loss. Terminally ill patients have come to terms with dying, and bereaved persons have accepted that the loved one is gone. For example, patients may write wills, complete advance directives, or plan funerals. A grieving spouse may finally decide to remove a deceased partner's clothing from a shared closet or to convert his or her office to a spare bedroom. Grieving family members can now move on to the growth stage, in which they adjust daily routines or become involved in new activities and relationships.

Although the stages of grief have been universally observed, each person dealing with loss grieves differently. Bereaved persons may not show their grief. A stage may be skipped or returned to repeatedly during the grieving process. A combination of all of the emotions just described may be felt at the same time.

Roberta Temes, PhD, also describes her perception of the distinctive behaviors of grief in her book, *Solace: Finding Your Way Through Grief and Learning to Live Again* (New York: Amacon Books, 2009). She discusses three stages as significant as one grieves:

1. Numbness, characterized by mechanical or rote functioning and social isolation.

2. Disorganization, where feelings of loss are so painful and disorienting one can't make plans or decide what to do next.

3. Reorganization, a return to one's previous, more normal and functional way of life.

While no one list of the stages of grief is useful for everyone, most touch on the types of behavior mentioned previously, which many people have experienced or observed at times of loss.

On the other hand, in *The Truth about Grief* (Simon & Schuster, 2011), Ruth Davis Konigsberg emphasizes that Kübler-Ross based her theory solely on interviews with terminally ill patients, and she was concerned primarily about the patients' feelings about their own approaching deaths. She did not ask them about her now famous stages of grief, because she conceived of the five stages later, after she had conducted the interviews. When Kübler-Ross's book was a surprise best seller, Konigsberg asserts, it marked the beginning of a new approach to death and dying, which "helped shatter the stoic silence that had surrounded death since World War I, and her ideas certainly raised the standard of care for dying people and their families. But she also ushered in a distinctly secular and psychological approach to death, one in which the focus shifted from the salvation of the deceased's soul . . . to the quality of his or her last days."

While Kübler-Ross's stages of grief have been applied to a wide range of experiences of loss, Konigsberg writes that they have also fostered certain misconceptions about grief, such as the following, as summarized in the January 24, 2011, edition of *Time:*

1. A person who has experienced loss or is facing death does not always grieve in stages, but rather experiences "a grab bag of symptoms that come and go and, eventually, simply lift."

2. Expressing grief helps some who experience it, but not all. In fact, a study published in the *Journal of Consulting and Clinical Psychology* in 2008 followed more than 2,000 people immediately after the events of 9/11 and for two more years, and found that some people who did not express their initial reactions showed fewer signs of distress later on.

3. When an individual loses his or her spouse, grief hits women harder than men. Several studies have shown that widows may show higher incidents of depression than widowers, but relatively speaking, men suffer more from the loss of a spouse.

4. Grief may never end. Researchers have found that the worst of grief is usually over within about six months. Thoughts and memories of those lost linger, of course, but the actual pain of loss does subside.

5. Counseling always helps those who grieve. Just as individuals grieve in different ways, for different lengths of time, some may find that counseling shortens the grieving period, while others come to terms with grief on their own.

The message for health care practitioners is to remain flexible in their expectations of other people's grief. That is, to realize that every person grieves in his or her own way, and some are resilient enough to get through grief on their own, while others may benefit from a combination of the helpful measures outlined in this chapter.

Finding Support

People who are grieving can find support from a variety of sources. They can read books on the subject, attend a bereavement support group sponsored by a hospital or hospice, visit a counselor, talk with a member of the clergy, or talk with family members and friends (Figure 12-7).

Health care practitioners can be excellent sources of support for terminally ill patients and their families. Talking and listening are the most helpful activities others can perform, the experts advise. Do not force a conversation, but make yourself available to talk. Do not respond in kind if patients are angry and resentful. Talking about distress helps relieve it, and sensitive listening is effective in itself. The following list of recommendations for talking to a dying patient is adapted from *"I Don't Know What to Say . . .": How to Help and Support Someone Who Is Dying* (Little, Brown, 1989), by oncologist Dr. Robert Buckman:

- Pay attention to setting. Sit down, relax, do not appear rushed, and act as though you are ready to listen.

- Determine whether or not the patient wants to talk. Ask, "Do you feel like talking?" before plunging into conversation.

> **Figure 12-7**

" Health care practitioners can be **caring sources of support** for grieving patients and for family members. **"**

- Listen well, and show that you are listening. Pay attention to the patient's words, without the distraction of planning your next remark.

- Encourage the patient to talk by saying, "What do you mean?" or "Tell me more."

- Remember that silence and nonverbal communication, such as grasping a hand or touching a shoulder, are also effective.

- Do not be afraid to describe your own feelings. It is permissible to say, "I find this difficult to talk about" or even, "I don't know what to say."

- Make sure you haven't misunderstood. You can ask, "How did it feel?" or say, "You seem angry."

- Do not change the subject. If you are uncomfortable, admit it. Don't try to distract the patient by changing the subject to something less threatening, such as the weather.

- Do not give advice early. The time may come when the patient asks your advice, but it is usually not prudent to offer unsolicited advice, because it stops the dialogue.

- Encourage reminiscence. Sharing memories can be a wrenching experience, but it can also encourage patients to look positively at the past.

- Respond to humor. Humor allows patients to express fears in a nonthreatening way. Do not try to cheer someone up with your own jokes, but if patients want to tell jokes or funny stories, humor them.

In short, the more you try to understand the feelings of others, the more support you will be able to give.

[CHAPTER SUMMARY]

LO 12.1 Which rituals surrounding death have survived to the present?

- Mourners wearing black.
- Halting traffic for a funeral procession.
- Wakes.
- Firing a rifle volley over the deceased.
- Funeral wreaths.

LO 12.2 What is the Uniform Determination of Death Act?

- A federal proposal that defines brain death as a means of determining when death actually occurs:
  - Circulation and respiration have irreversibly ceased.
  - The entire brain, including the brain stem, has irreversibly ceased to function.

What is the difference between a coma and a persistent vegetative state?

- Coma: A condition of deep stupor from which the patient cannot be roused by external stimuli.

- Persistent vegetative state (PVS): Severe mental impairment characterized by irreversible cessation of the higher functions of the brain, most often caused by damage to the cerebral cortex.

What tests may be performed to determine if death has occurred?

- Cannot breathe without assistance.

- No coughing or gagging reflex.

- No pupil response to light.

- No blinking reflex when cornea is touched.

- No grimace reflex when head is rotated or ears are flushed with ice water.

- No response to pain.

LO 12.3 What is the difference between palliative care and curative care?

- Palliative care: Treatment of a terminally ill patient's symptoms to make dying more comfortable—also called comfort care.

- Curative care: Treatment directed toward curing a patient's disease.

What is a hospice?

- A facility or program in which health care practitioners and volunteers provide a continuous environment that focuses on the physical, emotional, and psychological needs of the dying patient.

What is meant by the phrase *terminally* ill?

- A patient has six months or less to live.

What is *thanatology*?

- The study of death and psychological coping methods.

LO 12.4 What is the Uniform Rights of the Terminally Ill Act?

- A 1989 federal proposal to guide state legislatures in constructing laws concerned with advance directives.

What is euthanasia?

- Mercy killing of the hopelessly ill.

  - Active euthanasia: A conscious medical act that results in the death of a dying person.

  - Passive euthanasia: Allowing a dying patient to die without medical interference.

  - Voluntary euthanasia: Requires the patient's consent or the consent of the patient's legal representative to implement.

  - Involuntary euthanasia: The use of medical means to end a dying patient's life without his or her consent.

  - Physician-assisted suicide: Any of the previously listed methods in which a physician takes part in the patient's suicide.

What is the Patient Self-Determination Act?

- A federal act that requires hospitals and other health care providers to give written information to patients regarding their rights under state law to make medical decisions and to execute advance directives.

  - Living will: An advance directive that specifies a patient's end-of-life wishes.

  - Durable power of attorney: An advance directive that gives a designee authority to make a variety of legal decisions for a patient, including health care decisions.

  - Health care proxy: A durable power of attorney for health care decisions only.

  - Do-not-resuscitate order (DNR): The patient specifies in writing that he or she does not wish to be resuscitated if his or her heart stops.

What is the National Organ Transplant Act?

- A 1984 federal law that provides grants to qualified organ procurement organizations and that established an Organ Procurement and Transplantation Network (OPTN).

  - Established the United Network of Organ Sharing (UNOS) to administer the OPTN. The UNOS

    - Increases the effectiveness and efficiency of organ sharing and equity in the national system of organ allocation.

    - Increases the supply of donated organs available for transplant.

What is the Uniform Anatomical Gift Act?

- A federal proposal that states enact laws allowing anyone 18 or older, of sound mind, may make a gift of his or her body or certain organs to be used in medical research, transplantation, or storage in a tissue bank. The act recommends that

  - Donations made through a legal will are not to be held up by probate.

  - Except in autopsies, the donor's rights override those of others.

  - Survivors may speak for the deceased if no arrangements for donation were made prior to death, provided the deceased did not express an objection to donation before death.

  - Physicians who rely on donation documents for the acceptance of bodies or organs are immune from civil or criminal prosecution.

  - Hospitals, surgeons, physicians, accredited medical or dental schools, colleges and universities, and tissue banks or storage facilities may accept anatomical gifts for research, advancement of medical or dental science, therapy, or transplantation.

  - Time of death of the donor must be established by a physician who is not involved in transplanting the donor's designated organs, and the donor's attending physician cannot be a member of the transplant team.

  - Donors may revoke the gift, and gifts may be rejected.

What is grief?

- The human reaction to loss.

What are Elizabeth Kübler-Ross' stages of grief?

- Denial

- Anger

- Bargaining
- Depression
- Acceptance

What are Roberta Temes's stages of grief?

- Numbness
- Disorganization
- Reorganization

ETHICS ISSUES Death and Dying

Ethics ISSUE 1: Don Lundy, EMS director for Charleston County, South Carolina, says that DNR requests continue to be an ethical issue for EMTs. "The legal question has been answered," Lundy says, "but is it right or wrong [for EMTs] to support a DNR?" Most EMTs, Lundy explains, "would rather do too much than not enough."

Discussion Questions

1. Assume you are an emergency medical technician (EMT) responding to a 911 call at a grocery store. An elderly shopper has collapsed, and she is unconscious on the floor when you arrive. Her vital signs are weak. The woman is placed in the ambulance, where she arrests. You notice that the woman is wearing a bracelet that says "DNR," and a quick check of her purse reveals a signed and witnessed DNR order. What do you do?

   _____

   _____

2. EMTs reach the hospital with a patient who then arrests. The patient has been hospitalized before, and a DNR order is in place. The patient is middle-aged, and when his family arrives, his wife says, "I don't care what he says. Do everything to keep him alive." As a health care practitioner on the team assigned to care for this patient, what will you do?

   _____

   _____

Ethics ISSUE 2: In Maryland, according to EMS director Lundy, state law allows EMTs to do what is right for the patient when transporting them for care. In other states, the law may say you must obey the patient's instructions, regardless of what those instructions are.

Discussion Questions

1. As an EMT in Maryland, you are transporting a patient with chest pain, and you decide to transport her to a hospital with heart catheterization capabilities, even though the patient has expressed a desire to go to a less well-equipped hospital in the area. Legally and ethically, how will you respond?

   _____

   _____

2. You are an EMT in South Carolina, where state law says the patient has the last word. The patient has been injured in a car accident, and you want to take him to a hospital with a level 1 trauma center, but he says no, take him to a different hospital, without a level 1 trauma center. Legally and ethically, what will you do?

Ethics ISSUE 3: As a health care practitioner you are committed to acting in the patient's best interest, and you believe that the wishes of patients in end-of-life situations should be followed. Furthermore, professional codes of ethics generally state that the social commitment of health care practitioners is to sustain life and relieve suffering, and that when the performance of one duty conflicts with the other, the preferences of the patient should prevail.

Discussion Questions

1. A young mother who was severely injured in a car accident is brought into the hospital trauma center where you work. She belongs to the Jehovah's Witnesses church, and emphatically states that she refuses to have a blood transfusion. You know she risks death without a transfusion, but she believes her decision is a matter of her salvation. As a member of the patient's health care team, what will you do?

---

2. The patient in the car accident scenario is an elderly Jehovah's Witness and has no family. What will you do?

---

3. The female patient in the car accident scenario is unconscious, but her husband makes her wishes known regarding blood transfusions. Can you accept the husband's decision on the patient's behalf? Explain your answer.

Ethics ISSUE 4: Health care practitioners are ethically bound to respond to the needs of the patient at the end of life, but they are also ethically bound to preserve a patient's autonomy whenever possible.

Discussion Question

1. A mentally competent, elderly patient suffering from congestive heart failure presents a DNR order when admitted to the hospital. He also talks with his attending physician about his end-of-life care, asking for comfort care only. The physician concurs and records the patient's wishes on his chart. The patient's daughter arrives from out of state and loudly overrides her father's wishes. As a member of the man's health care team, what do you and others on the team do?

Ethics ISSUE 5: Your elderly aunt has asked you to take on her health care power of attorney. She makes the request while she is healthy and able to make her own decisions. You agree and sign the appropriate legal papers. She tells you at this time that she never wants "heroic measures" to be undertaken to save her life, if her quality of life would suffer.

Discussion Questions

1. Five years later your aunt is 86 and suffering from diabetes, coronary problems, and dementia. While in a long-term care facility, your aunt suffers a severe heart attack and is transported to the local hospital's emergency room. She is conscious when she reaches the emergency room, and when the attending physician asks her if she wants "all measures taken to preserve her life," she says yes. When you arrive at the hospital, your aunt is comatose and has been placed in the intensive care unit. Her physician says she cannot recover, but he could transport her to a larger hospital where physicians could "try" a pacemaker. How will you respond?

_____

_____

2. What ethical issues will influence your decision?

_____

_____

Ethics ISSUE 6: You are one of the health care practitioners involved in the care of a recently divorced, 55-year-old man with severe rheumatoid arthritis. He comes to the clinic where you work for a routine visit, complaining of insomnia. He requests a specific barbiturate, Seconal, as a sleep aid, asking for a month's supply. He says he wakes up every morning at four, tired but unable to go back to sleep. He admits that he rarely leaves his house during the day and says he has no interest in his previous enjoyable activities.

Discussion Question

1. What is an ethically appropriate course of action?

_____

Ethics ISSUE 7: A terminally ill patient you help care for in a hospice situation seems alienated from family members. The patient talks to you about her family situation, and asks you to intervene. You are uncomfortable with the request but do not know how to reply.

Discussion Question

1. What, in your opinion, is the ethically appropriate course of action?

_____

_____

Ethics ISSUE 8: A Jewish family wants to perform a *tarhara*—ceremony for washing a body—and bury a family member within 24 hours of his death in accordance with their religious beliefs.

Discussion Question

1. Should health care practitioners who treated the recently deceased help accommodate his family's wishes? If so, how?

_____

_____

Go to **www.mhhe.com/judson6e** to practice your case review skills. Then read on for more information.

KEY TERMS

active euthanasia
brain death
coma
curative care
do-not-resuscitate (DNR) order
durable power of attorney
health care proxy
hospice

involuntary euthanasia
living will
National Organ Transplant Act
palliative care
passive euthanasia
Patient Self-Determination Act
persistent vegetative state (PVS)

terminally ill
thanatology
Uniform Anatomical Gift Act
Uniform Determination of Death Act
Uniform Rights of the Terminally Ill Act
voluntary euthanasia

CHAPTER 12 REVIEW

Applying Knowledge

Circle the correct answer for each of the following questions.

LO 12.1

1. Before the twentieth century, death most likely occurred
   a. In a hospital
   b. In a hospice
   c. At home
   d. At work

2. Which of the following is a modern-day custom regarding death?
   a. Holding a funeral
   b. As a survivor, wearing sackcloth and ashes for several days
   c. As a survivor, wailing loudly at certain times in public places
   d. None of the above

3. Which of the following is true of death in the United States in the twenty-first century?
   a. Most deaths are occurring among teenagers.
   b. Most deaths occur in hospitals.
   c. All deaths result in autopsies.
   d. Infants seldom die.

LO 12.2

4. The purpose of the Uniform Determination of Death Act was to
   a. Define guidelines for determining when death actually occurs
   b. Teach caregivers how to prepare patients for death
   c. Teach caregivers how to use technology to prolong life
   d. None of the above

5. The Uniform Determination of Death Act defines _____ as a means of determining when death actually occurs.
   a. Cessation of breathing
   b. Brain death
   c. Blood pressure reading
   d. Cessation of ability to speak

6. *Coma* is best defined as
   a. A deep sleep
   b. Severe mental impairment
   c. Deep stupor from which the person cannot be roused by external stimuli
   d. Cessation of all brain function

7. Persons said to be in a *persistent vegetative state*
   a. Cannot breathe on their own
   b. Can be aroused by external stimuli
   c. Have severe brain damage
   d. Are in a deep coma

8. Technically, death results from
   a. Loss of oxygen
   b. Circulatory system collapse
   c. Coma
   d. None of the above

9. Before pronouncing a nonresponsive and unconscious patient dead, physicians may perform certain tests. Which of the following is *not* a prescribed test for determining death?
   a. Cannot breathe without assistance
   b. Cannot stand unaided
   c. Has no coughing or gagging reflex
   d. Pupils do not respond to light

10. Recent reports indicate a decline in the number of nonmandatory autopsies performed in hospitals. Which of the following is a probable reason for the decline?
    a. Fewer patients are dying.
    b. Family members of deceased patients are often reluctant to give permission for an autopsy.
    c. No one wants to perform them.
    d. The law does not allow hospitals to perform autopsies.

11. Recent reports also indicate a continuing decline in the number of all autopsies performed in the United States. Of what value is a nonmandatory autopsy performed after a hospital patient dies?
    a. Helps determine cause of death
    b. Helps advance medical knowledge about disease
    c. Helps reassure family members of the deceased that everything possible had been done for their loved one
    d. All of the above

LO 12.3

12. Care provided to relieve pain and make a patient's last days as comfortable as possible is referred to as
    a. ICU care
    b. Palliative care
    c. Curative care
    d. Hospital care

13. The Greek tern for "good death" is
    a. Palliative
    b. Thanatology
    c. Euthanasia
    d. DNR

14. If one has six months or less to live, he or she is said to be
    a. Under palliative care
    b. Eligible for curative care
    c. Terminally ill
    d. Not eligible for hospice care

15. The right to die movement is largely responsible for educating people about
    a. Advance directives
    b. Hospice care
    c. Palliative and curative care
    d. Wills

16. A document serving to appoint an individual, chosen by the patient, to represent the patient's interests is a(n)
    a. Advance directive
    b. Living will
    c. Durable power of attorney
    d. Guardian *ad litem*

17. An authorization in advance to withdraw artificial life support is
    a. Assault
    b. Battery
    c. An advance directive
    d. Uniform Anatomical Gift

18. Landmark events in the right to die movement include
    a. The *Karen Ann Quinlan* case
    b. The *Nancy Cruzan* case
    c. The *Terry Shiavo* case
    d. All of the above

19. Which of the following is *not* true of the Uniform Rights of the Terminally Ill Act?
    a. Recommended by the National Conference of Commissioners on Uniform State Laws
    b. Intended to guide state legislatures in constructing laws to address advance directives
    c. Was repealed in 1994
    d. None of the above are true

20. The Uniform Anatomical Gift Act does *not* include the provision(s) that
    a. Persons 18 and older and of sound mind may donate organs and tissues for transplantation
    b. Donations made through a will are not to be held up in probate
    c. Organs are not accepted from patients over 60 years of age
    d. Except in autopsies, the donor's rights override the rights of others

21. The Patient Self-Determination Act does *not* provide for
    a. Documenting the existence of an advance directive in the patient's medical record
    b. Nondiscrimination regarding whether or not a patient has an advance directive
    c. Compliance with state laws respecting advance directives
    d. Legal prosecution of health care practitioners who influence a patient's decision in preparing an advance directive

22. Physician-assisted suicide is legal:
    a. In all 50 states
    b. Only in Oregon and Washington
    c. Only when the patient agrees to be euthanized
    d. Never

23. A form of advance directive that allows hospital patients to tell health care practitioners not to revive them if breathing stops is called a
    a. Durable power of attorney
    b. Will
    c. Do-not-resuscitate order (DNR)
    d. Summons

24. Which legislation paved the way for organ transplantation in the United States?
    a. Patient Self-Determination Act
    b. Uniform Rights of the Terminally Ill Act
    c. Uniform Anatomical Gift Act
    d. Death With Dignity Acts

25. Which legislation established organ procurement and transplantation networks in the United States?
    a. Uniform Rights of the Terminally Ill Act
    b. Death With Dignity Acts
    c. DNR order
    d. National Organ Transplant Act

26. Which of the following is true of organ transplants?
    a. Organ donors or their families must pay if a transplant occurs.
    b. Only individuals under the age of 55 can serve as organ or tissue donors.
    c. Prospective donors should inform family members of their wishes.
    d. Only family members can donate certain organs for transplantation.

LO 12.6

27. Which of the following best describes grief?
    a. An emotion one feels when loss has occurred
    b. The wish to die
    c. An emotion that should be denied
    d. None of the above

28. Dr. Elisabeth Kübler-Ross's five stages of coping with a death or with a terminal illness do *not* include which of the following:
    a. Acceptance
    b. Bargaining
    c. Depression
    d. All of the above are included

29. Which of the following is *not* true of the stages of grief?
    a. All grieving people progress through the stages in order.
    b. Grieving people may not experience one or more of the stages of grief.
    c. A person may experience the second stage of grief before the first, or the third stage before the second.
    d. A person may go back and forth among the stages until resolution is accomplished.

30. Which of the following behaviors is probably most helpful to a dying person?
    a. Ignoring the fact that the person is dying
    b. Avoiding any discussion of future events
    c. Giving the person your attention and listening well
    d. Telling jokes

CASE STUDIES

Use your critical thinking skills to answer the questions that follow each case study.

LO 12.3

31. You are the health care practitioner assigned to speak with a deceased patient's family about permission to do an autopsy, and you find yourself feeling reluctant to do so. What reasons can you think of that might make one feel reluctant in such a situation?

_____

_____

32. How might you phrase a request to surviving family members to allow their deceased loved one's organs/tissues to be donated?

_____

_____

LO 12.3

You are a member of a hospital resource allocation committee that must decide which three out of seven critical patients will receive immediate live-saving surgery. The hospital has resources to save just three of the seven, but without surgery, all seven patients will die. The situation is further complicated by the fact that a blizzard is raging outside, and none of the patients can be transferred to another hospital. All seven are too critically ill to be moved by snowmobile.

33. Working alone or in a group, decide what criteria will be used to make the decisions (consider age, social standing, benefit to society, lifestyle, degree of physical deterioration, etc.).

_____

_____

34. Obtain a list of the seven patients from your instructor, and choose three patients to receive immediate life-saving surgery. Write your decisions, and/or discuss the rationale for your choices with the class

_____

_____

[INTERNET ACTIVITIES LO 12.4 and LO 12.6]

Complete the activities and answer the questions that follow.

35. Visit the Web site for Caring Connections at **www.caringinfo.org**. Download a living will and a health care power of attorney form, and compare the forms with those of a classmate from another state. Overall, how do the forms from another state differ from those for your state?

_____

_____

36. Visit the Hospice Patients Alliance at **www.hospicepatients.org/ hospic4.html**. List three recommendations offered at the site for choosing the right hospice for a dying family member.

_____

_____

37. Visit the Web site for Healing Resources at **www.webhealing.com**. List three grief links found at the site that might help the bereaved. Why might these resources prove helpful?

_____

_____

RESOURCES

Konigsberg, Ruth Davis. *The Truth about Grief*. New York: Simon & Schuster, 2011.

Kübler-Ross, Elisabeth. *On Death and Dying*. New York: Scribner, 1969.

Rafinski, Karen. "Easing Pain: Palliative Care Is Not What You Think." *AARP Bulletin* (June 2011), p. 14.

Temes, Roberta. *Solace: Finding Your Way through Grief and Learning to Live Again*. New York: Amacon Books, 2009.

Worden, W. *Grief Counseling and Grief Therapy*. New York: Springer, 1982.

Intervention and end-of-life care in ICU: **www.medscape.com/viewarticle/728356**.

Konigsberg's book synopsized in *Time*, January 24, 2011, pp. 42–46.

National organ transplant data: **http://optn.transplant.hrsa.gov/latestData/step2.asp?**

States with laws preventing/accepting assisted suicide: **www.euthanasia.com/bystate.html**.

Study on end-of-life care—physicians' religion: **http://religion.blogs.cnn.com/2010/08/26/study-doctors-religious-beliefs-affect-end-of-life-care/**.

Telephone interview November 10, 2007, with Don Lundy, EMS director for Charleston County, South Carolina.

U.S. Supreme Court upholds Oregon's right to die law: **http://abcnews.go.com/Politics/SupremeCourt/story?id=1514546**.

Washington's assisted-suicide law: **www.nytimes.com/2010/03/05/us/05suicide.html**.

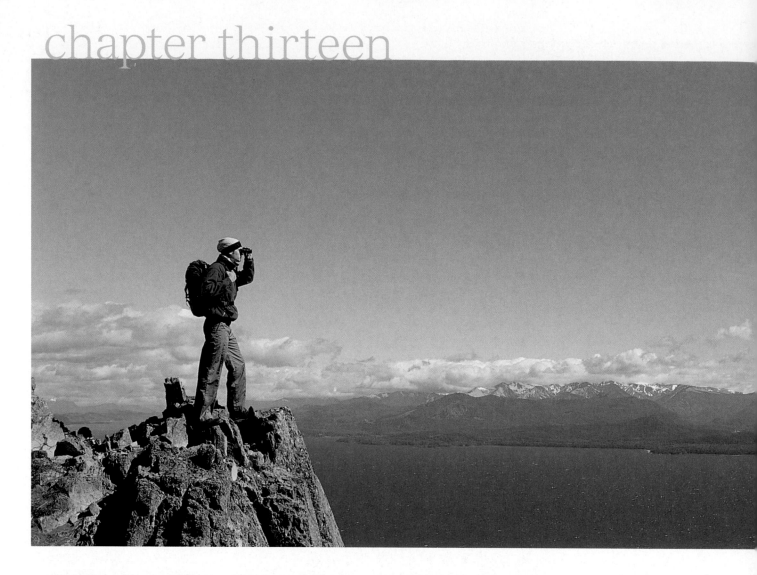

chapter thirteen

HEALTH CARE TRENDS AND FORECASTS

Learning Outcomes

After studying this chapter, you should be able to:

LO 13.1 Identify the major stakeholders in the U.S. health care system.

LO 13.2 Describe the major areas of concern to those stakeholders.

LO 13.3 Describe the major new trends that will affect health care in the United States in the next 20 years.

LO 13.4 Discuss former and ongoing attempts to reform the U.S. health care system.

from the perspective of . . .

CINDI, WHO works at a hospital in a southern state, began her career in health care as a certified nuclear medicine technologist. Her duties included administering radiopharmaceuticals (drugs containing radioactive isotopes) to patients, then monitoring the characteristics and functions of the tissues and organs where the radioactive drugs localized. Abnormal areas are characterized by higher-than-normal or lower-than-normal concentrations of the isotopes. Cindi took the certification test to specialize in PET (positron emission tomography), and she has progressed to a managerial position, where she supervises a PET imaging department. Her responsibilities also include payroll, budgeting, quality control for imaging, physician relations, and other supervisory duties.

PET scans are valuable diagnostic tools, Cindi emphasizes, because they produce 3-D images of organs and tissues that allow physicians to see inside patients' bodies for more accurate pinpointing of disease processes. "It's not [simply] anatomy," Cindi says. "These noninvasive procedures *show* how organs in the body work, for purposes of diagnosis, staging, and treatment which actually save the insurance companies money in the end."

The one thing Cindi dislikes most about her job, she says, is "insurances," because companies frequently see nuclear imaging as "medically unnecessary" and refuse payment. In addition, because of cutbacks to Medicare and other insurance payments in her state, "patients aren't getting what they need." For example, Cindi recalls a breast cancer patient who had a CT (computed tomography) scan first, but was denied authorization for the PET scan her physician ordered. "These scans are very expensive," Cindi explains, but they are such valuable diagnostic tools that insurance companies should be reimbursing for them. Another patient had a lung mass revealed in a CT scan, and his physician recommended surgery. The patient knew the value of a PET scan and insisted on one, which his physician finally reluctantly ordered. The PET scan showed widespread metastatic cancerous growths, which meant surgery was not recommended.

From Cindi's perspective, nuclear medicine provides valuable diagnostic and treatment tools that insurance companies should reimburse. Her attitude is summed up by her statement: "When patients don't get what they need, it's painful."

The patients Cindi sees probably appreciate her perspective, and apparently many recognize the value of PET scans in diagnosing and treating their illnesses.

Cindi opposes the perspective of "insurances" whose executives often see PET scans as too expensive to reimburse, thereby limiting the advanced diagnostic tools available to physicians.

As health care moves into the twenty-first century, insurance will become increasingly important and probably increasingly controversial. When technological tools such as nuclear medicine procedures are available, in your opinion should all insurance organizations reimburse for their use? Explain your answer.

Do you see a solution to the high cost of new health care treatments and procedures as we continue to develop them?

As you have progressed through *Law & Ethics for Medical Careers*, you have gained knowledge about legal issues affecting every health care practitioner. You have also learned that in addition to the law, ethics play a crucial role in health care decisions. This final chapter outlines major concerns all Americans have with the country's health care system, and offers a glimpse of possibilities for the future.

LO 13.1

Identify the major stakeholders in the U.S. health care system.

stakeholders Those who have a vested interest in the health care industry in the United States, and in any efforts to reform the industry.

Whom Does the Health Care System Serve?

Those who have a vested interest in the health care industry in the United States, and in any efforts to reform the industry, are called **stakeholders**. They include, but are not limited to, the following:

1. **The public.**

   The patients who use health care services will always be at the head of the list of stakeholders. When health problems arise, everyone wants the best medical care available, conveniently delivered, at an affordable cost.

2. **Employers.**

   Since employers often provide health care benefits for employees, they hope to contract with health care providers who can deliver quality services at reasonable cost.

3. **Health care facilities and practitioners.**

   As the providers of health care services, facilities such as hospitals, skilled nursing care organizations, physicians' practices, medical and dental clinics, laboratory and radiology services, rehabilitation hospitals, and many others influence the health care system in the quality, range, and cost of services provided.

4. **Federal, state, and local governments.**

   Governments help pay the cost of health care services through Medicare, Medicaid, Federal Employees Health Benefits Program, Military Health System, Veterans Health Administration, Indian Health Service, State Children's Health Insurance Program, and other state and federal government-financed programs. For that reason governments are near the top of the list of health care stakeholders.

5. **Managed care organizations.**

   Managed care organizations provide funds to help cover the costs of health care services for all the employees of a certain business or for other groups who have come together to buy coverage for health care at lower cost than each member of the group could get individually. As for-profit organizations, their focus is on the bottom line—helping reimburse health care providers while at the same time earning a profit.

6. **Private insurers.**

   Private insurance companies sell health care policies to individuals, agreeing to pay certain health care costs for policy holders for a fee. Fees are based on age, general state of health, preexisting medical conditions, and other factors that result in lower or higher rates, depending on each client's profile.

7. **Voluntary facilities and agencies that provide health care or influence health care policies.**

   Disaster relief agencies and nongovernmental volunteer organizations that provide health care or funds for health care are also important stakeholders in the national health care system.

8. **Health care practitioner training institutions.**

   Any training institution that prepares health care practitioners to administer health care has a huge stake in the health care system, and also influences the system proportionately according to the quality and quantity of practitioners they prepare.

9. **Professional associations and other health care industry organizations.**

   While each state's medical practice acts mandate licensing and/or certification for certain health care practitioners, professional associations and other industry organizations also establish and monitor health care practitioner ethics, and offer advice and support for members of their diverse groups.

10. **Medical, biotechnological, pharmaceutical, and other health care companies.**

   For-profit companies that develop treatments and cures for diseases and other medical conditions, which look at the business of health care to make a profit while serving the consumer, also have a vested interest in the health care system.

Cost, Access, and Quality

Key issues of concern to *stakeholders* within the American health care system are *cost, access,* and *quality.*

Cost refers to the amount individuals, employers, state and federal governments, managed care organizations, private insurers, and other stakeholders spend on health care in the United States. As explained in the section entitled "Access," the number of people who have **access** to health care services—that is, the number of people for whom the services are available and for which they as consumers can pay—also helps determine cost. In addition, the cost of health care services also directly affects the **quality,** or degree of excellence, of health care services offered.

Cost

Just as preparing a budget shows you how much of your income is spent on food (20 percent), housing (45 percent), clothing (15 percent), insurance (10 percent), and so on, the total cost of health care in the United States is often expressed as a percentage of the country's gross domestic product. The **gross domestic product (GDP)** represents the total value of all goods produced and services provided in a country in one year. The percentage of the GDP represented by health care spending was first determined in 1960, and it has been steadily increasing ever since. In 1960, health care spending accounted for slightly more than 5 percent of the GDP. In 2010, according to U.S. government figures, health care spending had risen to 17 percent of the GDP, or as stated in a Reuters report, $2.6 trillion—about $8,458 per person. The National Coalition on Health Care predicts that by 2015, the United States will most likely be spending 20 percent of the country's GDP on health care. The Health Care Financing Administration estimates that by 2025, if health care cost rises at 8 percent per year (the trend from 1960 to 1990), health care spending will exceed 25 percent of the GDP. By 2050, the Congressional Budget Office projects, health care spending could easily exceed 37 percent of the GDP—about $1.50 out of every $4 spent.

Why should health care stakeholders be concerned about the rising share of the GDP that health care expenditures consume? Because federal and state governments currently bear about 50 percent of the nation's health care costs, and higher health care spending is the main force expanding the federal budget. If the trend toward higher health care costs continues at the present rate of increase, the country could reach a point at which health care expenditures are so large that they overwhelm other important portions of government-spending allocations, such as schools, roads, parks, the environment, defense, and social welfare programs.

LO 13.2
Describe the major areas of concern to those stakeholders.

cost The amount individuals, employers, state and federal governments, HMOs, and insurers spend on health care in the United States.

quality The degree of excellence of health care services offered.

access The availability of health care and the means to purchase health care services.

gross domestic product (GDP) The total value of goods produced and services provided in a country during one year.

Figure 13-1 shows the government health care spending as a percentage of the GDP of the United States, as compared with other developed nations. Other developed nations spend less for health care on a per capita basis than the United States, yet ensure wider access to health care for their citizens. The United States is the only nation on the list that does not provide government-financed, universal health care to its citizens. (This is offered not as a judgment as to the desirability of universal health care, but simply as a matter of fact.)

As shown in Figure 13-2, most of federal spending goes toward defense, social security, and major health programs.

Harry Sultz and Kristina Young, social and preventive medicine experts, attribute increases in the cost of health care to the following factors:

- Application of more advanced and more types of technology.
- Growth in the population of older adults.
- Emphasis on specialty medicine.
- Increasing numbers of uninsured and underinsured.
- Labor intensity of health care services.
- Reimbursement system incentives.

Each of these factors is discussed in the following text.

New Health Care Technology

The availability of new computer-aided diagnostic and therapeutic tools, advanced surgical techniques and equipment, and an expanding array of medications are among many factors that have helped fuel the rise in health care costs.

Medical technologies currently in various stages of development that will be available, at a cost, in the future are discussed in the sections entitled "Medical Technologies" and "Health Information Technologies." Because both the equipment and the employee training needed to implement new medical technologies are expensive, the expanded use of advanced technologies in the future will continue to add to the cost of health care services.

Widespread adoption of health information technology (HIT) in the future will also add to rising health care costs, since hardware, software, and personnel trained in HIT are costly.

Growth in the Population of Older Adults

baby boom generation
Those individuals born between 1946 and 1964.

Much has been written about the effects of the baby boom generation on health care services in the United States. The **baby boom generation** is defined as those individuals born between 1946 and 1964. After American soldiers returned home from World War II in 1945 and 1946, the United States experienced an explosion of births (hence the name "baby boom") that continued for the next 18 years. In 1964, baby boomers made up 40 percent of all Americans. In the 1990s, about 76 million people were part of the baby boom generation, totaling 29 percent of the population in the United States. The baby boom population group is 70 percent larger than the generation born during the prior two decades, and baby boomers are expected to live longer than any previous generation. Baby boomers currently make up more than one-third of the U.S. population.

Because the baby boom generation is so large, its members have had a noticeable impact on all aspects of the nation's economy, including the health care industry, and as baby boomers age, they will continue to impact all health care services and costs.

Advances in medical technology have increased life spans for all Americans, including the baby boom generation. Consequently, there are more Americans aged 65 and older than at any other time in history. In fact, the

HEALTH CARE SPENDING WORLDWIDE, AS A PERCENTAGE OF EACH COUNTRY'S GPD

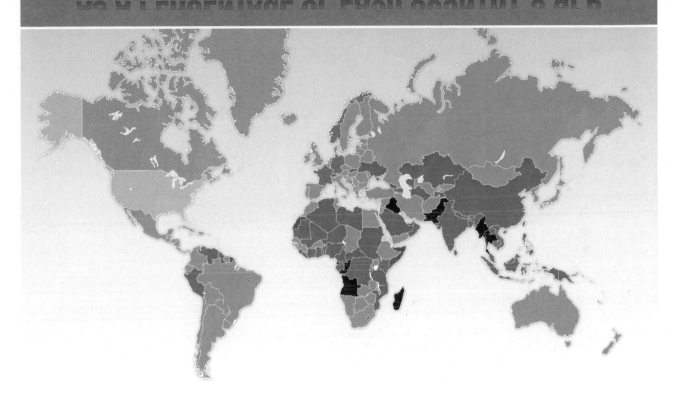

International Health Spending as Percentage of GDP

■ Less than or equal to 3	■ 3.1–5.0	■ 5.1–8.0
■ 8.1–10.0	■ 10.1–13.0	More than 13	■ No data

Highlights

- The U.S. spends the most on health care—16.2 percent of the GDP in 2007.

- Health spending in Germany, France, Austria, and Switzerland accounts for between 10.1 percent and 13.0 percent of GDP.

- In Canada, the United Kingdom, Australia, Norway, and Sweden, health spending accounts for between 8.1 percent and 10.0 percent of GDP.

- Japan and Finland spend between 5.1 percent and 8.0 percent of GDP on health care.

- In China health spending accounts for 4.7 percent of GDP.

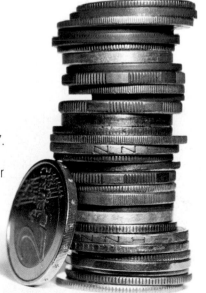

Source: **www.bcbs.com/blueresources/mcrg/chapter1/ch1_slide_1.html.**

Figure 13-2

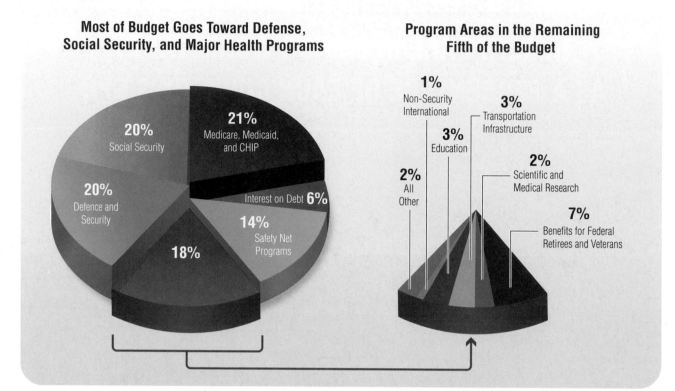

Most of Budget Goes Toward Defense, Social Security, and Major Health Programs

21% Medicare, Medicaid, and CHIP

20% Social Security

20% Defence and Security

18%

14% Safety Net Programs

Interest on Debt 6%

Program Areas in the Remaining Fifth of the Budget

1% Non-Security International

3% Education

3% Transportation Infrastructure

2% All Other

2% Scientific and Medical Research

7% Benefits for Federal Retirees and Veterans

Source: 2010 figures from Office of Management and Budget, FY 2012 Historical Tables.

Note: Percentages may not total 100 due to rounding.

Figure 13-3

Health Care Spending Chart U.S. from FY 1996 to FY 2016

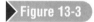

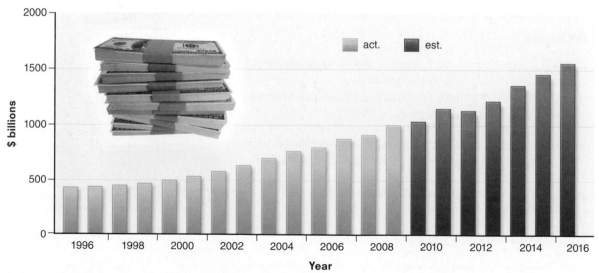

act. ☐ est. ☐

$ billions

Year

Source: **www.usgovernmentspending.com/health_care_chart_10.html.**

Figure 13-4

U.S. Census Projection for Population Growth by Age

Growth of the Population by Age, 1900–2030

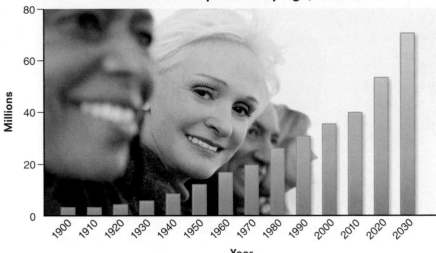

Source: U.S. Bureau of the Census, **www.census.gov/.**

age group of those 85 years and older is growing faster than any other age group in the United States. Figure 13-4 shows growth and projected growth of the U.S. population by age, from 1900 to 2030.

Not only do older people spend more on health care services than younger age groups, but they also use different services (Figure 13-5).

- Both older and younger health care consumers spend most of their health care dollars on hospital care and physician services, but health care expenses are greater for older Americans: $12,271 per person on average for people age 65 and older, versus $2,761 per person on average for people under age 65.

- Nursing home care takes a greater portion of the health care budget for the elderly: 22 percent of all health care spending per person over 65, versus 2 percent for people under 65.

Emphasis on Specialty Medicine

Medical students in the United States are more than three times more likely to specialize than to remain generalists or primary physicians. Since specialists are paid at higher rates than primary physicians, the tendency of Americans to see specialists more often is also adding to the cost of health care. Managed care organizations have sought to control costs by instituting "gatekeepers" to restrict clients to primary physicians for initial diagnosis and treatment, and limiting referrals to specialists, but the practice has met with resistance from both physicians and patients. Because of this public outcry, many legislative initiatives at state and federal levels have sought to preserve patients' rights to insurance reimbursement for specialty treatment.

As medical technology advances, new specialties will arise, with the potential of further adding to the spiraling cost of health care services in the United States.

Increasing Numbers of Underinsured and Uninsured

As health care costs rise, so, too, does the number of people who cannot afford health insurance. (People may be without health insurance coverage for a number of reasons, but cost is most often cited as the reason for

Figure 13-5

Elderly Individuals Spend More on Health Care Services

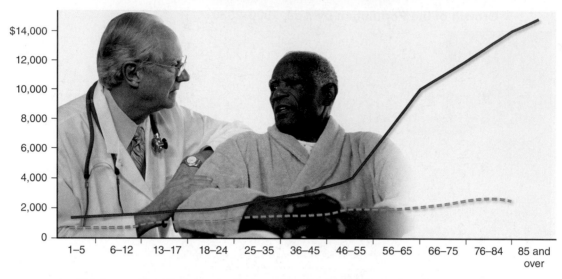

Source: U.S. Department of Health and Human Services, Agency for Healthcare Research and Quality, **www.ahrq.gov.**

no insurance or too little insurance.) According to the Centers for Disease Control and Prevention, in March 2010, 46.7 million Americans, or about 16 percent of the population, were without health insurance when surveyed.

Surveys of uninsured Americans consistently find that uninsured and underinsured people make more visits to emergency rooms than those who have health insurance, indicating that primarily because of cost, a large percentage of the population is not receiving sufficient health care to protect them in the event of major illnesses or injuries. Since costs are higher for emergency room services than for care provided in physicians' offices or medical clinics, uninsured and underinsured patients add significantly to the cost of health care delivery.

Health care costs are also affected by the fact that uninsured individuals do not see physicians regularly and are, therefore, more likely to develop medical conditions that lead to costly complications or hospitalizations.

Labor Intensity of Health Care Services

As one of the largest industries in the United States, in 2008 health care employed about 14.3 million workers (statistics from the U.S. Bureau of Labor Statistics) on a round-the-clock basis. About 40 percent were employed in hospitals; 21 percent worked in nursing and residential facilities; and 16 percent were in physicians' offices. Many of these workers have advanced educations and training, making labor an expensive component of total health care costs.

Technological advances and changing population demographics will contribute to the increasing health care services labor force, as new workers must be trained and new jobs created. In fact, U.S. Department of Labor forecasts for employment show that the health care industry will account for about 20 percent of all wage and salary jobs from 2008 through 2018. It follows that an increasingly skilled health services labor force will further add to health care costs.

Reimbursement System Incentives

Dating back to the 1930s, health insurance has been the primary source of health care reimbursement in the United States. Historically, when insurance

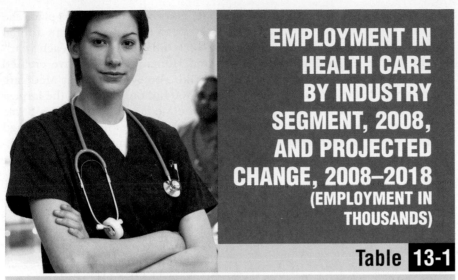

EMPLOYMENT IN HEALTH CARE BY INDUSTRY SEGMENT, 2008, AND PROJECTED CHANGE, 2008–2018 (EMPLOYMENT IN THOUSANDS)

Table 13-1

Industry Segment	2008 Employment	2008–2018 Percentage change
Health care, total	14,336.0	22.5
Hospitals, public and private	5,667.2	10.1
Nursing and residential care facilities	3,008.0	21.2
Offices of physicians	2,265.7	34.1
Home health care services	958.0	46.1
Offices of dentists	818.8	28.5
Offices of other health practitioners	628.8	41.3
Outpatient care centers	532.5	38.6
Other ambulatory health care services	238.5	6.8
Medical and diagnostic laboratories	210.5	39.8

Source: Bureau of Labor Statistics National Employment Matrix, 2008–2018, www.bls.gov/.

companies paid physicians, hospitals, and other health care providers, regardless of fees the providers charged, there was little incentive among providers for holding down fees. Over time, however, when reimbursement for health care costs—either through individual health insurance payments or through employer-provided health insurance payments—became routine, health care costs rose. Government financing mechanisms, such as Medicaid and Medicare, also added to health care costs.

Fraud Is Also Costly

Unfortunately, dishonest health care providers, pharmacies, and just plain criminals also add to the cost of health care. The National Health Care Anti-Fraud Association (NHCAA) estimates conservatively that 3 percent of all health care spending—or $78 billion using the figure $2.6 trillion for total spending in 2010—is lost to health care fraud. As stated on the NHCAA Web site in October 2010, "That's more than the gross domestic product of 120 countries, including Iceland, Ecuador, and Kenya.

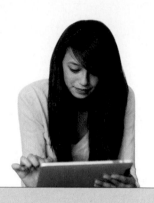

"Other estimates by government and law enforcement agencies place the loss due to health care fraud as high as 10 percent of our nation's annual health care expenditure—or a staggering $226 billion [and up]—each year."

The Justice Department and Health and Human Services have created a joint task force—the Medicare Fraud Strike Force—to combat Medicare fraud, which in 2009 totaled approximately $60 billion. In one of the largest arrests since the strike force was formed, the Medicare Fraud Strike Force announced in July 2010 that 94 people in several states had been charged with their alleged participation in schemes to collect more than $251 million in fraudulent claims to Medicare.

check your **progress**

1. Who are the major stakeholders in the American health care system?

2. What three issues are of primary concern to stakeholders within the American health care system?

3. Discuss how the three factors identified in question 2 are interrelated.

4. How do increasing levels of medical and health care information technologies add to health care costs?

5. Of what significance is the percentage of the gross domestic product represented by health care spending?

6. How does fraud add to health care costs?

In the 1980s, as health care costs continued to spiral upward, managed care organizations were formed as a means of containing costs. Under the managed care system, clients prepaid for health care services, and managed care organizations restricted reimbursement to health care providers according to certain guidelines. In most cases, for example, patients who belong to managed care organizations are required to see primary, or gatekeeper, physicians who control access to specialists. Furthermore, managed care organizations typically do not pay for medical treatments classified as experimental, and new treatments and procedures often fall within this category.

Managed care clients have often been dissatisfied with reimbursement restrictions, however, and their dissatisfaction has led to continually evolving reimbursement arrangements between health care providers and managed care payers.

Access

Access to health care is determined by availability as well as by the ability to pay for the service. The U.S. Department of Health and Human Services, Health Resources and Services Administration, has determined that 20 percent of the nation's population resides in areas where physicians, dentists, and other health care practitioners are in short supply. Shortages of medical facilities such as community clinics and hospitals are also a factor in determining access to health care. Medically underserved areas can include urban as well as rural areas, entire counties, sections within counties, groups of counties, and other designated areas. Medically underserved populations include groups of persons who face economic, cultural, or linguistic barriers to health care.

Government and employers are the largest purchasers of health care for a majority of working adults—but what happens when individuals are working for small employers who do not provide health care benefits, are too young for Medicare, are earning too much money for Medicaid but not enough to purchase private health insurance, are unemployed, or are otherwise ineligible for dependable health care benefits? Access to health care services, in these cases, is typically available only sporadically—through emergency room visits, free clinics, free immunizations, and so on—or not at all.

Some argue that access to health care services is a basic human right, and should not be denied to anyone, regardless of social or employment status. The fact remains, however, that health care services are not free—so who will pay the bill? This remains the crucial question for Congress and for all health care stakeholders as the twenty-first century progresses.

Quality

The **Agency for Healthcare Research and Quality (AHRQ)** is the lead federal agency responsible for tracking and improving the quality, safety, efficiency, and effectiveness of health care for Americans.

Since 2003, the AHRQ has studied the health care industry and tracked quality of health care. The agency's findings are published in an annual report, the National Healthcare Quality Report (NHQR). The first NHQR, issued in 2003, found certain key issues to be problematic, as listed in the following text. Findings from the most recent (2010) NHQR followed four themes that emphasize the need to accelerate progress if the United States is to achieve higher quality and more equitable health care in the future:

1. Health care quality and access are not as good as they could be, especially for minority and low-income people.

2. While quality is improving, there are still too many disparities in access and health care quality.

3. Urgent attention is needed in some areas, to ensure higher quality and access for some populations, geographical areas and services. These high priority areas include

   • Cancer screening.

   • Diabetes management.

   • Health care services in the central United States.

   • Services in inner cities and rural areas.

   • Disparities in preventative services and access to care.

4. Uneven progress in eight national priority areas

   • Two are improving in quality: (1) palliative and end-of-life care and (2) patient and family engagement.

   • Three are lagging: (3) population health, (4) safety, and (5) access.

   • Three require more data to assess: (6) care coordination, (7) overuse, and (8) health system infrastructure.

All eight priority areas showed disparities related to race, ethnicity, and socioeconomic status.

The NHQR has become an annual event, allowing for continuous tracking of certain health care measures. According to 2010 data, some areas merit urgent attention, including patient safety and hospital-based infections.

In hospitals, safety remains a significant problem. Of the 33 measures related to safety that are included in the report, more than half showed some improvement, but others remain lacking. Infections contracted in

Agency for Healthcare Research and Quality (AHRQ) The lead federal agency responsible for tracking and improving the quality, safety, efficiency, and effectiveness of health care for Americans.

Ranking the United States in Quality, Access, and Cost per Individual

Country Rankings

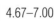

	1.00–2.33
	2.34–4.66
	4.67–7.00

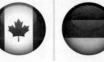 

	AUS	CAN	GER	NETH	NZ	UK	US
Overall Ranking (2010)	3	6	4	1	5	2	7
Quality Care	4	7	5	2	1	3	6
Effective Care	2	7	6	3	5	1	4
Safe Care	6	5	3	1	4	2	7
Coordinated Care	4	5	7	2	1	3	6
Patient-Centered Care	2	5	3	6	1	7	4
Access	6.5	5	3	1	4	2	6.5
Cost-Related Problem	6	3.5	3.5	2	5	1	7
Timeliness of care	6	7	2	1	3	4	5
Efficiency	2	6	5	3	4	1	7
Equity	4	5	3	1	6	2	7
Long, Healthy, Productive Lives	1	2	3	4	5	6	7
Health Expenditures/Capita, 2007*	$3,357	$3,895	$3,588	$3,837	$2,454	$2,992	$7,290

*Estimate. Expenditures shown in $US PPP (purchasing power parity).

Source: Calculated by The Commonwealth Fund based on 2007 International Health Policy Survey; 2008 International Health Policy Survey of Sicker Adults; 2009 International Health Policy Survey of Primary Care Physicians; Commonwealth Fund Commission on a High Performance Health System National Scorecard; and Organization for Economic Cooperation and Development, *OECD Health Data, 2009* (Paris: OECD, Nov. 2009).

THE COMMONWEALTH FUND

hospitals remain a concern, since rates of infection have not declined significantly since the last report.

The 2010 report continues to emphasize that greater improvement in health care quality in the United States is possible and crucial to extending life expectancy and maintaining a healthy quality of life for the nation's population.

(For more information contained in the 2010 NHQR, visit **www.ahrq.gov/qual/nhqr10/nhqr10.pdf.**)

Life Expectancy and Life Span

life expectancy The number of years an individual can expect to live, calculated from his or her birth.

life span The number of years an individual actually lives.

Life expectancy is the statistically probable number of years a newborn ought to live, based on environment, heredity, lifestyle, health practices, risk factors, and so on. **Life span** refers to the number of years an individual actually lives.

Life expectancy in the United States is currently about 78.11 years, placing the United States 49th when compared with other countries. As of 2010, residents of Macau, a small Vegas-style resort area in Asia, have the world's highest life expectancy, at 84.36 years, and residents of Angola, a country in south central Africa, have the lowest, at 38.20 years.

Access to universal health care is not necessarily a contributing factor to longer life expectancies. Factors that determine life expectancy vary greatly even within the United States, according to race, income level, geography, and such preventable risk factors as smoking, drug and alcohol abuse, obesity, high blood pressure, elevated cholesterol levels, poor diet, and physical inactivity.

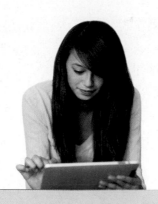

check your **progress**

7. Check the 10 amendments to the U.S. Constitution called the Bill of Rights at **www.archives. gov/exhibits/charters/bill_of_rights_transcript.html**. Is health care listed as a right for all Americans?

8. What are two areas of continuing concern revealed in the most current National Healthcare Quality Report (NHQR)?

9. What is the difference between life expectancy and life span?

10. In your opinion, why is the United States 49th on a list of life expectancies in various countries?

Health Care Trends

Experts predict that the key health care issues of cost, access, and quality will continue to be of concern for Americans within the health care system. As legislation is implemented changing the health insurance industry, a new group of issues will probably emerge. The Institute for the Future, an independent, nonprofit research group based in California, studies and issues forecasts concerning certain aspects of life in the United States, including:

LO 13.3

Describe the major new trends that will affect health care in the United States in the next 20 years.

- Work and daily life.
- Technology and society.
- Health and health care.
- Global business trends.
- Changing consumer society.

In 2009, the group's predictions about health care were detailed in the publication *Health & Health Care 2010: The Forecast, The Challenge.* Of special concern for the future were

- Security of benefits—ensuring that employees do not lose health care benefits when they lose their jobs or go to work for smaller employers.

- Monitoring and organizing increasing numbers of managed care organizations, insurers, intermediaries (case managers, provider partners, fee-for-service brokers, and safety-net funders) and providers.

- Including consumers in health care decision making.

- Determining responsibility for **medical management** (the management of patient care and populations to lower costs, ensure access, and increase quality of health care). Medical management will involve patients, providers, employers, health plans and governments, and will

medical management The management of patient care and populations.

consist of managing disease states for the acutely sick and chronically ill, as well as managing disease prevention in the generally well.

- Improving health behaviors of the American people.

Issues of concern will undoubtedly change as society moves further into the twenty-first century, when new health care legislation at federal and state levels changes the health care landscape.

The Institute of the Future's Health Horizons program now publishes trends and forecasts online. Reach Health Horizons at **www.iftf.org/ health** then review or download the forecast map for 2020 at **www.iftf. org/2020ForecastMap**.

- What are the three "What if" questions for the future of health care in the United States?
- List the six challenges focused on within the report.
- How does the map deal with forecasts for the six challenges?

As the health care landscape changes in the future, undoubtedly medical and health information technologies will continue to advance.

Medical Technologies

New medical technologies are a major driving force within the health care industry. According to *Health & Health Care 2010,* and other sources, advanced medical technologies that will affect patient care over the next decade include, but are not limited to, the following:

- Rational drug design—use of computers to create drugs designed to attack specific diseased cells or to otherwise pinpoint delivery and enhance efficacy.
- Continuing advancement in imaging equipment and techniques.
- Minimally invasive surgery such as highly developed arthroscopic and laparoscopic techniques, and robotic surgery.
- Genetic mapping and testing.
- Gene therapy.
- New and improved vaccines.
- Artificial blood.
- Xenotransplantation.
- Use of stem cells.
- Personalized medicine.

Rational Drug Design

Rational drug design refers to the use of increasingly powerful computers to develop new drugs by looking at the molecular structure and chemical composition of target cells and creating substances that will bind to certain molecules, affecting their function inside the body. For example, drugs now in development for antiviral use will prevent viruses from using the body's protease enzymes to chop up amino acids for viruses to use as building blocks for replicating. These new antiviral drugs may be used to combat such diseases as HIV, encephalitis, measles, and influenza.

Drugs are also in development that can bind with receptors for various neurotransmitters in the nervous system, helping to reduce symptoms in patients suffering from neurological and mental diseases.

Similarly, drugs in development to combat cancer will target cancer cells for destruction, but will not destroy normal cells in the body, thus eliminating many of the noxious side effects cancer patients often suffer during chemotherapy.

Advances in Imaging

The improvement of computers is also leading to advances in imaging equipment and techniques, as Cindi, quoted in the chapter's opening scenario can attest.

Energy sources currently used for imaging include X-rays, ultrasound, electron beams, positrons, magnets, and radio frequencies. By precisely pinpointing areas of the body to be imaged and closely focusing the energy source, new imaging devices will be better able to avoid damaging normal tissue. The use of concentrated ultrasound energy to destroy kidney stones is one example of a relatively new technique now in use.

Future imaging equipment will also take advantage of the trend toward smaller, yet more powerful, computerized devices. Smaller magnetic resonance imaging (MRI) machines, for example, will soon be available for use in orthopedics, neurology, and mammography, which developers predict will not only provide clearer, more detailed images, but also lower purchasing and operating costs.

Minimally Invasive Surgery

Minimally invasive surgery involves corrective surgical techniques that do not require large incisions into body cavities. Such techniques include arthroscopic knee surgery, some types of vascular and brain surgeries, coronary angioplasty, and laparoscopic surgeries such as appendectomy (Figure 13-7) and cholecystectomy (removal of the gall bladder).

As a result of minimally invasive surgery, ambulatory surgery centers will continue to increase in number. Since minimally invasive surgeries usually require short hospital stays or no stays at all, and recuperation times are shorter than with traditional surgical procedures, these techniques may also contribute significantly to lowering health care costs.

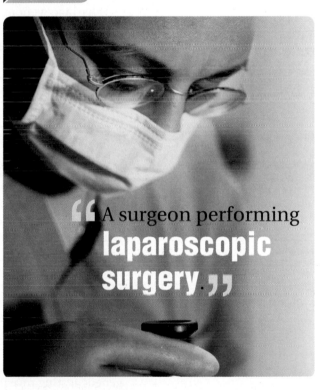

Figure 13-7

"A surgeon performing **laparoscopic surgery**."

Robotic Surgery

Surgical robots are also becoming increasingly common in hospitals across the country. In 2000, Mani Menon, a surgeon at the Henry Ford Hospital in Detroit, was the first surgeon in the United States to remove a cancerous prostate gland using a robot. Menon's revolutionary technique applied advances in laparoscopy to this delicate and complex operation. Because he could use smaller incisions, prostatectomy patients enjoyed shorter hospital stays, less pain, and quicker recoveries.

Then along came surgical robots, instruments designed for a U.S. Army–sponsored project in the 1980s for surgery on battlefields. Commercial applications soon became apparent, and in 1999 the first "Dr. Robots" were introduced as the futuristic phase of minimally invasive surgery.

As of January 2011, 1,000 hospitals and clinics in the United States were using a product called the da Vinci robot, and 400 facilities worldwide also used the product.

Genetic Mapping and Testing

The Human Genome Project, discussed in Chapter 11, launched an era of unprecedented interest in mapping the human genome. The project was begun in 1990 and progressed so quickly that it was ended ahead of schedule, in mid-2000. During that time, scientists identified approximately 20,000 to 25,000 genes present in human DNA. They also developed protocols for researching DNA, and passed on their acquired knowledge to other scientists.

pharmacogenomics The science that defines how individuals are genetically programmed to respond to drugs.

genometrics The science of determining how genes cause the expression of certain traits in individuals.

epigenetics The study of changes in gene activity that do not involve alterations to the genetic code, but are still passed down to at least one successive generation.

The project's results have led to applications in **pharmacogenomics,** the science that defines how individuals are genetically programmed to respond to drugs. The results have also speeded the development of specific tests for genes causing cancers of the breast, colon, and prostate, and have added to scientists' knowledge of how genes cause the expression of certain traits in individuals—a science called **genometrics.**

Also associated with advances in genometrics is a new field of research called **epigenetics,** or the study of changes in gene activity that do not involve alterations to the genetic code, but are still passed down to at least one successive generation. The process works like this: Certain cellular materials sit above the DNA in one's genome—hence the prefix epi-, which means "above"—and are responsible for telling genes when to switch completely or partially on and off. Through these epigenetic markers, a parent's bad habits, such as smoking, overeating, or not following a nutritious diet, can imprint genes so that undesirable characteristics are passed on to at least one generation. That means that the genes for obesity, for example, can express themselves too strongly in your offspring, or the genes for longevity to express themselves too weakly, thus causing your bad habits to affect your children through your DNA.

Pharmacogenomic research has led to genometric drug design—the process of using a person's DNA profile to design a drug specifically for that person. This procedure is showing promise for extending the lives of cancer patients. For example, Dendreon Corporation's drug Provenge was approved for use in April 2010 for patients suffering from incurable prostate tumors. The drug is not a "one-size-fits-all" cure but is similar to a vaccine, designed to train the immune system to fight prostate cancer cells. The drug is individually prepared using each patient's DNA profile and a protein found on most prostate cancer cells. Unfortunately, the price tag for a year's treatment with Provenge in 2010 was an astounding $93,000, and the drug does not cure the disease but may extend the life of patients an additional few months. Other cancer drugs designed for specific patients can run as much as $10,000 a month.

The future of such drugs seems promising, but cost then becomes an issue. If Medicare and private insurance plans pay for such drugs, will all enrollees share the cost in the form of higher premiums and fees? Since 85 percent of Americans earn less than $100,000 a year, will the price of such drugs limit their use and lead to rationing based on resources?

The Human Genome Project also revealed future ramifications of genetic testing, including social and ethical implications. If a health insurance company obtains a client's genetic testing results, for example, and learns that he or she is at risk to develop a genetic disease, can the company drop coverage for the client? Will reproductive rights of certain individuals be restricted if genetic testing reveals that their offspring are at risk for inherited disabilities or diseases? Will prenatal genetic testing result in "designer" children for many couples? Will self-administered genetic testing kits eventually become available, bypassing valuable genetic counseling for consumers?

Gene Therapy

Gene therapy, which involves correcting defective genes responsible for disease, is also on the horizon for the future. Researchers may use one of several approaches for correcting faulty genes:

- A normal gene may be inserted into a nonspecific location within the genome to replace a nonfunctional gene. This approach is most common.

- A normal gene could be substituted for an abnormal gene through an exchange of sections of chromosomes during meiosis.

- The abnormal gene could be repaired through selective reverse mutation, which returns the gene to its normal function.

- The regulation (the degree to which a gene is turned on or off) of a particular gene could be altered.

Both genetic testing and gene therapy are in evolving stages of development. Widespread utilization of the science will require practicing health care practitioners to acquire the knowledge and techniques necessary to practice genomic medicine—a field in which specialists are currently limited in number.

Utilizing gene therapy will undoubtedly also require testing in court. For example, in 1999, physician-researchers at the University of Pennsylvania conducted gene therapy experiments designed to treat a disease called ornithine transcarbamylase (OTC) deficiency, which inhibits the liver's ability to process proteins. Researchers sought out adult subjects for the study who were carriers of the disease (all carriers are women) or who exhibited milder forms of the disease. Jesse Gelsinger, an 18-year-old who allegedly fit the subject search, participated in the study and received treatment. On September 17, 1999, Gelsinger died, allegedly as a direct result of the gene therapy treatment. On September 18, 2000, Gelsinger's father filed a lawsuit against the University of Pennsylvania; researchers James M. Wilson, Steven E. Raper, and Mark L. Batshaw; Arthur Caplan, director of the university's Center for Bioethics; and others. The lawsuit was settled out of court in February 2005. Under the terms of the settlement, Wilson, Raper, and Batshaw did not admit any wrongdoing. The university and the Children's Hospital of Philadelphia, where Batshaw was affiliated, were to strengthen their research oversight and pay fines of $517,496 and $514,622, respectively. The case was settled, but terms were not officially reported, probably due to settlement agreements. Therefore, the case did not establish precedent.

The plaintiffs in the case also settled a second lawsuit which the U.S. Justice Department initiated, alleging breach of the False Claims Act. Under terms of this settlement, Wilson was required to wait until 2010 before again leading research on humans. In the meantime, he would also undergo training and education relating to research on human subjects, work under enhanced oversight and monitoring, and lecture and write an article on "lessons learned."

Since the *Gelsinger* case was settled, other ethical lapses have been alleged in additional lawsuits filed by study participants, including unreported deaths of monkeys given similar gene therapy treatments; failure to inform the FDA, as required, when patients became so ill from the treatment that the study should have been suspended; and researchers' failure to disclose opportunities to profit if the treatment were successful.

Improved Vaccines

The most common use of vaccines over time has been to prevent disease. Live or weakened forms of disease organisms are injected, and then stimulate the patient's immune system to produce antibodies against the disease organism. Infectious diseases such as whooping cough, diphtheria, measles, smallpox, polio, and influenza are prevented in this manner.

Another, more current, use of vaccines is to prevent the growth of small metastatic (spreading) tumors in cancer patients. Vaccinations to prevent various forms of cancer from developing are also in the works. For example, the vaccine for the human papillomavirus (HPV), which can cause cervical cancer, is now available for use, and is one example of a twenty-first-century vaccine that may significantly reduce cancer in the United States.

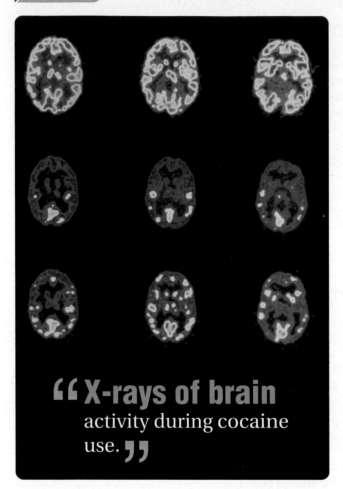

" X-rays of brain activity during cocaine use. **"**

Furthermore, recently two medical researchers from Baylor University in Houston, Texas, have reported progress in developing a vaccine to prevent or cure an addiction to cocaine (Figure 13-8). Inactivated drug molecules are bonded with inactivated cholera molecules and injected into the body. The body releases antibodies against the cholera molecule, which also act to prevent the drug from entering the brain, where it can activate an addiction response. The liver metabolizes the drug molecules and they are excreted from the body. When the drug no longer produces a high, addicts may lose interest and stop taking the drug. Scientists theorize that if the FDA approves the vaccine, it may also be developed to cure addiction to other drugs, such as nicotine.

Artificial Blood

When a patient loses a large volume of blood, the loss is significant on two fronts:

1. Loss of plasma, the liquid portion of the blood that consists mostly of water and carries nutrients, hormones, and waste, causes reduced blood volume.

2. Loss of the formed elements in blood—including red and white blood cells, platelets that aid in clotting, and parts of cells that float in the plasma—means that oxygen is not reaching the damaged tissue, and the tissue can die.

For the millions of traumatic brain injury (TBI) and spinal cord injury patients that are rushed to emergency rooms every year, tissue death is especially drastic because it usually causes paralysis, coma, or even death. Physicians treating such patients have found that administering an artificial blood substitute can restore oxygen circulation to damaged tissue faster than transfusing whole blood, without the necessity for cross-typing or screening for disease organisms.

Pharmaceutical companies developed several varieties of artificial blood in the 1980s and 1990s, but early formulas were abandoned when they caused heart attacks, strokes, and deaths in human trials. Some early formulas also caused capillaries to collapse and blood pressure to rise. Recent research, however, has led to several blood substitutes classified into two types: hemoglobin-based oxygen carriers (HBOCs) and perfluorocarbons (PFCs), which are entirely synthetic and have the highest gas-dissolving capacity of any liquid. Some of these blood substitutes are already in use, and others are nearing the end of their FDA-required testing phases and may soon be available to hospitals.

Xenotransplantation

As discussed in Chapter 11, xenotransplantation involves transplanting animal tissue into human patients.

Two documented cases of xenotransplantation in the 1980s and 1990s involved the use of baboon organs. In 1984, Dr. Leonard Bailey transplanted a baboon's heart into Baby Fae, a newborn with a severe heart defect known as left hypoplastic heart. Bailey had theorized that the baby's underdeveloped immune system would not attack the foreign tissue. Baby Fae did well for a few days; then her body mounted a massive immune reaction to the baboon heart that subsequently caused her death.

A baboon was the organ source again in 1992, when surgeons at the University of Pittsburgh Medical Center replaced a man's diseased liver with a healthy baboon liver. The patient had hepatitis B and was not considered a good transplant prospect because the disease was likely to occur in the new, healthy liver as well. Surgeons hoped the baboon liver would survive because baboons are not susceptible to the hepatitis B virus. Again, however, the patient died from a massive immune reaction.

The most successful uses of xenotransplantation to date have involved transplanting into human patients certain pig tissues, such as skin and nervous tissue. Pigs have been chosen as an object of study for possible xenotransplantation of whole organs, various tissues, and cells, since the sizes of their organs and cells closely match those of humans.

A strain of genetically engineered pigs has been raised that lacks the gene responsible for alpha-1,3-galactosyltransferase (GT), a sugary substance normally present in the pig vascular system. Since humans have natural, preformed antibodies to GT, transplants of pig tissue have, in the past, often resulted in immediate rejection. Scientists are hopeful that tissues and organs in the genetically engineered pigs will more readily be accepted by human transplantation patients.

Use of Stem Cells

The largest barrier to using stem cells to treat disease has been political objection, on religious and ethical grounds, to the destruction of human embryos that are most useful in stem cell research. President George W. Bush felt so strongly about this issue that his administration prohibited federal funding of embryonic stem cell research, which slowed the progress of such research.

In 2007, however, researchers announced that human skin cells had been used to produce the stem cells that might someday be useful to patients with spinal cord injuries, Parkinson's disease, diabetes, damaged hearts, and other diseases or conditions. Skin and bone cells have been among the initial cell-building successes, but the potential for large-scale stem cell use is huge. Political and ethical issues seem the most formidable barriers to use of stem cell technology in the future.

Progress in growing stem cells from tissues other than embryos has continued, and as of 2011, through a process called tissue engineering, scientists have been able to grow functioning bladders, urethras, and even heart and lung tissue from a person's own cells. Using cells taken from an individual, an organ such as a bladder is grown over a scaffold. The bladder can be transplanted into that same individual without the fear of rejection, since the recipient's own cells were used to grow the bladder. Once transplanted, the scaffold disintegrates, and the bladder adapts to its new location. To date, several individuals have received such transplants, and the laboratory-grown bladders have functioned successfully. So far, tissue-engineered hearts and lungs are still in the experimental stage.

Wake Forest University Medical Center in Winston-Salem, North Carolina, pioneered the world's first lab-grown bladder, and it remains at the forefront of the organ-growing field. Wake Forest is the world's largest regenerative medicine research center, and its current research is in growing 22 different types of tissue: heart valves, muscle cells, arteries, and even fingers.

Personalized Medicine

Imagine that sometime in the near future you visit your doctor for your annual physical. On your first visit, the medical facility's lab analyzed your genome, so your physician is aware that you carry genes for certain gastrointestinal disorders and for late-onset breast cancer. You have not yet developed symptoms of any disorder, but your physician orders all

proteomics The study of the proteins that genes create or "express."

personalized medicine The products and services that leverage the science of genomics and proteomics and capitalize on the trends toward wellness and consumerism to enable tailored approaches to prevention and care.

appropriate tests. You have lost 10 pounds since your last visit, making your weight now appropriate for your height and age, so your physician recommends that you continue with the wellness activities outlined during your first visit. Since scientists estimate that one gene can trigger the manufacture of as many as 1,000 proteins responsible for various bodily functions—both normal and abnormal—your physician also orders a protein panel. (The study of the proteins associated with one's genome is called **proteomics**.) After she completes her physical examination and all laboratory results are in, your physician prescribes a regimen of care that includes wellness recommendations and perhaps a medication tailored especially for you. This is **personalized medicine,** and it's coming to a medical facility near you.

Although still in its infancy, the concept of personalized medicine continues to grow as a trend in the United States. PriceWaterhouseCoopers, a global accounting and business consulting firm, defines it as "the products and services that leverage the science of genomics and proteomics (directly or indirectly) and capitalize on the trends towards wellness and consumerism to enable tailored approaches to prevention and care."

The personalized medicine industry includes nutrition and wellness components—made up of complementary and alternative medicine, health clubs, organic care, and the medical retail establishment—and unique-to-each-patient aspects that include telemedicine, electronic and personal health records, tests to analyze DNA, and target therapeutics to help providers find the right therapy at the right time. PriceWaterhouseCoopers estimates that this was a $225 billion industry in 2009.

The hope with personalized medicine is that there will be better patient outcomes, not just in disease management, but in maintaining wellness and improving each patient's participation in his or her own care. Most experts believe that personalized medicine can only become reality with coordination of services and long-term business strategies consistent among all of the players.

Diabetes, Obesity, and the Future

In October 2010 the Centers for Disease Control and Prevention issued a report predicting that one in three people may develop diabetes in the next 40 years. According to the CDC, diabetes is presently the number one cause of adult blindness, kidney failure, and limb amputation and is seventh on the list of diseases that cause death in the United States. The 2009 costs for diabetes and related problems were $116 billion.

The predicted increase in diabetics is partially because people are living longer with the disease. However, there is some evidence to suggest that obesity and diabetes are related, and obesity has become epidemic in the United States. According to a report released by the CDC in June 2010, approximately 34 percent of adults 20 years old and over are obese—that is, these individuals are at least 20 percent over their ideal body weight. Additionally, approximately 10 percent of children 2 to 5 years old are obese. Twenty percent of children 6 to 11 years old are obese and 18 percent of children 12 to 20 years old are obese. Obesity is a medical condition in which excess body fat has accumulated to the point that it has an adverse effect on health, and may shorten one's life expectancy.

Health Information Technologies

Polls indicate that most Americans believe that their health care providers routinely use computer technology for storing and managing their medical records. Unfortunately, too often this is not the case. The health care industry has lagged behind other industries in adopting technology for performing

Figure 13-9

Trends in Overweight, Obesity, and Extreme Obesity

Trends in overweight, obesity, and extreme obesity among adults aged 20 years and over: United States, 1988–2008

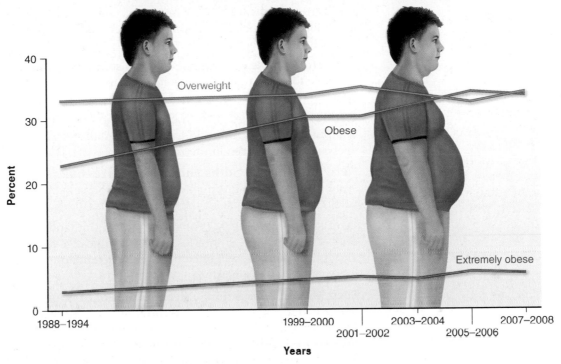

NOTES: Age adjusted by the direct method to the year 2000 U.S. Census Bureau estimates, using the age groups 20–39, 40–59, and 60 years and over. Pregnant females were excluded. Overweight is defined as a body mass index (BMI) of 25 or greater but less than 30; obesity is a BMI greater than or equal to 30; extreme obesity is a BMI greater than or equal to 40.

Source: CDC/NCHS, National Health and Nutrition Examination Survey III 1988–1994, 1999–2000, 2001–2002, 2003–2004, 2005–2006, and 2007–2008.

Source: Centers for Disease Control and Prevention, **www.cdc.gov/NCHS/data/hestat/obesity_adult_07_08/obesity_adult_07_08.pdf.**

Figure 13-10

U.S. Population with Diagnosed Diabetes, 1958–2008

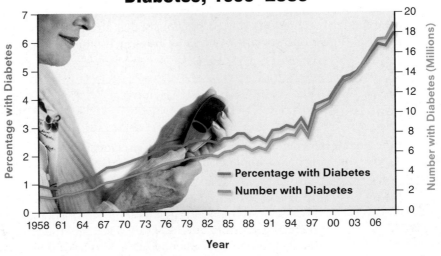

daily business chores. For instance, many physician offices still keep reams of paper patient files, filled with hastily scrawled notes, test results, X-rays, illegible copies of prescriptions written, and other materials that are subject to fire, flood (witness the Katrina disaster), rot, and other natural forces.

Over the next decade, advances in these areas of communications and information technology will significantly affect the health care industry:

Computer hardware. Faster microprocessors and larger memory capabilities will make managing health care information faster and easier for HCI specialists.

Data storage. Nearly unlimited digital storage capabilities will make it possible to store a population's health care data in smaller and smaller spaces.

Wireless technology. Health care practitioners currently use handheld computers as study aids and to access digitalized patient records, and such use will increase in the future.

Networking bandwidths and data compression. Faster networking systems with larger information transmission capabilities will be the rule, increasing the use of these technologies.

Data storage retrieval. Programs that can find and retrieve information—from digitalized libraries, search engines, government collections, and other sources—will become more efficient and easier to use, thus increasing their popularity.

Security and encryption. Privacy of health care information is a major concern as information technology becomes more sophisticated and more widely used. HIPAA's requirements concerning electronic health care records have spurred hospitals and other medical facilities to move toward digital transmission and storage, and the movement will progress as security and encryption methods become more reliable.

Internet. The Internet and the World Wide Web are currently popular sources for medical information, and the trend will continue as the Internet continues to evolve.

3-D computing. Interior designers, architects, car and equipment designers, animated movie makers, and others in various design fields have access to computer programs, called computer-aided design

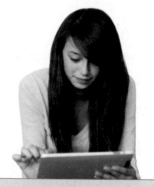

check your **progress**

Choose three of the medical technologies listed previously that are forecast to improve or otherwise change in the future, and give one specific example of how each might be applied in medical situations.

11. _____

12. _____

13. _____

Choose three of the health information technologies listed previously that are forecasted to improve in the future, and give one specific example of how each might be applied in medical situations.

14. _____

15. _____

16. _____

(CAD) programs, that let them work in 3-D. In the future, CAD programs will become more readily available to health care practitioners, as a means both of visualizing medical procedures and of displaying large amounts of information at one time.

Database software. Already used extensively in business, database software will evolve into new classes that will increase the capacity to store, present, sort, and analyze data.

Sensors. Just as implanted pacemakers and insulin pumps sense when a patient's heart rate or insulin levels must be adjusted, future devices will allow health care practitioners to monitor and adjust a wider range of patient symptoms and events.

As all of these devices and systems become less expensive, larger numbers of health care practitioners and facilities will adopt them for routine use.

Government Attempts to Reform Health Care

LO 13.4
Discuss former and ongoing attempts to reform the U.S. health care system.

Presidents Truman, Nixon, and Carter said that health care reform was a priority for their administrations, but no reforms were passed during their years in office. Legislation to substantially reform the American health care industry was introduced during the Clinton presidential administration, in the form of the Health Security Act of 1993. The act included the following provisions:

- It guaranteed health insurance benefits to all Americans, with no lifetime limits on coverage.

- It provided a comprehensive package of medical services delivered in hospitals, clinics, professional offices, and other sites.

- It provided for one uniform, comprehensive benefit package that would replace hundreds of different insurance products on the market.

- Health insurance premiums would pay the cost of the new system, but enforceable caps would be placed on the rate of increase in premium prices.

The structure of the proposed new health care system consisted of an independent National Health Board that would act as the board of directors for the health care system, setting national standards and overseeing implementation of reform. It also provided for alliances—state, regional, corporate, and health plan alliances—that would offer a choice of health insurance plans, including traditional fee-for-service arrangements, preferred provider organizations, and health maintenance organizations.

The Health Security Act of 1993 failed to pass, and there were many reasons for its failure. Among them were these:

- Medicare was in place to provide help with health care costs for seniors, and Medicaid provided aid for lower-income and unemployed individuals; therefore, the public and their congressional representatives did not see the need for drastic health care reform.

- The act's basis for reform was *managed competition:* a complicated concept that combined market forces and government regulations. The concept had a narrow bloc of backers among members of Congress and the health care provider community.

- The act mandated that everyone have health insurance, with employed individuals paying 80 percent of the cost and employers paying 20 percent. (The government would pay for low-income and unemployed individuals' coverage.)

As first mentioned in Chapter 3, President Barack Obama, who took office in January 2009, promised that his administration, with the cooperation of a Democrat-controlled Congress, would restructure the American health care system. The overhaul of the system began in earnest in 2010 with passage of the Patient Protection and Affordable Care Act (PPACA) and the Health Care and Education Reconciliation Act, which amended the original PPACA.

The many provisions of the law were scheduled to take effect over eight years. They included expanding Medicaid eligibility, which was intended to extend health insurance to many individuals who were uninsured, as well as establishing state-run health insurance exchanges, also intended to make health insurance coverage available to many consumers who had previously been uninsured or underinsured. The act also provided for expanding medical research, and ensuring that health insurance companies could no longer impose preexisting condition exclusions on children, could not deny coverage based on unintentional mistakes on applications, and could not set lifetime limits on coverage or raise premium charges beyond certain limits. The act's provisions were to be paid for by new taxes and fees contained within its 1,000-plus pages.

Tables 13-2 and 13-3 show how the act's major provisions were scheduled to take effect, from 2010 through 2018.

PPACA PROVISIONS EFFECTIVE IN 2010

Table 13-2

Issue	Effect
Temporary high-risk insurance pool	Creates a national pool to provide health coverage for individuals with preexisting conditions who have been uninsured for six months.
Preexisting conditions	Prevents insurance companies from denying coverage to children with preexisting medical conditions.
Adult children	Insurance companies must cover dependent children up to age 26.
Coverage limits	Insurance plans cannot place lifetime limits on coverage and cannot rescind coverage except for fraud.
Tanning salons	A 10 percent tax is imposed on indoor tanning services.
Preventive care	Insurance plans must cover preventive services such as vaccinations for children and cancer screening for women.
Medicare recipients	Some Medicare patients receive a $250 rebate to help cover the cost of medications.
Tax credit for business	Small businesses with 25 or fewer employees can receive tax credits for the 2010 tax year to help pay for offering employees health insurance.

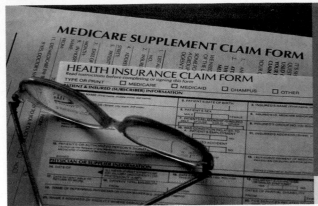

PPACA PROVISIONS EFFECTIVE IN 2014 THROUGH 2018

Table 13-3

Year	Issue	Effect
2014	Health insurance exchanges	State-run health care exchanges for uninsured individuals and small businesses are created.
	Individual mandate	Everyone must have health insurance or pay a fine. Companies with 50 or more employees will pay a fine if any of their full-time workers qualified for federal subsidies.
	Medicaid expansion	Income eligibility is increased for those under 65.
	Federal subsidies	Federal subsidies will help lower-income people buy insurance.
	Annual insurance company fees	Annual fees are imposed on health insurance companies.
2015–2016	Individual mandate	Penalties for not carrying insurance are increased each year.
	Annual insurance company fees	Annual fees imposed on health insurance companies are increased.
2017–2018	Annual fee on drug manufacture	Annual fee on pharmaceutical manufacturers is increased each year.
	Annual insurance company fees	Annual fees imposed on health insurance companies are increased each year.
	Excise tax on high-cost insurance plans	A 40 percent excise tax is imposed on the more expensive health care plans.

Changes scheduled for implementation in 2011 concerned annual fees imposed on pharmaceutical manufacturers, tax changes on health care savings accounts, closing the Medicare "doughnut hole" for seniors who experience a gap in drug coverage, paying bonuses through Medicare fees to primary care doctors and general surgeons practicing in underserved areas, funding community health centers for low-income people, and requiring insurance companies to pay rebates to enrollees if they spent less than 80 to 85 percent of premium dollars on health care as opposed to administrative costs.

In 2012 and 2013, a voluntary long-term care program would be created, the annual fee on drug makers would increase, limits would be placed on contributions to health care savings accounts, the threshold for out-of-pocket medical expenses on income tax forms would increase, and the Medicare tax rate would increase.

Since the PPACA was unpopular with some American citizens, and faced opposition from many newly elected politicians after the 2010 midterm elections, some of these provisions may have been revised or repealed since the publication of *Law & Ethics for Medical Careers,* sixth edition.

Some states have taken the initiative in health care reform, but at the national level, because many of the stakeholders in the health care industry do not want change, reform has been an unpopular issue. With passage of the Patient Protection and Affordable Care Act in 2010, however, health care reform seemed inevitable. The act followed some of the following suggestions for reform, coming from national organizations, policy analysts, and presidential and congressional candidates, and was intended to cover cost, access, and quality:

- Charge Medicare beneficiaries more. (Probably inevitable as costs continue to rise.)

- Create a dedicated federal health tax to cover all government health spending, such as Medicare and Medicaid. The tax could be an energy tax, a payroll tax, or an income surtax. If health spending rose, the tax would increase. (The PPACA provides for several taxes and fees to help pay for health care coverage for more Americans.)

- Eliminate the income tax exclusion for employer-paid insurance and replace it with a tax credit of lesser value. (Also probably inevitable, either under the PPACA, or other legislation passed to address health care costs.)

- Provide access to health insurance through public financing for Americans living at or below poverty levels.

- Provide extensive education to consumers concerning living a healthy lifestyle.

- Disclose and reward quality-based medical practice.

- Support and reinvigorate through government financing the nation's deteriorating public health system.

- Require all Americans to have health insurance coverage, available through public and private plan options made available through state-run exchanges, where citizens could obtain coverage at a reasonable cost, or through government subsidies.

State Children's Health Initiative Program (SCHIP) A program enacted by the Balanced Budget Act of 1997 to help low-income children under 19 who are not covered by Medicaid.

The **State Children's Health Initiative Program (SCHIP)** was enacted by the Balanced Budget Act of 1997 to help ensure health care for low-income children under 19 who are not covered by Medicaid. SCHIP is jointly financed by the federal and state governments and is state-administered. Within broad federal guidelines, each state determines the design of its program, eligibility groups, benefit packages, payment levels for coverage, and administrative and operating procedures. SCHIP provides a capped amount of funds to states on a matching basis for federal funds. Variations of the SCHIP program are in effect in all 50 states, but Congress must periodically pass legislation reauthorizing federal funding, and the president must sign the reauthorization laws to keep the program funded.

As a health care practitioner, not only is it your responsibility to offer patient-centered, thoughtful, professionally competent care; it is also your duty to stay abreast of current trends in the health care industry and to know what is forecast for the future.

[CHAPTER SUMMARY]

LO 13.1 Who are health care *stakeholders*?

- Anyone with a vested interest in the health care industry.

Who are the major stakeholders in the United States health care industry?

- The public.
- Employers.
- Health care facilities and practitioners.
- Federal, state, and local governments.
- Managed care organizations.
- Private insurers.
- Volunteer facilities and agencies.
- Health care practitioner training institutions.
- Professional associations and other health care industry organizations.
- Medical and pharmaceutical research groups.

LO 13.2 What are the key issues of concern to health care industry stakeholders?

- Cost: The amount individuals, employers, state and federal governments, HMOs, and insurers spend on health care in the United States.
  - Health care costs as a percentage of gross national product (GDP) rise yearly.
  - GDP: Total value of all goods produced and services provided in American for one year.
  - Factors adding to health care costs annually include
    - Application of more advanced and more types of technology.
    - Growth in the population of older adults.
    - Emphasis on specialty medicine.
    - Increasing numbers of uninsured and underinsured.
    - Labor intensity of health care services.
    - Reimbursement system incentives.
    - Fraud.
- Access: The availability of health care and the means to purchase health care services.
  - Government attempts to reform the health care system have been intended, largely, to increase access and lower costs—the latest attempt at reform was the Patient Protection and Affordable Care Act (PPACA) of 2010.
- Quality: The degree of excellence of health care services offered.
  - What is the Agency for Healthcare Research and Quality (AHRQ)?
    - The lead federal agency responsible for tracking and improving the quality, safety, efficiency, and effectiveness of health care for Americans.
  - Latest AHRQ report shows
    - Access to quality care still not universal.
    - Access to quality care often depends on individuals' type of health insurance.
    - Matters of urgent concern are hospital safety and hospital infections.

LO 13.3 What health care advances have been forecast for the near future?

- Rational drug design—use of computers to create drugs designed to attack specific diseased cells or to otherwise pinpoint delivery and enhance efficacy.

- Continuing advancement in imaging equipment and techniques.
- Minimally invasive surgery, such as highly developed arthroscopic and laparoscopic techniques, such as robotic surgery.
- Genetic mapping and testing.
- Gene therapy.
- New and improved vaccines.
- Artificial blood.
- Xenotransplantation.
- Use of stem cells.
- Personalized medicine.

What are three additional areas where we should see improvement/advancement in the near future?

- Use of stem cells.
- Tissue engineering.
- Health information technologies (HITs).

LO 13.4 What health care system reforms have often been proposed, and may be inevitable in the near future?

- Charge Medicare beneficiaries more.
- Create a dedicated federal health tax to cover all government health spending, such as Medicare and Medicaid.
- Eliminate the income tax exclusion for employer-paid insurance and replace it with a tax credit of lesser value.
- Provide access to health insurance through public financing for Americans living at or below poverty levels.
- Provide extensive education to consumers concerning living a healthy lifestyle.
- Disclose and reward quality-based medical practice.
- Support and reinvigorate through government financing the nation's deteriorating public health system.
- Require all Americans to have health insurance coverage, available through public and private plan options made available through state-run exchanges, where citizens could obtain coverage at a reasonable cost, or through government subsidies.

[ETHICS ISSUES Health Care Trends and Forecasts]

Jean Connor of Cambridge, Massachusetts, was the 2007–2008 president of the Chicago-based American Dental Hygienists' Association (ADHA). At the time, she also worked as a practicing dental hygienist. Connor, who said she especially liked the variety of patients she saw, emphasized that dental hygienists work under the supervision of their dentist-employers. "We may not agree with the dentist's opinions, but they are the opinions that count," she said. "State dental boards may help us with ethical dilemmas, but these types of issues are so subjective, it's often difficult to resolve them.

"It helps if the office where you work has set procedures and standards that you can rely on," Connor continued. Don't take a job just because there was an opening; check the policy and procedures manual before you agree to work for an employer, to be sure you and the potential employer are a good fit.

Ethics ISSUE 1: You are an LPN employed in a medical office. Medicare payments to the physicians who work in the clinic have been cut, so policy has changed to "no new Medicare patients will be accepted."

Discussion Questions

1. Do you believe this policy is ethical? Why or why not?

_____

_____

2. You are accompanying an older relative visiting the clinic for the first time, and your relative has been turned away as a patient. What is your reaction to the clinic's stated policy?

_____

_____

3. Imagine that *you* are the older person visiting the clinic for the first time, and you are turned away as a patient. Will your reaction be the same as in question 2? Explain your answer.

_____

_____

Ethics ISSUE 2: Higher health insurance costs limit wage and salary gains because as insurance costs go up, employers who provide health care benefits raise the amount employees must pay for health insurance.

Discussion Question

1. Do you believe it is ethical for employers to increase employees' share of health insurance premiums when health care costs rise? Explain your answer.

_____

_____

Ethics ISSUE 3: Health insurance costs rise when health care becomes more costly. Patients who cannot afford to pay more for health insurance may then become underinsured or uninsured.

Discussion Question

1. Do you believe health care practitioners have an ethical obligation to hold down or reduce the fees they charge, considering the millions of people in the United States who are underinsured or uninsured? Why or why not?

_____

_____

Ethics ISSUE 4: Connor, the dental hygienist quoted earlier, said that her association is concerned that access to the care dental hygienists provide is decreasing. One reason is lack of insurance coverage, but another is that dental hygienists who retire or leave the profession early are not being replaced.

Discussion Question

1. Do you believe the health care industry has an ethical obligation to actively recruit health care practitioners who are in short supply? Explain your answer.

_____

_____

Ethics ISSUE 5: Laura Swisher, an associate professor in the physical therapy department at the University of South Florida, says physical therapists are moving toward more autonomy, which creates new ethical issues. For example, in the past it was unethical for physical therapists to diagnose a patient. Now, however, patients have direct access to physical therapists, who often diagnose conditions and refer patients to physicians.

Discussion Question

1. Since a physical therapist may see a patient before he or she visits a physician, does the PT have an ethical obligation to ask this patient about health (e.g., Do you get regular physical exams? Are your immunizations up to date? Have you had health problems in other areas lately?)? Explain your answer.

_____

_____

Ethics ISSUE 6: The trend in hospital staffing is to hire many temporary workers. This, according to Swisher, raises the continuity of care issue.

Discussion Questions

1. What is the responsibility for continuity of care for the patients a temporary health care worker sees, when that worker may be gone tomorrow?

_____

_____

2. Do you see an ethical solution to the continuity of care issue regarding temporary health care practitioners? Explain your answer.

_____

_____

Go to **www.mhhe.com/judson6e** to practice your case review skills. Then read on for more information.

[KEY TERMS]

access	genometrics	pharmacogenomics
Agency for Healthcare Research and Quality (AHRQ)	gross domestic product (GDP)	proteomics
	life expectancy	quality
baby boom generation	life span	stakeholders
cost	medical management	State Children's Health Initiative Program (SCHIP)
epigenetics	personalized medicine	

Applying Knowledge

Circle the correct answer for each of the following questions.

LO 13.1

1. Those who have a vested interest in the American health care industry are called
   a. Employers
   b. The public
   c. Stakeholders
   d. Insurers

2. What is the term for the total value of all goods produced and services provided in America for one year?
   a. Stakeholders
   b. Gross domestic product
   c. Net income
   d. Gross income

LO 13.2

3. Three key issues of concern to everyone within the American health care industry are
   a. Cost, access, quality
   b. Cost, availability, insurance
   c. Competition, education, quality
   d. Cost, access, hospitalization

4. What is the main force expanding the federal budget?
   a. Price of oil
   b. Health care costs
   c. Foreign aid
   d. Construction industry

5. Which of the following has *not* added to the cost of health care in the United States?
   a. Advances in medical technology
   b. Increasing numbers of older Americans
   c. Longer hospital stays for patients
   d. A highly educated health care labor force

6. What is most often cited as the reason for being uninsured or underinsured?
   a. Physicians won't accept Medicare
   b. Costs
   c. Advanced technology
   d. Refused insurance

7. The largest purchasers of health care for most working adults are
   a. Parents
   b. Single individuals
   c. Government and employers
   d. Insurance companies

8. "Baby boom" generation refers to the group of Americans born
   a. To low-income parents
   b. In hospitals
   c. From 1946 to 1964
   d. While fathers were in the military

9. What is the name of the lead federal agency responsible for tracking and improving the quality, safety, efficiency, and effectiveness of health care for Americans?
   a. AHRQ
   b. HIPAA
   c. PPACA
   d. NHQR

10. High-quality health care is *not*
    a. Possible
    b. Expensive
    c. Universal
    d. Practical

LO 13.3

11. According to the 2010 NHQR data, what two significant concerns remain for hospital patients?
    a. Safety and infections
    b. Diabetes education and obesity
    c. Death from strokes and heart attacks
    d. Death from tuberculosis related symptoms

12. What health care area continues to lag behind treatment for illness?
    a. Washington, DC
    b. Diabetes
    c. Prevention
    d. Exercise

13. What is the term for the statistically probable number of years a newborn ought to live, based on environment, heredity, lifestyle and health practices, risk factors, and so on?
    a. Lifetime
    b. Life expectancy
    c. Life span
    d. Adulthood

14. What is the number of years an individual actually lives called?
    a. Life span
    b. Life expectancy
    c. Adulthood
    d. Childhood

15. The science that defines how individuals are genetically programmed to respond to drugs is
    a. Pharmacology
    b. Genetics
    c. Pharmacogenomics
    d. Genometrics

16. The science of determining how genes cause the expression of certain traits in individuals is
    a. Advanced genetics
    b. Pharmacology
    c. Pharmacogenomics
    d. Genometrics

17. What is the process called that involves correcting defective genes responsible for disease?
    a. Genetics
    b. Genomics
    c. Pharmacology
    d. Gene therapy

18. Transplanting animal tissue into human patients is referred to as
    a. Genomics
    b. Xenotransplantation
    c. Gene therapy
    d. Genometrics

19. _____ is the federal government's most recent attempt to reform health care.
   a. HIPAA
   b. NHQR
   c. AHRQ
   d. PPACA

20. _____ is a federal program designed to provide health insurance for children.
   a. Genomics
   b. PPACA
   c. SCHIP
   d. HIPAA

LO 13.1 to LO 13.4

Answer the following questions in the spaces provided.

An article by Robert J. Samuelson in the December 10, 2007, issue of *Newsweek* stated, "The politics of health care rests on a mass illusion: Most Americans think that someone else pays for their care."

21. As an employee working in a job with health care benefits, who pays for your care?

_____

_____

22. Who pays for the health care of the uninsured?

_____

_____

23. As the number of people 65 and older increases, who will pay for higher Medicare spending?

_____

_____

24. In your opinion, what are the implications for future health care practitioners in the United States if health care costs continue to rise?

_____

_____

25. How can the major stakeholders in the American health care system work to improve the system?

_____

_____

26. How do increasing numbers of uninsured Americans add to health care costs?

_____

_____

[CASE STUDIES]

Use your critical thinking skills to answer the questions that follow each case study.

LO 13.3

Medical tourism is a recent trend in health care. Patients go to a different country for either urgent or elective medical procedures. The procedures are the same procedures being done in U.S. hospitals and outpatient surgery centers, often by American-trained physicians who have moved back home. Medical tourism is fast becoming a worldwide, multibillion-dollar industry. In fact, some insurance companies are paying for the cost of the procedures, as costs are far less than those charged in the United States. Sometimes the insurance company even pays for the plane fare and hotel costs—so a patient gets a vacation in addition to the needed surgical procedure. The reasons patients travel for treatment vary from the lower costs (for Americans) to shorter waiting times (for those in countries where there is national health insurance). There is no regulation by the U.S. government of medical tourism. Many patients come back enthusiastic about not only the success of their treatment, and the integrity and skill of all the providers, but also the high-class hotel-like accommodations while in the foreign hospital. India is one of the major countries advertising these services.

27. If other countries are able to do similar procedures as those done in the United States for lower fees, and with the same or better outcomes, why can't the United States offer the same services?

_____

_____

_____

28. If your insurance company wanted you to go to another country for a procedure because it was less expensive, would you do it? Explain your answer.

_____

_____

_____

In 2007, American patients with recurring head and neck cancers were traveling to China to receive gene therapy via a drug designed to activate the p53 gene, which is supposed to turn off cells that multiply abnormally, but often malfunctions, letting cancerous tumors grow. Since the drug was not FDA-approved in the United States, patients traveled to China to receive it, at a cost of $20,000 for the two-month treatment. No studies had yet been conducted to determine the efficacy of the treatment, but many patients believed their tumors were receding. A genetic research company in the United States was threatening to sue the Chinese company manufacturing the drug, alleging patent infringement.

29. In your opinion, should American patients be prohibited from traveling to foreign countries to receive unproven and possibly dangerous medical treatment? Explain your answer.

_____

_____

_____

30. In your opinion, was it ethical for the Chinese company to charge $10,000 per month for the treatment? Explain your answer.

_____

_____

Complete the activities and answer the questions that follow.

31. Visit **http://statesnapshots.ahrq.gov/snaps09/index.jsp** to see how well your state is doing in health care quality, as measured by the National Healthcare Quality Report. In which area does your state excel? Where does your state still lag behind?

_____

_____

32. Visit the Kaiser Family Foundation Web site (**www.kff.org**) or the Commonwealth Health Foundation Web site (**www. commonwealthfund.org**). Select "New and Noteworthy" at the Kaiser site, or a topic listed on Commonwealth Fund's home page. Select a current topic to summarize and present to your class. Are the reports at these Web sites easy to understand and summarize? Explain your answer.

33. Visit the Centers for Disease Control and Prevention, National Center for Health Statistics Web site (**www.cdc.gov/nchs**). List those reports that you think might be helpful to you if you had to prepare a report on the latest trends in health care.

_____

_____

RESOURCES

The Body: **www.thebody.com/content/art13091.html**.

Cloud, John. "Why Your DNA Isn't Your Destiny." *Time,* January 6, 2010, online ed., pp. 1–6, **www.time.com/time/health/article/0,8599,1951968,00.html**.

Institute for the Future. *Health & Health Care 2010, The Forecast, The Challenge.* 2nd ed. Princeton, NJ: Jossey-Bass, 2003. Reprinted with permission from Wiley.

Sultz, Harry A., and Kristina M. Young. *Health Care USA: Understanding Its Organization and Deliver.* 6th ed. Sudbury, MA: Jones and Bartlett, 2009.

Von Drehle, David. "Meet Dr. Robot." *Time,* December 13, 2010.

Agency for Healthcare Research and Quality: **www.ahrq.gov/**.

Agency for Healthcare Research and Quality data sources: **www.ahrq.gov/data/dataresources.htm**.

Agency for Healthcare Research and Quality links: **www.ahrq.gov/data/dataresources.htm**.

Government spending charts: **www.usgovernmentspending.com/**.

Health care employee statistics: **www.bls.gov/oco/cg/cgs035.htm**.

Health Care Financing Administration: **www.hcfa.org/**.

Health care jobs/U.S. government: **www.bls.gov/oco/cg/cgs035.htm**.

Health care spending as a percentage of GDP: **www.bcbs.com/blueresources/mcrg/chapter1/ch1_slide_1.html**.

Holder quote: **www.justice.gov/opa/pr/2010/July/10-ag-821.html**.

Institute of Medicine reports: **www.iom.edu/Reports.aspx**.

Institute for the Future/4 health care system scenarios/videos: **www.hc2020.org/**.

Interview 10/11/2010 with Cindi Luckett-Gilbert, MBA.

Job description for nuclear medicine technician: **www1.salary.com/Nuclear-Medicine-Technician-salary.html**.

List of life expectancies: **www.cia.gov/library/publications/the-world-factbook/rankorder/2102rank.html**.

Medicare fraud cases: **www.justice.gov/opa/pr/2010/July/10-ag-821.html**.

Medicare fraud total for 2009: **www.cbsnews.com/stories/2009/10/23/60minutes/main5414390.shtml**.

National Center for Health Statistics: **www.cdc.gov/nchs/**.

National Center for Policy Analysis, health care information: **www.ncpa.org/healthcare**.

National Healthcare Anti-Fraud Association NHCAA, cost of health care fraud: **www.nhcaa.org/eweb/DynamicPage.aspx?webcode=anti_fraud_resource_centr&wpscode=TheProblemOfHCFraud**.

No health insurance: **www.cdc.gov/nchs/data/nhis/earlyrelease/insur201009.htm**.

Nuclear medicine technologists: **www.mshealthcareers.com/careers/nuclearmedicinetechnologist.htm**.

Nuclear Medicine Technology Certification Board: **www.nmtcb.org/exam/instructions.php**.

Occupational Outlook Handbook, 2010–2011: **www.bls.gov/oco/oco2003.htm**.

PBS Newshour Web site, $2.5 trillion (2010 health care cost): **www.pbs.org/newshour/rundown/2010/09/health-spending-may-jump-new-report-says.html**.

Reuter's.com figures: **www.reuters.com/subjects/healthcare**.

Telephone interview November 15, 2007, with Laura Swisher, PhD, associate professor in the physical therapy department of University of South Florida.

Telephone interview November 16, 2007, with Jean Connor, RDH, president American Dental Hygienists' Association.

Tissue engineering: **www.wakehealth.edu/Research/**.

Total spent for health care: **www.kaiseredu.org/Issue-Modules/US-Health-Care-Costs/Background-Brief.aspx**.

2010 National Health Care Quality Report: **www.ahrq.gov/qual/nhqr10/nhqr10.pdf**.

U.S. government spending century chart: **www.usgovernmentspening.com/us_20th_century_chart.html**.

GLOSSARY

A

access   The availability of health care and the means to purchase health care services.

accreditation   Official authorization or approval for conforming to a specified standard.

active euthanasia   A conscious medical act that results in death.

administer   To instill a drug into the body of a patient.

administrative law   Enabling statutes enacted to define powers and procedures when an agency is created.

affirmative action   Programs that use goals and quotas to provide preferential treatment for minority persons determined to have been underutilized in the past.

affirmative defenses   Defenses used by defendants in medical professional liability suits that allow the accused to present factual evidence that the patient's condition was caused by some factor other than the defendant's negligence.

Agency for Healthcare Research and Quality (AHRQ)   The lead federal agency responsible for tracking and improving the quality, safety, efficiency, and effectiveness of health care for Americans.

agent   One who acts for or represents another. In performing workplace duties, the employee acts as the agent, or authorized representative, of the employer.

allopathic   Literally, "different suffering"; referring to the medical philosophy that dictates training physicians to intervene in the disease process, through the use of drugs and surgery.

alternative dispute resolution (ADR)   Settlement of civil disputes between parties using neutral mediators or arbitrators without going to court.

Amendments to the Older Americans Act   A 1987 federal act that defines elder abuse, neglect, and exploitation, but does not deal with enforcement.

American Medical Association Principles   A code of ethics for members of the American Medical Association written in 1847.

amniocentesis   A test whereby the physician withdraws a sample of amniotic fluid (the fluid surrounding the developing fetus inside the mother's womb) from the uterus of a pregnant woman. The fluid is then tested for genetic or other conditions that may lead to abnormal development of the fetus.

artificial insemination   The mechanical injection of viable semen into the vagina.

associate practice   A medical management system in which two or more physicians share office space and employees but practice individually.

assumption of risk   A legal defense that holds the defendant is not guilty of a negligent act, since the plaintiff knew of and accepted beforehand any risks involved.

autonomy (or self-determination)   The word *autonomy* comes from the Greek words *auto* (self) and *nomos* (governance). It is generally understood as the capacity to be one's own person, to make decisions based on one's own reasons and motives, not manipulated or dictated to by external forces.

autopsy   A postmortem examination to determine the cause of death or to obtain physiological evidence, as in the case of a suspicious death.

B

baby boom generation   Those individuals born between 1946 and 1964.

beneficence   Refers to the acts health care practitioners perform to help people stay healthy or recover from an illness.

bioethicists   Specialists who consult with physicians, researchers, and others to help them make difficult ethical decisions regarding patient care.

bioethics   A discipline dealing with the ethical implications of biological research methods and results, especially in medicine.

brain death   Final cessation of bodily activity, used to determine when death actually occurs; circulatory and respiratory functions have irreversibly ceased, and the entire brain (including the brain stem) has irreversibly ceased to function.

breach of contract   Failure of either party to comply with the terms of a legally valid contract.

C

case law Law established through common law and legal precedent.

categorical imperative This principle means that there are no exceptions (categorical) from the rule (imperative). The right action is one based on a determined principle, regardless of outcome.

certification A voluntary credentialing process whereby applicants who meet specific requirements may receive a certificate.

checks and balances The system established by the U.S. Constitution that keeps any one branch of government from assuming too much power over the other branches.

Chemical Hygiene Plan The Standard for Occupational Exposures to Hazardous Chemicals in Laboratories, which clarifies the handling of hazardous chemicals in medical laboratories.

Child Abuse Prevention and Treatment Act A federal law passed in 1974 requiring physicians to report cases of child abuse and to try to prevent future cases.

chromosome A microscopic structure found within the nucleus of a plant or animal cell that carries genes responsible for the organism's characteristics.

civil law Law that involves wrongful acts against persons.

Clinical Laboratory Improvement Act (CLIA) Also called Clinical Laboratory Improvement Amendments. Federal statutes passed in 1988 that established minimum quality standards for all laboratory testing.

clone An organism begun asexually, usually from a single cell of the parent.

cloning The process by which organisms are created asexually, usually from a single cell of the parent organism.

code of ethics A system of principles intended to govern behavior—here, the behavior of those entrusted with providing care to the sick.

code set Under HIPAA, terms that provide for uniformity and simplification of health care billing and record keeping.

coma A condition of deep stupor from which the patient cannot be roused by external stimuli.

common law The body of unwritten law developed in England, primarily from judicial decisions based on custom and tradition.

common sense Sound practical judgment.

comparative negligence An affirmative defense claimed by the defendant, alleging that the plaintiff contributed to the injury by a certain degree.

compassion The identification with and understanding of another's situation, feelings, and motives.

confidentiality The act of holding information in confidence, not to be released to unauthorized individuals.

Confidentiality of Alcohol and Drug Abuse, Patient Records A federal statute that protects patients with histories of substance abuse regarding the release of information about treatment.

consent Permission from a patient, either expressed or implied, for something to be done by another. For example, consent is required for a physician to examine a patient, to perform tests that aid in diagnosis, and/or to treat for a medical condition.

consequence-oriented (or teleological) theories Consequence-oriented or teleological theories judge the rightness of a decision based on the outcome or predicted outcome of the decision.

constitutional law Law that derives from federal and state constitutions.

contract A voluntary agreement between two parties in which specific promises are made for a consideration.

contributory negligence An affirmative defense that alleges that the plaintiff, through a lack of care, caused or contributed to his or her own injury.

Controlled Substances Act The federal law giving authority to the Drug Enforcement Administration to regulate the sale and use of drugs.

coroner A public official who investigates and holds inquests over those who die from unknown or violent causes; he or she may or may not be a physician, depending on state law.

corporation A body formed and authorized by law to act as a single person.

cost In this context, the amount individuals, employers, state and federal governments, HMOs, and insurers spend on health care in the United States.

courtesy The practice of good manners.

covered entity Health care providers and clearinghouses that transmit HIPAA transactions electronically, and must comply with HIPAA standards and rules.

covered transactions Electronic exchanges of information between two covered-entity business partners using HIPAA-mandated transaction standards.

criminal law   Law that involves crimes against the state.

critical thinking   The ability to think analytically, using fewer emotions and more rationality.

curative care   Treatment directed toward curing a patient's disease.

cybermedicine   A form of telemedicine that involves direct contact between patients and physicians over the Internet, usually for a fee.

D

damages   Monetary awards sought by plaintiffs in lawsuits.

defendant   The person or party against whom criminal or civil charges are brought in a lawsuit.

de-identify   To remove all information that identifies patients from health care transactions.

denial   A defense that claims innocence of the charges or that one or more of the four Ds of negligence are lacking.

deontological (or duty-oriented) theory   Focuses on the essential rightness or wrongness of an act, not the consequences of the act.

deposition   Sworn testimony given and recorded outside the courtroom during the pretrial phase of a case.

designated record set   Records maintained by or for a HIPAA-covered entity.

discrimination   Prejudiced or prejudicial outlook, action, or treatment.

dispense   To deliver controlled substances in some type of bottle, box, or other container to a patient.

DNA (deoxyribonucleic acid)   The combination of proteins, called nucleotides, that is arranged to make up an organism's chromosomes.

doctrine of informed consent   The legal basis for informed consent, usually outlined in a state's medical practice acts.

doctrine of professional discretion   A principle under which a physician can exercise judgment as to whether to show patients who are being treated for mental or emotional conditions their records. Disclosure depends on whether, in the physician's judgment, such patients would be harmed by viewing the records.

do-not-resuscitate (DNR) orders   Orders written at the request of patients or their authorized representatives that cardiopulmonary resuscitation not be used to sustain life in a medical crisis.

Drug Enforcement Administration (DEA)   A branch of the U.S. Department of Justice that regulates the sale and use of drugs.

durable power of attorney   An advance directive that confers on a designee the authority to make a variety of legal decisions on behalf of the grantor, usually including health care decisions.

duty of care   The obligation of health care professionals to patients and, in some cases, nonpatients.

duty-oriented (or deontological) theory   See *deontological (or duty-oriented) theory.*

E

e-health   Term used for the use of the Internet as a source of consumer information about health and medicine.

electronic data interchange (EDI)   The use of uniform electronic protocols to transfer business information between organizations via computer networks.

electronic health record (EHR)   Contains the same information as any medical record, but in electronic form.

electronic transmission   The sending of information from one network-connected computer to another.

emancipated minors   Individuals in their mid- to late teens who legally live outside their parents' or guardians' control.

employment-at-will   A concept of employment whereby either the employer or the employee can end the employment at any time, for any reason.

encryption   The scrambling or encoding of information before sending it electronically.

endorsement   The process by which a license may be awarded based on individual credentials judged to meet licensing requirements in a new state.

epigenetics   The study of changes in gene activity that do not involve alterations to the genetic code, but are still passed down to at least one successive generation.

ethics   Standards of behavior, developed as a result of one's concept of right and wrong.

ethics committee   Committee made up of individuals who are involved in a patient's care, including health care practitioners, family members, clergy, and others, with the purpose of reviewing ethical issues in difficult cases.

ethics guidelines   Publications that detail a wide variety of ethical situations that professionals (in this case, health care practitioners) might face in their work and offer principles for dealing with the situations in an ethical manner.

etiquette   Standards of behavior considered to be good manners among members of a profession as they function as individuals in society.

executive order   A rule or regulation issued by the president of the United States that becomes law without the prior approval of Congress.

expressed contract   A written or oral agreement in which all terms are explicitly stated.

F

Fair Debt Collection Practices Act (FDCPA) A federal statute prohibiting certain unfair and illegal practices by debt collectors and creditors. It prohibits certain methods of debt collection, including harassment, misrepresentation, threats, dissemination of false information about the debtor, and engagement in unfair or illegal practices in attempting to collect a debt.

Federal False Claims Act   A law that allows for individuals to bring civil actions on behalf of the U.S. government for false claims made to the federal government, under a provision of the law called *qui tam* (from Latin meaning "to bring an action for the king and for oneself").

federal preemption   A doctrine that can bar injured consumers from suing in state court when the products that hurt them had met federal standards.

federalism   The sharing of power among national, state, and local governments.

felony   An offense punishable by death or by imprisonment in a state or federal prison for more than one year.

fiduciary duty   A physician's obligation to his or her patient, based on trust and confidence.

firewall   Hardware, software, or both designed to prevent unauthorized persons from accessing electronic information.

Food and Drug Administration (FDA)   A federal agency within the Department of Health and Human Services that oversees drug quality and standardization and must approve drugs before they are released for public use.

forensics   A division of medicine that incorporates law and medicine and involves medical issues or medical proof at trials having to do with malpractice, crimes, and accidents.

fraud   Dishonest or deceitful practices in depriving, or attempting to deprive, another of his or her rights.

G

gatekeeper physician   The primary care physician who directs the medical care of HMO members.

gene   A tiny segment of DNA found on a chromosome in a cell. Each gene holds the formula for making a specific enzyme or protein.

gene therapy   The insertion of a normally functioning gene into cells in which an abnormal or absent element of the gene has caused disease.

General Duty Clause   A section of the Hazard Communication Standard that states that any equipment that may pose a health risk must be specified as a hazard.

genetic counselor   An expert in human genetics who is qualified to counsel individuals who may have inherited genes for certain diseases or conditions.

genetic discrimination   Differential treatment of individuals based on their actual or presumed genetic differences.

genetic engineering   Manipulation of DNA within the cells of plants and animals, through synthesis, alteration, or repair, to ensure that certain harmful traits will be eliminated in offspring and that desirable traits will appear and be passed on.

genetics   The science that accounts for natural differences and resemblances among organisms related by descent.

genome   All the DNA in an organism, including its genes.

genometrics   The science of determining how genes cause the expression of certain traits in individuals.

Good Samaritan acts   State laws protecting physicians and sometimes other health care practitioners and laypersons from charges of negligence or abandonment if they stop to help the victim of an accident or other emergency.

gross domestic product (GDP)   America's total value for all goods and services produced.

group practice   A medical management system in which a group of three or more licensed physicians share their collective income, expenses, facilities, equipment, records, and personnel.

H

Hazard Communication Standard (HCS)   An OSHA standard intended to increase health care practitioners' awareness of risks, to improve work practices and appropriate use of personal protective equipment, and to reduce injuries and illnesses in the workplace.

Health Care and Education Reconciliation Act (HCERA)   Enacted in 2010, a federal law that added to regulations imposed on the insurance industry by the Patient Protection and Affordable Care Act.

Healthcare Integrity and Protection Data Bank (HIPDB)   A national health care fraud and abuse data collection program established by HIPAA for the reporting and disclosure of certain adverse actions taken against health care providers, suppliers, or practitioners.

health care practitioners   Those who are trained to administer medical or health care to patients.

health care proxy   A durable power of attorney issued for purposes of health care decisions only.

Health Care Quality Improvement Act (HCQIA) of 1986   A federal statute passed to improve the quality of medical care nationwide. One provision established the National Practitioner Data Bank.

health information technology (HIT)   The application of information processing, involving both computer hardware and software, that deals with the storage, retrieval, sharing, and use of health care information, data, and knowledge for communication and decision making.

Health Insurance Portability and Accountability Act (HIPAA) of 1996   A federal law passed in 1996 to protect privacy and other health care rights for patients. The act helps workers keep continuous health insurance coverage for themselves and their dependents when they change jobs, and protects confidential medical information from unauthorized disclosure and/or use. It was also intended to help curb the rising cost of health care fraud and abuse.

health maintenance organization (HMO)   A health plan that combines coverage of health care costs and delivery of health care for a prepaid premium.

heredity   The process by which organisms pass on genetic traits to their offspring.

heterologous artificial insemination   The process in which donor sperm is mechanically injected into a woman's vagina to fertilize her eggs.

Hippocratic oath   A pledge for physicians, developed by the Greek physician Hippocrates circa 400 B.C.E.

homologous artificial insemination   The process in which a husband's sperm is mechanically injected into his wife's vagina to fertilize her eggs.

hospice   A facility or program (often carried out in a patient's home) in which teams of health care practitioners and volunteers provide a continuing environment that focuses on the emotional and psychological needs of the dying patient.

Human Genome Project   A scientific project funded by the U.S. government, begun in 1990 and successfully completed in 2000, for the purpose of mapping all of a human's genes. This Web site is an excellent resource: **www.ornl. gov/sci/techresources/Human_Genome/home. shtml.**

I

implied contract   An unwritten and unspoken agreement whose terms result from the actions of the parties involved.

implied limited contract   A contract created when a physician or other health care worker treats a patient in an emergency situation. The agreement does not extend to the relationship after the emergency ends.

indemnity   A traditional form of health insurance that covers the insured against a potential loss of money from medical expenses resulting from an illness or accident.

individual (or independent) practice association (IPA)   A type of HMO that contracts with groups of physicians who practice in their own offices and receive a per-member payment (capitation) from participating HMOs to provide a full range of health services for HMO members.

infertility   The failure to conceive for a period of 12 months or longer due to a deviation from or interruption of the normal structure or function of any reproductive part, organ, or system.

intentional tort   *See tort.*

interrogatory   A written set of questions requiring written answers from a plaintiff or defendant under oath.

in vitro fertilization (IVF)   Fertilization that takes place outside a woman's body, literally, "in glass," as in a test tube.

involuntary euthanasia   The act of ending a terminal patient's life by medical means without his or her permission.

J

jurisdiction   The power and authority given to a court to hear a case and to make a judgment.

just cause   An employer's legal reason for firing an employee.

justice   What is due an individual.

L

law   Rule of conduct or action prescribed or formally recognized as binding or enforced by a controlling authority.

law of agency   The law that governs the relationship between a principal and his or her agent.

legal precedents   Decisions made by judges in the various courts that become rule of law and apply to future cases, even though they were not enacted by legislation.

liability insurance   Contract coverage for potential damages incurred as a result of a negligent act.

liable   Legally responsible or obligated.

libel   Expressing through publication in print, writing, pictures, or signed statements that injure the reputation of another.

licensure   A mandatory credentialing process established by law, usually at the state level, that grants the right to practice certain skills and endeavors.

life expectancy   The number of years an individual can expect to live, calculated from his or her birth.

life span   The number of years an individual actually lives.

limited data set   Protected health information from which certain specified, direct identifiers of individuals have been removed.

litigious   Prone to engage in lawsuits.

living will   An advance directive that specifies an individual's end-of-life wishes.

M

malfeasance   The performance of a totally wrongful and unlawful act.

managed care   A system in which financing, administration, and delivery of health care are combined to provide medical services to subscribers for a prepaid fee.

mature minors   Individual in their mid- to late teens, who, for health care purposes, are considered mature enough to comprehend a physician's recommendations and give informed consent.

medical boards   Bodies established by the authority of each state's medical practice acts for the purpose of protecting the health, safety, and welfare of health care consumers through proper licensing and regulation of physicians and other health care practitioners.

medical ethicists   Specialists who consult with physicians, researchers, and others to help them make difficult ethical decisions regarding patient care.

medical examiner   A physician who investigates suspicious or unexplained deaths.

medical management   The management of patient care and populations.

medical practice acts   State laws written for the express purpose of governing the practice of medicine.

medical record   A collection of data recorded when a patient seeks medical treatment.

Medical Waste Tracking Act   The federal law that authorizes OSHA to inspect hazardous medical wastes and to cite offices for unsafe or unhealthy practices regarding these wastes.

mentally incompetent   Unable to fully understand all the terms and conditions of a transaction, and therefore unable to enter into a legal contract.

minimum necessary   Term referring to the limited amount of patient information that may be disclosed, depending on circumstances.

minor   Anyone under the age of majority: 18 years in most states, 21 years in some jurisdictions.

misdemeanor   A crime punishable by fine or by imprisonment in a facility other than a prison for less than one year.

misfeasance   The performance of a lawful act in an illegal or improper manner.

moral values   One's personal concept of right and wrong, formed through the influence of the family, culture, and society.

multipotent stem cells   Stem cells that can become a limited number of types of tissues and cells in the body.

mutation   A permanent change in DNA.

mutual assent   An understanding and consent to the terms of an agreement by both parties for the contract to be legally valid.

N

National Childhood Vaccine Injury Act   A federal law passed in 1986 that created a no-fault compensation program for citizens injured or killed by vaccines, as an alternative to suing vaccine manufacturers and providers.

National Vaccine Injury Compensation Program (VICP)   A no-fault federal system of compensation for individuals or families of individuals injured by childhood vaccination.

National Organ Transplant Act   Passed in 1984, a statute that provides grants to qualified organ procurement organizations and established an Organ Procurement and Transplantation Network (OPTN).

National Practitioner Data Bank (NPDB) A repository of information about health care practitioners, established by the Health Care Quality Improvement Act of 1986.

needs-based motivation: Human behavior is based on specific human needs that must often be met in a specific order. Abraham Maslow is the best-known psychologist for this theory.

negligence An unintentional tort alleged when one may have performed or failed to perform an act that a reasonable person would not or would have done in similar circumstances.

nonfeasance The failure to act when one should.

nonmaleficence As paraphrased from the Hippocratic oath, means the duty to "do no harm."

Notice of Privacy Practices (NPP) A written document detailing a health care provider's privacy practices.

O

Occupational Exposure to Bloodborne Pathogen Standard An OSHA regulation designed to protect health care workers from the risk of exposure to bloodborne pathogens.

Occupational Safety and Health Administration (OSHA) Established by the Occupational Safety and Health Act, the organization that is charged with writing and enforcing compulsory standards for health and safety in the workplace.

occurrence insurance A type of liability insurance that covers the insured for any claims arising from an incident that occurred, or is alleged to have occurred, during the time the policy is in force, regardless of when the claim is made.

open access plan A managed care feature whereby subscribers may see any in-network health care provider without a referral.

P

palliative care Treatment of a terminally ill patient's symptoms to make dying more comfortable; also called comfort care.

parens patriae A legal doctrine that gives the state the authority to act in a child's best interest.

partnership A form of medical practice management system whereby two or more parties practice together under a written agreement specifying the rights, obligations, and responsibilities of each partner.

passive euthanasia The act of allowing a patient to die naturally, without medical interference.

Patient Protection and Affordable Care Act (PPACA) A federal law enacted in 2010, to expand health insurance coverage and otherwise regulate the health insurance industry. Many provisions of the law were scheduled to take effect in 2014 and 2015.

Patient Self-Determination Act A federal law passed in 1990 that requires hospitals and other health care providers to provide written information to patients regarding their rights under state law to make medical decisions and execute advance directives.

permissions Reasons under HIPAA for disclosing patient information.

persistent vegetative state (PVS) Severe mental impairment characterized by irreversible cessation of the higher functions of the brain, most often caused by damage to the cerebral cortex.

personalized medicine The products and services that leverage the science of genomics and proteomics and capitalize on the trends toward wellness and consumerism to enable tailored approaches to prevention and care.

pharmacogenomics The science that defines how individuals are genetically programmed to respond to drugs.

physician-hospital organization (PHO) A health care plan in which physicians join with hospitals to provide a medical care delivery system and then contract for insurance with a commercial carrier or an HMO.

plaintiff The person bringing charges in a lawsuit.

pluripotent stem cells Stem cells that can become almost all types of tissues and cells in the body.

point-of-service (POS) plan A health care plan that allows members to seek health care from nonnetwork physicians but pays the highest benefits for care when it is given by the primary care physician (PCP) or via a referral from the PCP.

precedent Decisions made by judges in the various courts that become rule of law and apply to future cases, even though they were not enacted by a legislature; also known as case law.

preferred provider organization (PPO) A network of independent physicians, hospitals, and other health care providers who contract with an insurance carrier to provide medical care at a discount rate to patients who are part of the insurer's plan. Also called preferred provider association (PPA).

prescribe To issue a medical prescription for a patient.

primary care physician (PCP) The physician responsible for directing all of a patient's medical care and determining whether the patient should be referred for specialty care.

principle of utility Requires that the rule used to make a decision bring about positive results when generalized to a wide variety of situations.

privacy Freedom from unauthorized intrusion.

prior acts insurance coverage A supplement to a claims-made policy that can be purchased when health care practitioners change insurance carriers.

privileged communication Information held confidential within a protected relationship.

procedural law Law that defines the rules used to enforce substantive law.

prosecution The government as plaintiff in a criminal case.

protected health information (PHI) Information that contains one or more patient identifiers.

proteomics The study of the proteins that genes create or "express."

protocol A code prescribing correct behavior in a specific situation, such as a situation arising in a medical office.

public policy The common law concept of wrongful discharge when an employee has acted for the "common good."

Q

quality The degree of excellence of health care services offered.

quality assurance See *quality improvement (QI)*.

quality improvement (QI) A program of measures taken by health care providers and practitioners to uphold the quality of patient care. Also called quality assurance.

R

reasonable person standard That standard of behavior that judges a person's actions in a situation according to what a reasonable person would or would not do under similar circumstances.

reciprocity The process by which a professional license obtained in one state may be accepted as valid in other states by prior agreement without reexamination.

registration A credentialing procedure whereby one's name is listed on a register as having paid a fee and/or met certain criteria within a profession.

release of tortfeasor A technical defense to a lawsuit that prohibits a lawsuit against the person who caused an injury (the tortfeasor) if he or she was expressly released from further liability in the settlement of a suit.

res ipsa loquitur Literally, "the thing speaks for itself"; a situation that is so obviously negligent that no expert witnesses need be called. Also known as the doctrine of common knowledge.

res judicata Literally, "the thing has been decided"; legal principle that a claim cannot be retried between the same parties if it has already been legally resolved.

respondeat superior Literally, "let the master answer." A doctrine under which an employer is legally liable for the acts of his or her employees, if such acts were performed within the scope of the employees' duties.

revocation The cancellation of a professional license.

right-to-know laws State laws that allow employees access to information about toxic or hazardous substances, employer duties, employee rights, and other workplace health and safety issues.

risk management The taking of steps to minimize danger, hazard, and liability.

role fidelity All health care practitioners have a specific scope of practice, for which they are licensed, certified, or registered, and from which the law says they may not deviate.

rule A document that includes the HIPAA standards or requirements.

S

safe haven laws State laws that allow mothers to abandon newborns to designated safe facilities without penalty.

security The use of policies and procedures to protect electronic information from unauthorized access.

self-determination (or autonomy) See *autonomy*.

self-insurance coverage An insurance coverage option whereby insured subscribers contribute to a trust fund to be used in paying potential damage awards.

Smallpox Emergency Personnel Protection Act (SEPPA) A no-fault program to provide benefits and/or compensation to certain individuals, including health care workers and emergency responders, who are injured as the result of the administration of smallpox countermeasures, including the smallpox vaccine.

sole proprietorship A form of medical practice management in which a physician practices alone, assuming all benefits and liabilities for the business.

stakeholders Those who have a vested interest in the health care industry in the United States, and in any efforts to reform the industry.

standard A general requirement under HIPAA.

standard of care The level of performance expected of a health care worker in carrying out his or her professional duties.

State Children's Health Initiative Program (SCHIP) A program enacted by the Balanced Budget Act of 1997 to help low-income children under 19 who are not covered by Medicaid.

state preemption If a state's privacy laws are stricter than HIPAA privacy standards, state laws take precedence.

statute of frauds State legislation governing written contracts.

statute of limitations That period of time established by state law during which a lawsuit may be filed.

statutory law Law passed by the U.S. Congress or state legislatures.

stem cells Cells that have the potential to become any type of body cell.

subpoena A legal document requiring the recipient to appear as a witness in court or to give a deposition.

subpoena *duces tecum* A legal document requiring the recipient to bring certain written records to court to be used as evidence in a lawsuit.

substantive law The statutory or written law that defines and regulates legal rights and obligations.

summary judgment A decision made by a court in a lawsuit in response to a motion that pleads there is no basis for a trial.

summons A written notification issued by the clerk of the court and delivered with a copy of the complaint to the defendant in a lawsuit, directing him or her to respond to the charges brought in a court of law.

surety bond A type of insurance that allows employers, if covered, to collect up to the specified amount of the bond if an employee embezzles or otherwise absconds with business funds.

surrogate mother A woman who becomes pregnant, usually by artificial insemination or surgical implantation of a fertilized egg, and bears a child for another woman.

T

tail coverage An insurance coverage option available for health care practitioners: When a claims-made policy is discontinued, it extends coverage for malpractice claims alleged to have occurred during those dates that claims-made coverage was in effect.

technical defenses Defenses used in a lawsuit that are based on legal technicalities.

telemedicine Remote consultation by patients with physicians or other health professionals via telephone, closed-circuit television, or the Internet.

teleological (or consequence-oriented) theories See *consequence-oriented (or teleological) theories.*

terminally ill Referring to patients who are expected to die within six months.

tertiary care settings Those care settings providing highly specialized services.

testimony Statements sworn to under oath by witnesses testifying in court and giving depositions.

thanatology The study of death and of the psychological methods of coping with it.

third-party payer contract A written agreement signed by a party other than the patient who promises to pay the patient's bill.

tort A civil wrong committed against a person or property, excluding breach of contract.

tortfeasor The person guilty of committing a tort.

transaction Transmission of information between two parties for financial or administrative activities.

treatment, payment, and health care operations (TPO) A HIPAA term for qualified providers, disclosure of PHI to obtain reimbursement, and activities and transactions among entities. Treatment means that a health care provider can provide care; payment means that a provider can disclose PHI to be reimbursed; health care operations refers to HIPAA-approved activities and transactions.

U

Unborn Victims of Violence Act Also called Laci and Conner's Act, a federal law passed in 2004 that provides for the prosecution of anyone who causes injury to or the death of a fetus in utero.

Uniform Anatomical Gift Act A national statute allowing individuals to donate their bodies or body parts, after death, for use in transplant surgery, tissue banks, or medical research or education.

Uniform Determination of Death Act   A proposal that established uniform guidelines for determining when death has occurred.

Uniform Rights of the Terminally Ill Act
A federal statute passed in 1989 to guide state legislatures in constructing laws to address advance directives.

unintentional tort   See *tort*.

utilitarianism   A person makes value decisions based on results or a rule that will produce the greatest balance of good over evil, everyone considered.

V

veracity   Truth telling.

verification   The requirement under HIPAA to verify any request as legitimate before protected health information is released.

virtue ethics   Focuses on the traits, characteristics, and virtues that a moral person should have.

vital statistics   Numbers collected for the population of live births, deaths, fetal deaths, marriages, divorces, induced terminations of pregnancy, and any change in civil status that occurs during an individual's lifetime.

void   Without legal force or effect.

voidable   Able to be set aside or to be revalidated at a later date.

voluntary euthanasia   The act of ending a patient's life by medical means with his or her permission.

W

workers' compensation   A form of insurance established by federal and state statutes that provides reimbursement for workers who are injured on the job.

wrongful death statutes   State statutes that allow a person's beneficiaries to collect for loss to the estate of the deceased for future earnings when a death is judged to have been due to negligence.

wrongful discharge   A concept established by precedent that says an employer risks litigation if he or she does not have just cause for firing an employee.

X

xenotransplantation   Transplantation of animal tissues and organs into humans.

PHOTO CREDITS

Design Elements

Progress icon: © Blend Images/Veer

Chapter 1

Opener: © Stockbyte/Getty RF; **p. 3:** © Shanna Baker/ Getty Images; **p. 9:** © Image Source/Getty RF; **p. 10:** © Jon Feingersh/Getty RF; **1-2:** © Ryan McVay/Getty RF; **1-3:** © Karen Moskowitz/Getty Image; **1-4:** © Comstock Images/PictureQuest RF; **1-5:** © Royalty-Free/Corbis.

Chapter 2

Opener: © Tim Roberts/Getty Image; **p. 33:** © Thinkstock/ Getty RF; **2-1a** (*bottom left*): © BananaStock/age fotostock RF; **2-1b** (*bottom right*): © Plush Studios/ BrandX/JupiterImages RF; **2-1c** (*top right*): © Stockbyte/ Getty RF; **2-1d** (*top left*): © Mark Scott/Getty RF; **2-3:** © Tim Pannell/Corbis RF; **p. 41:** © Paul Harizan/Getty Image; **p. 43:** © C Squared Studios/Getty RF.

Chapter 3

Opener: © Jon Feingersh/Blend Images RF; **p. 55:** © BananaStock/Punchstock RF; **p. 58:** © Karen Moskowitz/Getty Image; **p. 62:** © Jeff Hamilton/ Getty RF; **p. 64** (*classroom*): © Tetra images/Getty RF; (*athletes*): © Howard Kingsnorth/Getty RF; (*audiologist*): © Jupiterimages RF; (*dental*): © Scott T. Baxter/Getty RF; (*diet*): © Duncan Smith/Getty RF; (*EMT*): © liquidlibrary/ PictureQuest RF; **p. 65** (*fitness*): © ColorBlind Images/ Blend Images RF; (*technician*): © Image Source/ JupiterImages RF; (*LPN*): © Mike Powell/Getty RF; (*massage*): © Ingram Publishing/SuperStock RF; **p. 66** (*transcriptionist*): © JGI/Daniel Grill/Blend Images/ Getty RF; (*nursing assistant*): © Jose Luis Pelaez Inc/ Blend Images RF; (*therapy*): © Royalty-Free/Corbis; (*optometrist*): © SPL/Getty RF; (*personal fitness*): © image100/Corbis RF; **3-2:** © Martin Heitner—The Stock Connection/Getty; **p. 67** (*registered nurse*): © Jose Luis Pelaez Inc./Getty RF; (*blood bank*): © Keith Brofsky/ Getty RF; **3-3:** © Hans Neleman/Getty; **p. 68** (*surgeons*): © Getty Images/OJO Images RF; **p. 74:** © The McGraw-Hill Companies, Inc./Jill Braaten, photographer.

Chapter 4

Opener: © Ryan McGinnis/Flickr/Getty RF; **p. 91:** © Dynamic Graphics/JupiterImages RF; **4-2:** © Jupiterimages/Comstock Images/Alamy RF; **p. 94:** © Eyewire (Photodisc)/PunchStock RF; **4-3:** © Royalty-Free/Corbis; **p. 99** (*left*): © Jack Hollingsworth/Getty RF; (*middle*): © Comstock Images/PictureQuest RF; (*right*):

© Darrenwise/iStock/Getty RF; **p. 100** (*top*): © John Lund/Sam Diephuis/Getty RF; (*bottom*): © C Squared Studios/Getty RF; **p. 101:** © Peter Dazeley/Getty Images; **4-4:** © Michael Grimm/Getty RF; **p. 104:** © Photodisc Collection/Getty RF; **4-6:** © Creatas/PunchStock RF; **p. 110:** © Ingram Publishing/Alamy RF.

Chapter 5

Opener: © Fuse/Getty RF; **p. 129:** © Erik Dreyer/Stone/ Getty; **p. 130:** © Creative Crop/Getty RF; **5-1:** © Keith Brofsky/Getty RF; **p. 132:** © PhotoDisc/Getty RF; **p. 133:** © Thomas Northcut/Getty RF; **p. 134** (*top*): © Jonathan Selig/Getty; (*bottom*): © Asia Images Group/Getty RF; **p. 135:** © Stockbyte/Getty RF; **p. 138:** © Allison Michael Orenstein/Getty; **5-2:** © Hill Street Studios/Getty RF; **p. 140:** © Alan Thornton/Getty; **p. 141** (*top*): © Comstock/Alamy RF; (*middle*): © TRBfoto/Getty RF; (*bottom*): © TRBfoto/Getty RF; **p. 142:** © Keith Brofsky/ Getty RF; **5-3:** © Image Source/Getty RF; **p. 143** (*middle*): © Ryan McVay/Getty RF; (*bottom*): © OJO Images/Getty RF; **p. 146** (*top*): © Stockbyte/Getty RF; (*bottom*): © Getty RF; **p. 147:** © Jeffrey Hamilton/ Getty RF; **p. 148:** © Royalty-Free/Corbis.

Chapter 6

Opener: © Martin Poole/Getty; **p. 165:** © Karen Moskowitz/Getty Images; **6-2:** © Dynamic Graphics/ JupiterImages RF; **p. 169:** © Jim Arbogast/Digital Vision/ Getty RF; **p. 170:** © Photographer's Choice/Getty RF; **p. 171:** © Sean Justice/Getty; **6-3:** © Fuse/Getty RF; **p. 176:** © Gen Pettersen/Getty RF; **p. 177:** © Andersen Ross/Getty RF; **p. 178:** © JupiterImages/Corbis RF; **p. 179:** © Science Photo Library/Getty RF; **p. 181:** © Ed Morris/Getty.

Chapter 7

Opener: © Chris Ryan/OJO Images/Getty RF; **p. 195:** © Charles Gullung/Getty Images; **7-1:** © OJO Images/ Getty RF; **p. 199:** © Magictorch/Getty RF; **p. 201:** © PhotoDisc/Getty RF; **7-2:** © Heath Corvola/Getty RF; **p. 205:** © ERproductions Ltd/Getty RF; **p. 206:** © C Squared Studios/Getty RF; **p. 207:** © Stockdisc/ Punchstock RF; **p. 208:** © Image Source/Getty RF; **7-3:** © Stockbyte Platinum/Alamy RF; **p. 211:** © Science Photo Library/Getty RF.

Chapter 8

Opener: © Image Source/Jupiterimages RF; **p. 228:** © The McGraw-Hill Companies, Inc./Christopher

Kerrigan, photographer; **p. 229:** © F. Schussler/
PhotoLink/Getty RF; **8-2:** © Jupiterimages/Imagesource
RF; **p. 243:** © Image Source/Getty RF; **p. 249:** © Digital
Vision/PunchStock RF; **p. 250:** © Dynamic Graphics/
JupiterImages RR.

Chapter 9

Opener: © Janis Christie/Getty RF; **p. 267:** © TRBfoto/
Getty RF; **p. 274** (*top*): © Blend Images/Jupiterimages
RF; (*middle*): © Photodisc Collection/Getty RF; (*bottom*):
© Burke/Triolo Productions/Getty RF; **9-3:** Centers
for Disease Control and Prevention; **9-4:** © C Squared
Studios/Getty RF; **p. 278** (*top*): © Jeffrey Hamilton/Getty
RF; (*middle*): CDC/Jim Gathany; (*bottom*): © Image
Source/Getty RF; **9-6:** CDC/Public Health Image
Library; **p. 283:** © Peter Dazeley/Getty Images;
p. 284: © Steve Allan/Getty RF; **p. 288:** © Comstock
Images/PictureQuest.

Chapter 10

Opener: © Andersen Ross/Getty; **p. 301:** © Steve Allan/
Getty RF; **p. 302:** © Andersen Ross/Photodsic/Getty
RF; **10-1:** © Andy Sotiriou/Getty RF; **p. 306:** © Image
Source/Getty RF; **10-2:** © ERproductions Ltd/Getty RF;
10-3: © Karen Judson; **10-4:** © Karen Judson.

Chapter 11

Opener: © Stephen Marks/Getty Images; **11-2:** © Randy
Allbritton/Getty RF; **11-3:** © Rhea Anna/Getty Images;
p. 342: © Steve Glass/Getty RF; **p. 345:** © Steve Taylor/
Getty Images.

Chapter 12

Opener: © David Sacks/Getty; **p. 357:** © Rob Lewine/
Getty Images; **12-1:** © Royalty-Free/Corbis; **12-2:**
© Ryan McVay/Getty RF; **12-3:** © Stockbyte/Getty RF;
p. 365 (*top*): © Ruse/Getty RF; (*bottom*): © Ocean/Corbis
RF; **p. 366:** © Gerard Fritz/Getty Images; **12-4a:**
© Ryan McVay/Getty RF; **12-4b:** © Ryan McVay/Getty RF;
12-4c: © Royalty-Free/Corbis; **p. 376:** © Rubberball/
Getty RF; **12-7:** © Image Source/JupiterImages RF.

Chapter 13

Opener: © Javier Pierini/Getty RF; **p. 393:** © Mark
Harmel/Getty Images; **13-1:** © BrandX/Getty RF; **13-3:**
© Comstock Images/Alamy RF; **13-4:** © Glow Images/
Getty RF; **13-5:** © Brooklyn Production/Corbis RF;
p. 401: © Purestock/Getty RF; **13-7:** © Royalty-Free/
Corbis; **13-8:** © Brookhaven National Laboratory/Getty
RF; **13-10:** © Royalty-Free/Corbis; **p. 416:** © PhotoDisc/
Getty RF; **p. 417:** © Kent Knudson/PhotoLink/Getty RF.

COURT CASES
in Alphabetical Order Index

COURT CASES by Subject Index

INDEX

Note: 'f' indicates a figure; 't' indicates a table.

A

Aarskog syndrome, 331t
Abandoned infants, 341–342
Abortion
    court cases, 206, 207
    minors seeking, 343–344
    state laws 2010, 208t
Abuse, identification, 284–286
Acceptance, Kübler-Ross grief stage,
    376–377, 381
Access, health care, 395,
    402–403, 419
Accessory to crime, 96–97
Accident reports, workplace
    hazards, 312
Accreditation, 56, 81
Accrediting Bureau of Health
    Education Schools
    (ABHES), 56
Act utilitarianism, 38, 46
Action Dismissed Due to Statute
    of Limitations (*Bala*
    v. Maxwell), 181
Active euthanasia, 368t
Addiction, vaccine research, 410
Administration consent form,
    vaccination, 276
Administrative law, 96
Adoption, 339–341
Adoption Assistance and Child
    Welfare Act (1980), 339
Advance directives, 366, 369
Advertising
    ethics issues, 117–118
    fraud case study, 88–89
Affirmative action, 305
Affirmative defenses, medical
    malpractice, 175–178
Against medical advice (AMA), 112
    case study, 124
    letter, 113f
Age Discrimination in Employment
    Act (ADEA) (1967), 305
Agency for Healthcare Research
    and Quality (AHRQ), 112,
    403, 419
Agent, 114
Agreement, 103–104
Aicardi syndrome, 331t
Alcoholism, staff ethical
    decision, 33, 38
Allied Health Education Programs,
    CAAHEP, 64t–68t
Allopathic medicine, 58
Alper, Joseph S., 332, 355

Alternative dispute resolution
    (ADR), 152, 154
    agreement, 153f
Alternatives and implications
    consideration, critical thinking
    skill, 18–19
Alzheimer's disease, 327, 329,
    330, 331t
    therapeutic stem cell use, 335
Ambulatory care setting, 56
Amendments to the Older Americans
    Act (2000), 283
American Academy of Family
    Practice, vaccination
    recommendations, 277, 278t
American Academy of Pediatrics
    child health care shared
    responsibility, 348
    on MMR vaccine, 279
    vaccination recommendations,
    277, 278t
American Arbitration Association
    (AAA), 152
    website, 163
American Association of Medical
    Assistants (AAMA), Code of
    Ethics, 11, 14
American Board of Medical
    Specialties (ABMS), 58
American Health Information
    Management Association,
    Code of Ethics, 11
American Institute of Life-
    Threatening Illness and
    Loss, 364
American Medical Association (AMA)
    Code of Medical Ethics, 11,
    187, 318
    website, 13
American Medical Association
*   Principles of Medical*
*   Ethics*, 13
American Medical Informatics
    Association (AMIA),
    website, 224
American Medical Student
    Association (AMSA), 59
    death and dying interest
    group, 363
American Nurses Association, Code
    for Nurses, 11
American Recovery and
    Reinvestment Act (ARRA)
    (2009), 231, 233t
    enforcement and penalties, 247
    individual privacy rights, 246–247

American Society of
    Anesthesiologists, Committee
    on Professional Liability, 171
American Society of Radiologic
    Technologists, Code of
    Ethics, 11
American Tort Reform Association
    (ATRA), website, 192
Americans for Better Care of the
    Dying (ABCD), 364
Americans with Disabilities Act
    (ADA) (1990)
    genetic discrimination,
    332, 333
    Titles I and V, 305
Amniocentesis, 330
Anesthesiologist assistant, 64t
Anger, Kübler-Ross grief stage,
    376, 381
Animal cloning, 333–335, 334f
Animals, research use, 15
Antibiotic samples, ethics
    issue, 24
Anti-Kickback Law, 77
Appeals phase, lawsuit, 150
Arbitration, 152
Archer v. Warren (2003), 175
Aristotle, 39
Artificial blood, 410
Artificial insemination, 338
Assault, 98, 99t
Associate practice, 72
Association of American Medical
    Colleges, death and dying
    courses, 363
Association of Organ Procurement
    Organizations, website, 372
Assumption of Risk Defense
    Denied (*Conrad-Hutsell v.*
    Colturi), 178
Assumption of risk, 177
    court case, 178
Athletic trainer, 64t
Attorney–client, privileged
    communication, 136
Attorney Guilty of Unauthorized
    Disclosure of Medical
    Information (*Hageman v.*
    Southwest General Health
    Center), 43
Attorneys, 103
Audiologist, 64t
Authorization, PHI disclosure, 242
    medical records release
    rules, 202
Autism, and vaccinations, 279

Commonwealth Health Foundation, website, 427

Communication
  medical malpractice prevention, 166f, 167, 171, 172t
  TJC safety standards, 143

Comparative negligence, 176

Compassion, 17

Compensatory justice, 42

Competence, medical malpractice prevention, 166f, 167

Competency, 40
  and informed consent, 205–206
  court case, 206

Complications, patient communication recommendations, 172t

Computers
  and confidentiality, 214–215
  hardware advances, 414

Conceptual Models of Law and Ethics, 44f

Concrete operational stage of development, 35f

Confidential information, ethics issue, 48

Confidentiality, 4, 42, 136–138, 154
  court cases, 201
  medical records, 200–203
  and privacy, 256
  technology use guidelines, 214–215
  waivers, 139

Confidentiality of Alcohol and Drug Abuse, Patient Records, 202

Conflicts of interest, ethics issue, 83

Congress, powers of, 91–92

Connor, Jean, 420, 429

Conrad-Hutsell v. Colturi (2002), 178

Consent, 4, 203. See also Informed consent
  court cases, 205, 206
  sample form, 204f

Consent to Release Information, 139f

Consequence-oriented ethics reasoning, 38, 46

Consequential award, 146t

Consideration, 104

Constitution Protects the Right to Privacy (Griswold v. Connecticut), 228

Constitutional law, 92

Consultation Did Not Establish a Duty of Care (Ranier v. Grossman), 135

Consumer precautions, telemedicine, 80

Consumer Protection Act (1968), 106–107

Contempt of court, 149

Contract, 103, 115–116
  payment fulfillment, 105–106, 118
  termination, 105, 118

Contractual capacity, 104

Contributory negligence, 176

Controlled substances
  drug schedules, 288t, 292
  regulations, 286–287, 291–292

Controlled Substances Act (1970), 286, 287, 289

Conventional morality, Kohlberg, 36

Conversion, 99t

Copayment, 73

Coroner, 270

Corporation, 72

Cost (health care), 395–396, 398f, 419
  fraud, 401–402
  genometric drugs, 408
  international health care spending, 397f
  labor, 400–401
  specialty medicine, 399
  U.S. health care spending, 398f

County Liable in Ambulance Delay (Koher v. Dial), 6

Court clerks, 103

Court Finds It Improper to Blame Patient (Brady v. McNamara), 177

Court reporters, 103

Court Rules Consulting Physician Owes No Duty to Patient (Irvin v. Smith), 135

Court systems, 101, 102f
  players, 102–103

Courtesy, defined, 16

Courtroom conduct, 151–152

Covered entities, HIPAA, 234–235

Covered transactions, HIPAA, 235

Credentialing, 182

Criminal law, 96

Critical thinking skills, 18, 21

Cruz v. Agelides (1991), 201

Cruzan v. Director, Missouri Department of Health (1990), 365

CT (computed tomography) scan, 393

Cultural diversity, 11

Curative care, 360, 380

Curtis, J. Randall, 363

Cybermedicine, 79

Cystic fibrosis, 331t

Cytotechnologist, 64t

D

Damages
  awards, 145, 146t
  four Ds of negligence, 142

Dangerous care, ethics issue, 23–24

Darling v. Charleston Community Memorial Hospital (1965), 140

Data compression, advances, 414

Data storage and retrieval, advances, 414

Database software, advances, 415

Dating ethics issue
  colleague, 83–84
  patient, 24, 39

Davis v. Weiskopf (1982), 134

Death
  attitudes toward, 357–358
  determination of, 359
  ethics issues, 381–384
  reporting, 268, 270
  rituals, 358, 379

Death certificates, 268, 270, 271f

Deceit, 99t

Deductible amounts, 72

Defamation of character, 98, 99t

Defective health care products, 7

Defendant, 5, 103, 148

Defenses
  affirmative, 175–178
  ethics issues, 186–188
  technical, 178–181

DeGrazea, David, 53, 89

De-identification, HIPAA, 235, 242

Dempsey v. Pease (2001), 104

Dendreon Corporation, 408

Denial
  Kübler-Ross grief stage, 376, 381
  liability defense, 175

Dental hygienist, 64t

Deontological (duty-oriented) theory, 38

Depew v. Burkle (2003), 180

Deposition, 149

Depositions in lieu of trial, 150

Depressed patient, ethics issue, 24

Depression, Kübler-Ross grief stage, 376, 381

Dereliction, four Ds of negligence, 142

Designated records set, HIPAA, 235

Diabetes, future trends, 412, 413f

Diagnostic medical sonographer, 64t

Diagnostic testing, genetic diseases, 330

Dias v. Brigham Medical Associates, Inc., 2002, 71

Diphtheria, tetanus and pertussis (DTP) vaccination, 278
  VIS information, 280f–281f

Direct cause, four Ds of negligence, 142

Disaster relief agencies/organizations
  health care system stakeholders, 394
  PHI disclosure, 240

Disclosures, HIPAA, 239–241

Discovery depositions, 150

Discrimination, workplace, 302–303, 314

Dismissals, medical malpractice evidence, 174

Disorganization, Temes grief stage, 377, 381